Methadone Matters:
Evolving Community Met
Treatment of Opiate Addi

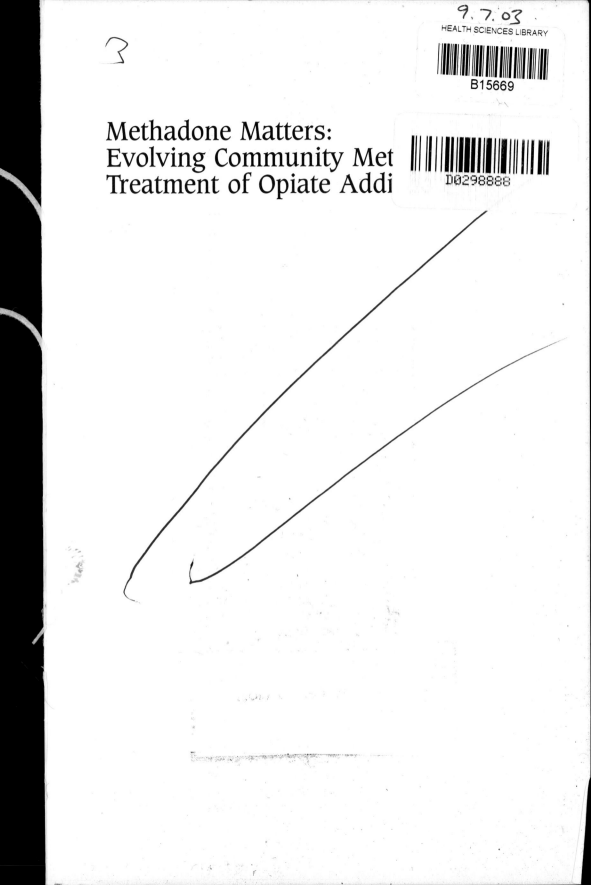

Methadone Matters: Evolving Community Methadone Treatment of Opiate Addiction

Edited by

Gillian Tober
Head of Training
and Deputy Clinical Director
Leeds Addiction Unit
Leeds, UK

John Strang
Director, National Addiction Centre
Institute of Psychiatry and
South London and Maudsley NHS Trust
London, UK

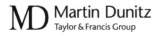

Martin Dunitz
Taylor & Francis Group

First published in the United Kingdom in 2003
by Martin Dunitz, an imprint of theTaylor & Francis Group,
11 New Fetter Lane, London EC4P 4EE

Tel.:   +44 (0) 20 7583 9855
Fax.:   +44 (0) 20 7842 2298
E-mail: info@dunitz.co.uk
Website: http://www.dunitz.co.uk

A CIP record for this book is available from the British Library.

Hardback ISBN 1 84184 365 2
Paperback ISBN 1 84184 159 5

Distributed in the USA by
Fulfilment Center
Taylor & Francis
10650 Tobben Drive
Independence, KY 41051, USA
Toll Free Tel.: +1 800 634 7064
E-mail: taylorandfrancis@thomsonlearning.com

Distributed in Canada by
Taylor & Francis
74 Rolark Drive
Scarborough, Ontario M1R 4G2, Canada
Toll Free Tel.: +1 877 226 2237
E-mail: tal_fran@istar.ca

Distributed in the rest of the world by
Thomson Publishing Services
Cheriton House
North Way
Andover, Hampshire SP10 5BE, UK
Tel.:   +44 (0)1264 332424
E-mail: salesorder.tandf@thomsonpublishingservices.co.uk

Composition by ᴛ Tek-Art
Printed and bound in Great Britain by Biddles Ltd, Guildford and King's Lynn

Contents

Section C: The special case of injectables

Section D: The risks

Section E: Service delivery

Section F: Special cases

Section G: Methadone studies

Section H: In conclusion

Editors

Dr Gillian Tober is Deputy Clinical Director and Head of Training at the Leeds Addiction Unit, and Associate Lecturer at the University of Leeds. She was Principal Investigator for Training in the United Kingdom Alcohol Treatment Trial. Her research is in the process of treatment delivery, the effectiveness of addiction treatment, the nature and measurement of substance dependence. Her clinical work includes development of and supervision in the use of treatment manuals.

Professor John Strang is Director of the National Addiction Centre, leading the clinical developments in addiction services at the South London and Maudsley NHS Trust, whilst also directing the addiction research and training work within the Institute of Psychiatry. His involvement with the Department of Health has covered the period of the introduction of harm reduction initiatives, and also the preparation of the 'Orange Guidelines'; in both, a more competent use of methadone treatment is charted.

Contributors

Dr Gerald Bennett is Consultant Clinical Psychologist in Addictions for Dorset Healthcare NHS Trust, Bournemouth, UK, and his publications focus on interventions for addiction problems in the community.

Dr David Best is Senior Lecturer in the Addictions at the National Addiction Centre/Institute of Psychiatry and Head of Research for the Police Complaints Authority. He has an undergraduate degree in psychology and philosophy, a Masters in Criminology and a PhD in explanation seeking and attributions related to substance use. His main areas of research interest are around the relationship between drugs and crime, developmental aspects of addiction careers and lifestyle issues for drug users in contact with treatment services.

Dr Judy Bury is Primary Care Facilitator (HIV/Drugs) for NHS Lothian, based in Edinburgh. She leads a team which offers support to GPs and other members of the primary care team in caring for drug users and caring for people with HIV infection. She previously worked in general practice and then in the Community Drug Problem Service in Lothian and was involved in setting up a scheme for supporting GP practices caring for drug users and for supervising methadone consumption in Lothian.

Mike Cummins has been working for the NHS since 1986 and specialized in addiction treatment since 1993. Between 1997 and 2001 he was the specialist nurse who supervised, on a day-to-day basis, the on-site self-injection clinic for methadone maintenance clients in the Lambeth and Southwark boroughs of London. He is now Team Leader for a community drug service in Bromley.

Dr Michael Farrell is Senior Lecturer and Consultant Psychiatrist at the Maudsley Hospital and National Addiction Centre, Institute of Psychiatry, Kings College London. He is responsible for a community based drug and alcohol service as well as inpatient services. His research interests include treatment evaluation, with a particular focus on the treatment of drug dependence, and psychiatric co-morbidity. He has been a senior policy adviser to the Department of Health in England. He has worked as a consultant with the World Health Organization and is a member of the WHO Expert Advisory Committee on Drug Dependence and Alcohol Problems.

Dr Emily Finch is Consultant Psychiatrist and Honorary Senior Lecturer at the National Addiction Centre and the South London and Maudsley NHS Trust. She runs the methadone maintenance clinic at the Maudsley, the community drug services for Croydon and a drug treatment and testing order programme.

Her research interests include the outcome of treatment for opiate misusers, drug using parents and coercive treatment in the criminal justice system.

Dr Jane Fountain is Principal Lecturer (Research) at the Ethnicity and Health Unit, University of Central Lancashire, and has been researching aspects of drug use for twelve years. She previously worked as a researcher at the National Addiction Centre and is involved in qualitative research projects on drug use for the European Monitoring Centre for Drugs and Drug Addiction (EMCDDA) and the Council of Europe's Pompidou Group.

Dr Eilish Gilvarry is Lead Clinician for the Addiction Services in Newcastle upon Tyne and Co-director of the Centre for Alcohol and Drug Studies. She has published widely, particularly in the field of youth substance abuse, and leads a review of the Health Advisory Service Report on this subject.

Professor Michael Gossop is Head of Research in the Addictions Directorate at the Maudsley Hospital in London, and a leading researcher in the National Addiction Centre at the London University Institute of Psychiatry. He is the Director of NTORS, the National Treatment Outcome Research Study. He is the founding Editor of *Addiction Abstracts*, and his publications include more than 300 works. These include 6 books. *Living with Drugs* first appeared in 1982 and has been continuously in print since that time; it has been published in five editions.

Dr Laurence Gruer is Consultant in Public Health Medicine. He has played a major role in planning and building services for drug users in Glasgow since 1988. He was responsible for setting up the Greater Glasgow Drug Misuse Clinic Scheme and the Glasgow Drug Problem Service in 1994 and managed the Scheme for its first seven years. He has been a member of the UK Advisory Council on the Misuse of Drugs since 1996.

Professor Wayne Hall is Professorial Research Fellow and Director of the Office of Public Policy and Ethics, Institute for Molecular Bioscience, University of Queensland. He was formerly Executive Director of the National Drug and Alcohol Research Centre and Professor of Drug and Alcohol Studies at the University of New South Wales. His past research interests included: the epidemiology of drug and alcohol use, the effectiveness of drug treatment, and the health effects of amphetamine, cannabis and heroin use. He is Australasian Regional Editor of Addiction (since May 1999) and has been an Adviser to the World Health Organization and a Member of the WHO Expert Advisory Panel on Drug Dependence and Alcohol Problems (since May 1996).

Dr Jane Jay has been Clinical Director of the Glasgow Drug Problem Service since 1999. Before that she was a hospital physician. Her main research interest is drug deaths.

Dr Olawale Lagundoye is Consultant Psychiatrist in Substance Misuse at the Community Health Sheffield NHS Trust. He qualified from medical school and undertook junior psychiatric training in Nigeria, before transferring to the UK. As well as having a general interest in transcultural psychiatry, he is involved with research projects in dual diagnosis and methadone pharmacokinetics.

Dr Susanna Lawrence is GP Principal at St Martins Practice, an inner city group practice in Leeds. St Martin's Practice also runs a Drug and Alcohol Service, delivering secondary care in a primary care setting. The Drug and Alcohol Service was awarded NHS Beacon status in 1991. She designed, taught and led training programmes for GP's and other primary care personnel in the management of problem drug users in primary care. She was Chair of Leeds Health Authority and is a Non-Executive Director of the National Institute for Clinical Excellence.

Robert Lilly worked at the Centre for Research on Drugs and Health Behaviour (Imperial College) for two years. He undertook qualitative research into methadone treatment focusing and publishing on staff/client relationships. He has since worked as a researcher for the Office for National Statistics and the Department for Work and Pensions.

Dr Jim McCambridge is Health Services Research Co-ordinator at the National Addiction Centre. His main interests are in the application of brief motivational interventions among young people. He is also involved in addiction intervention studies more broadly and is interested in various aspects of the epidemiology of drug use among young people.

Dr John Marsden is Senior Lecturer in Addictive Behaviour at the Institute of Psychiatry, London and a senior member of the National Addiction Centre. He has co-ordinated the National Treatment Outcome Research Study since 1995 and holds research grants from the Department of Health, the Home Office and various charitable foundations. He is a consultant for the National Treatment Agency for Substance Misuse, the WHO's Substance Abuse Department and the UN's Drug Control Programme. He is also a member of the UK Advisory Council on the Misuse of Drugs.

Lynda Mays has a career in addictions which has spanned 17 years, commencing in the field of research with the University of London. Following this, as Nurse Specialist (Drugs), she was involved in developing services in Gwent. For the past 9 years she worked as a manager in the Community Drug Problem Service in Edinburgh and more recently in the Fife NHS Addiction Services.

Andrew Preston worked as GP Liaison Nurse for community drug services for 10 years. He is now a full time harm reduction writer, trainer and activist and has written many books and other publications on drugs and related issues.

Dr Alan Quirk is a research sociologist, employed as Research Fellow at the Royal College of Psychiatrists Research Unit in London. He previously worked at the Centre for Research on Drugs and Health Behaviour (CRDHB),

Imperial College, where he was involved in a qualitative study of the process of methadone treatment and qualitative research into the negotiation of sexual safety by illicit drug users. He was Series Editor of CRDHB's *Executive Summary* series from 1992–98.

Dr Duncan Raistrick is Consultant Psychiatrist and the Clinical Director of the Leeds Addiction Unit. He has extensive clinical and teaching experience, is Associate Lecturer at the University of Leeds and his research interests include the nature of dependence, therapist effects on treatment and measurement of treatment outcomes. He is co-author of the RESULT information system.

Dr Tim Rhodes is Deputy Director of the Centre for Research on Drugs and Health Behaviour at Imperial College, University of London, and Editor of *The International Journal of Drug Policy*. His research interests focus on HIV prevention, injecting drug use, and qualitative research in the field of illicit drug use. He currently manages a number of HIV prevention research and intervention projects in the Russian Federation.

Gayle Ridge is Senior Clinical Researcher at the National Addiction Centre and the South London and Maudsley NHS Trust, where she has carried out local needs assessments for treatment services and manages a randomized controlled trial investigating the impact of treatment waiting time on treatment uptake in drug patients. She is working on a PhD assessing changing patient motivation in the period around treatment initiation.

Kay Roberts is Area Pharmacy Specialist in Drug Misuse in Greater Glasgow and National Pharmacy Specialist Drug Misuse, Scotland. She is a member of the Advisory Council on the Misuse of Drugs and the Scottish Advisory Committee on Drug Misuse.

Dr Nicholas Seivewright is Consultant Psychiatrist in Substance Misuse at the Community Health Sheffield NHS Trust. He undertook his postgraduate psychiatric training and doctorate in Nottingham, then for 6 years was Consultant and Senior Lecturer in Drug Dependence in Manchester before moving to his present post. He combines substantial research involvement in personality and neurotic disorders, psychopharmacology, and dual diagnosis with full-time clinical studies in addictions.

Dr Louise Sell is Consultant Psychiatrist specializing in drug dependence. She works in the drug service for the city of Salford, Manchester, UK and in a regional drug clinic where most referrals are for consideration of injectable prescribing and where many long-term patients are managed. She is pursuing research into injectable opiate prescribing.

Professor Janie Sheridan is Associate Professor of Pharmacy Practice at the University of Auckland, New Zealand. She trained as a pharmacist in the UK and worked in community pharmacy for a number of years. Since 1995 she has been working at the National Addiction Centre, Institute of Psychiatry/Maudsley Hospital in London, undertaking national and local research into the role of community pharmacists and GPs with regard to services for drug misusers. She has been part of local service development initiatives and is also regularly involved in training GPs and pharmacists in aspects of shared care for drug misusers.

Duncan Stewart is a sociologist and has been at the National Addiction Centre since 1995. His principal role is as a researcher on the National Treatment Outcome Research Study (NTORS). NTORS is the first prospective, multi-site treatment outcome investigation of drug users to be conducted in the UK.

Professor Gerry Stimson is Professor of the Sociology of Health Behaviour, Director for the Centre for Research on Drugs and Health Behaviour and Head of Department of Social Science and Medicine at Imperial College of Science, Technology and Medicine. His research spans epidemiology, public health and clinical management of substance misuse.

Dr Ann Walker is Lead Clinician at the Leeds Addiction Unit for the pregnant women who abuse drugs. Her background is in general practice. Over the last five years she has been instrumental in developing the integrated Pregnancy Addiction Service.

Professor James Walker is Specialist in High Risk Obstetrics at St James University Hospital. He is Lead Obstetrician in the Pregnancy Addiction Service working closely with the Leeds Addiction Unit.

Dr Fiona Watson trained in general practice first, in Tayside, then switched to Psychiatry. She developed an interest in substance misuse as a Registrar and subsequently secured training and practice opportunities. She took up her consultant post in 1993 and has been Clinical Director for Substance Misuse in the Lothian Primary Care NHS Trust since 1999.

Dr Richard Watson is a General Practitioner and a Trainer in Glasgow. He cares for over a hundred patients on methadone in his own practice and has been involved in the development of methadone prescribing in the city for the past ten years. He has published several papers and organized and spoken at many events.

John Witton is currently Health Services Research Co-ordinator at the National Addiction Centre in London. His research interests include drug prevention, criminal justice interventions and cannabis as well as drug treatment. He was formerly Head of Information Services at the Institute for the Study of Drug Dependence (ISDD) (now Drugscope).

Dr Kim Wolff is Senior Lecturer at the National Addiction Centre, Institute of Psychiatry. She has 15 years' experience in the addictions/investigation biological indicators of drug addiction and the pharmacokinetics of methadone. She is also currently Programme Leader for the MSc in Clinical and Public Health Aspects of Addiction and Vice-Chair of the Institute Teaching Committee.

Acknowledgements

Our thanks to Christine Weatherill for her early role in organizing the editorial management process and to Melanie Barker for her hours of tireless and patient attention in ensuring the completion of this book.

We also wish to acknowledge how much we owe to the patients and colleagues who have, over the years, stimulated our interest in, and expanded our understanding of the important contributory role of methadone in this field.

Abbreviations used

AA	Alcoholics Anonymous
ACMD	Advisory Council on the Misuse of Drugs
AIDS	Acquired Immune Deficiency Syndrome
APA	American Psychiatric Association
APC	Area Pharmaceutical Committee
ASI	Addiction Severity Index
CBT	Cognitive Behavioural Therapy
CDPS	Community Drug Problems Service
CPR	Cardiopulmonary Resuscitation
DAT	Drug Action Team
DDU	Drug Dependency Unit
DOH	Department of Health
DSM	Diagnostic and Statistical Manual (of Mental Disorders)
EDDP	2-ethylidene-1.5-dimethyl-3.3-disphenylphrrolidine
EMCDDA	European Monitoring Centre for Drugs and Drug Addiction
ER	Extraction Rate
GDPS	Glasgow Drug Problem Service
GGHB	Greater Glasgow Health Board
GP	General Practitioner
HIV	Human Immunodeficiency Virus
ICD	International Classification of Diseases
ICP	Integrated Care Pathways
IUGR	Intra Uterine Growth Restriction
LAAM	Levo-alpha-acetylmethadol
LAU	Leeds Addiction Unit
LDQ	Leeds Dependence Questionnaire
MAP	Maudsley Addiction Profile
MMT	Methadone Maintenance Treatment
MRT	Methadone Reduction Treatment
MUG	Methadone Users Group
NA	Narcotics Anonymous
NAS	Neonatal Abstinence Syndrome
NDTMS	National Drug Treatment Monitoring System
NHS	National Health Service
NTORS	National Treatment Outcome Research Study
OTI	Opiate Treatment Index
PCFT	Primary Care Facilitator Team
RESULT	Routine Evaluation of the Substance Use Ladder of Treatments

SCODA	Standing Conference on Drug Abuse
SIDS	Sudden Infant Death Syndrome
SSRI	Selective Serotonin Re-uptake Inhibitors
TDI	Treatment Demand Indicator
TEDS	Treatment Episode Data Sets
TOPS	Treatment Outcome Prospective Study
UK	United Kingdom
UKADCU	United Kingdom Anti-Drugs Coordination Unit
WHO	World Health Organization

Section A: Introduction, background and scope

1
Methadone: panacea or poison?

John Strang and Gillian Tober

Methadone heals, but it also harms. It is a life-saving treatment, but it is also a life-threatening poison. The challenge is how to confer the benefit without incurring the damage and that is what this book is all about.

Methadone is by far the most widely prescribed drug in the treatment of heroin addiction, and yet, all too often, we are clumsy in our use of it. To improve methadone treatment and to maximize its benefits, we need to address important questions: how much of the observed benefit is to do with methadone itself? Does dose matter? How important are the psychosocial components of care? How can problems of poor compliance be addressed? Is supervised consumption feasible, and, if so, is it justifiable and beneficial? What is the purpose of prescribing injectable methadone? When is it prescribed, for whom, and how? And what about the dangers of methadone? When methadone itself can be the actual drug of overdose, how successful have efforts been to restructure methadone treatment to prevent overdose deaths? How can the problems of diversion to the illicit market be kept to a minimum?

The scope of this book

There are ways of using methadone constructively, and there are also ways that leave wide open its destructive potential. There are ways of doing it well, and there are also ways of doing it badly; the task of differentiating between the two is the idea behind this book.

Before proceeding with the rich variety of individual contributions, it is appropriate to take stock of why 'methadone matters' so much. In this introductory chapter, let us first take note of why methadone treatment is so particularly special and where UK methadone treatment fits into an international context. Secondly, let us look at the extent to which it matters whether the treatment is provided in one way or another and finally let us check on our objective – to bring together evidence of good practice, those evidence-based components of care that should be the essential elements of methadone treatment in a wide variety of contexts.

Why is methadone so special?

Is a book that is solely about methadone justified? If our interest in methadone related purely to the drug itself, then it is doubtful whether the subject would merit a whole book. However, methadone treatment is about more than just the drug. A serious examination of treatment with methadone requires us to look at organizational aspects of methadone treatment programmes, the structuring of the therapeutic relationship between clients and carers, the psycho-social components of the overall therapeutic interaction, as well as more orthodox drug-related issues such as dosing and dispensing protocols and the use of different available formulations of the drug.

Response to a growing problem

The importance of methadone treatment at the level of public policy has grown with the expansion of the heroin problem. The ever-growing demand for this treatment and the resulting service expansion need to be matched by improvements in the nature and quality of investigations into optimal methods of its delivery. At the time of great public concern about heroin addiction in the 1960s, a 'crisis' was sparked off by the sudden emergence of about 2000 young heroin addicts in the UK (mainly in the London area) – a crisis indeed for a system that was not used to dealing with any more than a handful of opiate addicts, many of whom were middle-aged, middle-class and professionals, and had come into contact with opiates from either therapeutic necessity or from occupational access (for example medical practitioners). The system was ill-prepared for the very different demands of a new young addict population. Let us bring a sense of perspective to the increased scale of the heroin addiction problem. By the beginning of the twenty-first century, the 1960s' figure of 2000 had grown about 100 times, with estimates of 200,000 heroin addicts across the UK; greater geographical diversity was accompanied by a spread across the age groups and involvement of a wider range of demographic and ethnic groups.

This growth in the size of the problem has a direct bearing on the importance that should be attached to the subject by a wide variety of people – not just staff working in addiction treatment centres. The general public, health care planners and purchasers, public health physicians, accident and emergency staff, general practitioners in their positions as custodians of the health care for the general public, and many others are called to address the problem. For the individual patient, the benefits derived from methadone may be no greater than in earlier decades, but at a population level, the overall importance of high quality methadone treatment to society now matters a great deal more.

The dominant position of methadone

The question could reasonably be asked, why have we chosen methadone in particular as the focus of this book? Our position is this: it is not that we believe that methadone has any particular unassailable advantage over any other potential drug treatment in this field, and it is not because we believe that the drug itself is all-important. Rather it is that we are mindful of the need to recognize the current dominant position of methadone.

Methadone occupies 90% of the substitute opiate-prescribing market in the UK. Of course the other 10% also matters, and there can be a lively debate about whether this 10% should be greater or smaller, about whether this 10% should comprise more or less of drug A or drug B, and so on. But 90% indicates an extraordinary dominance of the market place, and so getting it right with methadone matters greatly. Get it wrong with methadone, and it is almost irrelevant whether the 10% is being delivered competently or dangerously. Get it right with methadone, and you are 90% of the way to getting it right for the whole field – indeed you are far more than 90% of the way since many of the changes that you have introduced to improve your methadone treatment will be similarly applicable to substitute prescribing with the other drugs in the remaining 10%.

Methadone's dominant position is also evident in many other countries, and the extent of use of methadone is increasing rapidly. Across Europe over the 1990s, for example, there was a seven-fold increase (between 1993 and 2000) in the number of opiate addicts being treated with methadone (see Figure 1.1).

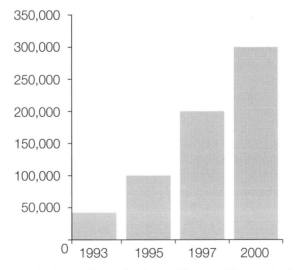

Figure 1.1 Increase in the numbers of opiate addicts receiving methadone in the 15 EU member states (1993–1997) (European Monitoring Centre for Drugs and Drug Addiction 2000).

An extremely well-studied treatment

Methadone treatment is extraordinarily well studied. Excellent substantial text books now exist, such as the Australian book from Jeff Ward, Richard Mattick and Wayne Hall (Ward *et al.* 1997), which gives a comprehensive overview of the extensive research literature dealing with oral methadone maintenance.

We owe a lot to the USA for their recognition, from the mid-1960s onwards, of the need for a good scientific base for this particular type of treatment – a treatment for a patient population who were seen by a large proportion of the general public as having no legitimate health care needs. Up to this point, the problem of heroin addiction in the USA was seen almost entirely as a criminal justice problem, with no legitimate contribution from treatment needed, apart from the need to manage any withdrawal syndrome that might occur at the time of imprisonment. Interestingly, it is precisely because methadone maintenance was being proposed in such a hostile environment that it was so necessary to establish whether there was indeed an adequate scientific evidence base for such a controversial approach to treatment. If this public and professional hostility had not been so strong, it is almost certain that our research evidence base to date would not be so robust.

Today, we have available to us the results of several thousand published studies covering various aspects of methadone maintenance. Admittedly, the number of randomized controlled trials is still very low, but there is a wealth of comparative and descriptive studies which give us a very good picture of how, when and in what way methadone maintenance can be delivered – and with what consequent results.

Warning – apparently strong evidence base is limited in its coverage

The strong scientific endorsement is not necessarily universally applicable. Champions of methadone maintenance are sometimes much too cavalier in their assertion that there is an unassailable evidence base for methadone treatment. An important qualification needs to be added. Virtually the entire international evidence base concerns structured oral methadone maintenance programmes. The fact that this evidence base specifically relates to maintenance programmes means it is of unknown relevance to the more arbitrary slow tapering doses that are commonly used in the UK. Similarly, as the evidence base is about the benefit of methadone being provided in the context of structured programmes, it remains uncertain to what extent it would also be applicable to the common UK practice of prescribing methadone in less structured settings and without the same amount of ancillary care. Finally, as the evidence is entirely about treatment with oral methadone, it has questionable relevance to the exclusively UK interest in the use of injectable methadone. We would still be wise to look carefully at the international research evidence base about methadone maintenance, but we must not be so naive as to presume that the findings will be universally and directly applicable to methadone treatment as it is delivered in different settings and according to different protocols.

Methadone treatments – but treatment for what?

As medicines go, methadone is unusual in many ways. Not least is the extraordinarily wide range of benefits that are seen with methadone treatment. There are predictable benefits, such as the relief of withdrawal distress, and modification of the extent of craving for opiates. Secondly, there is a very clear benefit in the temperance of the urge to seek and to use heroin; this includes the observed reductions in the extent of use of non-prescribed opiates as well as observed reductions in the extent of injecting. Thirdly, there are general improvements in the individual's well-being, improvements in the physical, psychological and social well-being of the opiate addict who has commenced treatment. Finally, and surely most remote of all from the actual pharmacological effect of the methadone itself, there is the reduction of criminal behaviour, which is presumably an expression of the reduced drive to raise income, by any means possible, to buy further supplies of the illicit drug.

Different ideologies, different postulated mechanisms

Given the above statements about the strong scientific evidence base, the reader would be forgiven for thinking that there would be a uniform view on the nature of the disorder being treated and on the mechanism by which methadone exerted its beneficial effect. The reality of the situation could not be more different.

At one end of the spectrum, there stand the champions of the new science of methadone maintenance treatment, with their explanations of the distinctive pharmacological properties of methadone and how it exerts a specific anti-craving effect. This explanation for the mechanism by which methadone exerts its effect also includes the proposal that there is a specific effect at the level of the opiate receptor with a consequent 'narcotic blockade' as a result of which, any heroin that might be self-administered is unable to find a vacant receptor site at which to exert a drug effect. The view put forward is that the patient on effective methadone maintenance is protected by the methadone-induced blockade.

At the other end of the spectrum, there are those who hold on to the long-standing view that any provision of drugs to the addict is just prolonging the addiction and should not be regarded as treatment because it is ultimately counterproductive. At the extreme, Thomas Szasz criticized methadone maintenance treatment as being 'not the solution, but the very epitome of the problem' and that 'treating heroin addiction with methadone is like treating Scotch addiction with bourbon'. He held that drug-taking behaviour has nothing whatsoever to do with disease or treatment: 'Misbehaviours of all sorts are now defined as medical problems. Unwanted behaviour, exemplified by the use of illegal drugs, is, by fiat [government decree], a disease. The concepts of disease and treatment have thus become politicised' (Szasz 1975).

And then there is a 'middle way'. For many practitioners, especially across the UK, much of Europe and Australasia, the arguments put forward at both of these two extremes seem fundamentally at odds with the situation before them. It seems simplistic to equate methadone maintenance treatment with insulin treatment for diabetes, and it seems equally simplistic and absurd to ignore the clear benefits that could result from timely methadone treatment – for the individual heroin addict as well as for society. And so a pragmatic middle way is trod, with the clinician and the policy maker being open to negotiation with the heroin addict to bring about a valuable change in their addictive behaviour in the context of a treatment programme, where explicit key behaviour changes are part of the expected outcome of the treatment.

This pragmatic middle way has been a central feature of much prescribing practice in the UK, and became a key part of recommendations in the wake of HIV. Thus, in a chapter exploring 'the roles of prescribing' in the new age of HIV consciousness, four positive possible roles for prescribing were identified (for relief of withdrawal, as bait to capture, as an adhesive to improve retention and as promoter of change) as well as two negative possible roles for prescribing (as an obstruction to change and as an end state in itself) (Strang 1990).

UK methadone treatment – connected to, or independent of Europe and the rest of the world?

Since the 1960s, there has been a major increase in the size of the heroin problem in the UK, as outlined earlier in this chapter. In fact a growth in the heroin problem, though on a much larger scale, has occurred in most European countries, although the precise timing and various expressions of the heroin addiction problem have differed from one country to the next. National data are often of little value since they sometimes represent little more than the attempt by officialdom to appear 'on top of things', when in reality they have very little information about this essentially hidden behaviour.

Since we are particularly interested, in this book, in the methadone data, we are fortunately able to look at more concrete evidence than is the case with the heroin addiction problem itself. In the year 2000, the situation with regard to methadone substitution treatment across the European Union was reviewed by Michael Farrell and colleagues (European Monitoring Centre for

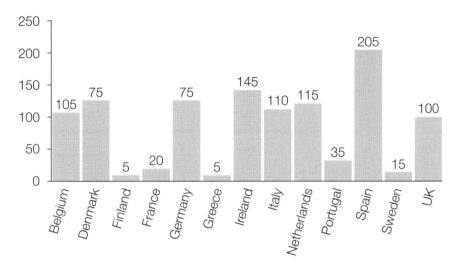

Figure 1.2 National annual number of individuals receiving methadone across Europe, 1997 (per 100,000 population aged 16–60) (European Monitoring Centre for Drugs and Drug Addiction 2000).

Drugs and Drug Addiction 2000). They found that, between 1993 and 1999, the number of persons in treatment roughly tripled and, in 2000, an estimated 300,000 drug users (in the countries of the European Union) were receiving substitution treatment – mostly methadone (see earlier Figure 1.1). However, there were huge variations from one country to the next, as shown in Figure 1.2. In Spain, for example, once correction had been made for the difference in population levels of the different countries, there were more than twice the number of drug users in methadone substitution treatment compared with virtually all of the other countries in the European Union. In contrast, extremely low proportions of the population were in methadone treatment in several other European countries.

 Another way of looking at the national patterns of methadone prescribing is to look at the amounts (weight) of methadone consumed by each country, since these data are recorded by the International Narcotics Control Board. Here again, major national variations can be seen, although with some puzzling (and, as yet, lacking adequate explanation) differences between the recorded amounts of methadone and the actual reported numbers of individuals receiving treatment (see Figure 1.3).

 One further point should be made about these national methadone data, and this relates to the apparently quiet or blank areas, areas which would often attract little attention owing to the presumption that there was little in the way of a heroin problem. In some instances, this may reflect the fact that it is a different type of drug that is providing the main problem in this country. This may be the explanation for the lower levels of methadone prescribing in several of the Scandinavian countries, where stimulant drug problems have historically

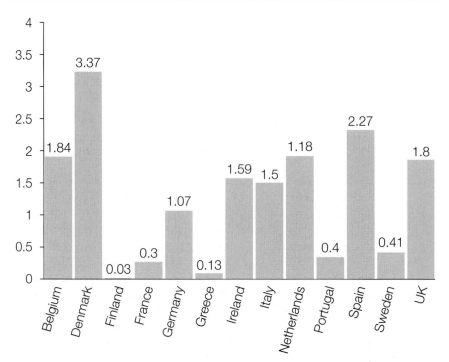

Figure 1.3 National annual methadone consumption (kg) across Europe, 1997 (per 100,000 population aged 16–60) (European Monitoring Centre for Drugs and Drug Addiction 2000).

been more prominent. However, for many of the other apparently quiet countries (quiet insofar as very little methadone is being prescribed), this would be an inadequate explanation. For such other countries with minimal methadone prescribing (including France, Germany, Russia and other parts of the former Soviet Union, India and China) the absence or low level of methadone prescribing is directly the result of overt opposition, or a disagreement regarding the potential health contribution of methadone maintenance treatment. For some of these countries, such as Germany and France, the situation has changed significantly in recent years, and it remains to be seen whether this change is maintained and extended, and whether a similar change occurs in other countries which have, as yet, not introduced methadone maintenance treatment.

The diversity of the UK

Which features of methadone prescribing in the UK are distinct from the practice of methadone treatment in other countries? At this stage, we are not making a judgement as to whether these differences represent good or bad variations – rather we are first wishing to recognize those aspects of practice in the UK which are at odds with practice elsewhere. Such differences can broadly be considered as: variations in the forms and formulations of methadone, different approaches to requirements for consumption to be supervised, conditions determining take-home doses, and the major role played by primary care physicians (general practitioners (GPs)) in the provision of methadone treatment in the UK.

Only in the UK is methadone available in injectable form. The whole notion of injectable methadone is incompatible with the beliefs of many of those who champion oral methadone maintenance, since it is clearly impossible for the prevention of injecting to be an objective of such treatment. Maybe there is great strength in the availability of injectable methadone maintenance as one of the options in the treatment tool kit for the UK practitioner; or maybe it just destroys the very feature of methadone which makes it so valuable. One way or another, it is crucial to be clear about the reasons behind injectable methadone maintenance, if such reasons can be identified and applied effectively. Several chapters in this book specifically examine injectable methadone prescribing.

Anything goes, as far as pick-up arrangements are concerned in the UK – or so it must look to an observer visiting many parts of the country. In some areas, practice would immediately be recognizable as similar to that of other countries. Elsewhere, either we are dangerously lax, or we are bravely emancipated in our disregard of the usual precaution of supervision of methadone consumption, precautions that are universally required in virtually every other country (certainly during the early stages of methadone treatment). Outside the UK, take-home facilities are seen as a sought-after privilege that can be 'earned' by demonstrating progress towards agreed treatment goals such as quitting injecting and quitting non-prescribed drug use.

The third, distinctly UK, feature is the major reliance on primary care physicians for the provision of methadone treatment to the heroin addict. From the mid-1980s onwards, it is probable that about one-half of all heroin addicts in treatment received this treatment from their general practitioner. This is a radical departure from the approach used in most other countries where there has been a deliberate concentration of this form of treatment in clearly identified methadone clinics, with both the associated facilities and the stigma usually linked with a specialist clinic. A growing interest in the utilization of general practitioners in the UK can be seen in the exploratory projects introducing 'office-based practice' in the USA and Australia, for example. However, so far, little has been published about the changes required in the practice of the typical GP and the extent to which they are willing to extend their treatment repertoire in this way. Several chapters in this book explore this important UK feature.

Doing good, instead of just wishing well

Being well-intentioned is no longer good enough. An excessive readiness to rely on instinct and intuition is one of the reasons why do-gooders can do harm. We now work in a field where, at least with methadone treatments, we have available a substantial evidence base, and much of it is discussed in this book. Where possible, the following chapters gather together the available evidence for review and as a backdrop to the practice described; and where evidence is missing or weak, this is labelled as such.

Methadone treatments in the UK today are markedly different from those provided in many other countries; it is unclear why these differences originally occurred and why they now persist. Exploration of some of these unique practices is one of the important functions of this book. We hope that it will promote carefully considered judgement about whether to move to greater conformity with international practice or, alternatively, to encourage greater attention to selected UK aspects of methadone treatment so that they can be the subject of further examination and study.

Conclusions

Methadone heals, but it also harms. Our practice (at least in part) determines which impact occurs. Within this book, the reader can examine the evidence and the methods described and consider applying them in their own practice settings. Presentation of this material is designed to assist in the making of informed choices on optimal implementation of methadone treatment. As clinicians in this important area, the decisions we make can have a profound influence on the well-being of our patients and clients. This book is about helping to make these crucial decisions.

References

European Monitoring Centre for Drugs and Drug Addiction (2000) *Reviewing Current Practice in Drug-substitution Treatment in the European Union* (Insights no. 3). Luxembourg: Office for the Official Publications of the European Committees.

Strang, J. (1990) The roles of prescribing. In: Strang, J., Stimson, G., eds. *AIDS and Drug Misuse: The challenge for policy and practice in the 1990s.* London: Routledge.

Szasz, T. (1975) *Ceremonial Chemistry.* New York: Routledge.

Ward, J., Mattick, R. & Hall, W. (1997) *Methadone Maintenance Treatment and Other Opioid Replacement Therapies.* London: Harwood Academic.

2
The history of methadone and methadone prescribing

Andrew Preston and Gerald Bennett

The German origins of methadone

Methadone was first synthesized during the course of the methodical search for effective opiate-like drugs. Having recognized that it was possible to isolate some of the effects of diamorphine and to produce particular drugs to fulfil particular functions, the pharmaceutical company I G Farbenindustrie pursued a research programme at Hoechst-Am-Main in Germany to develop effective analgesics that did not have the dependence potential of diamorphine. The scientists who discovered methadone were developing further the work of colleagues Eisleb and Schaumann who, in 1939, had patented an effective opioid analgesic drug, which was numbered 'Hoechst 8909' in the catalogue of newly discovered substances, and called Dolantin (Preston 1996). This drug is known as pethidine and it is still widely used today for pain relief. As with diamorphine before, and buprenorphine since, the early hopes of having discovered a new non-addictive analgesic were mistaken. However, the powerful analgesic action of pethidine was much needed by the Germans during the Second World War, and it was rapidly brought into commercial production. At the height of the conflict, in 1944, it was being manufactured at the rate of 1600 kg per year.

Max Bockmühl and Gustav Ehrhart took this work forward and were working on compounds with a similar structure to Dolantin. They were hoping to find hypnotic substances that were water-soluble, effective drugs to slow the gastrointestinal tract to make surgery easier (Payte 1991) and effective analgesics that were structurally dissimilar to morphine in the hope that they would be non-addictive and escape the strict controls on opiates. There has been no hard evidence to support the often-repeated assertion that they were working as part of a specific German attempt, directed by Hitler, to replace opium supplies that had been cut off by the war. During 1937 and the spring and summer of 1938, Bockmühl and Ehrhart's systematic manipulation of the compounds resulted in the creation of another new substance which they labelled 'Hoechst 10820' and later 'Polamidon'. A patent application was filed on 11 September 1941 (Preston 1996).

In the autumn of 1942, after it had been determined through animal experiments that the drug was both an analgesic and a spasmolytic, it was handed over to the military for further testing under the code name 'Amidon'. However, there was no attempt to get the new drug into commercial production, and construction continued on a new pethidine production plant (Bäumler 1968). One explanation for this was offered by Dr KK Chen, an American doctor, who did much of the early clinical research work after the war. He reported that a former employee of I G Farbenindustrie had told him in personal correspondence that they had discounted its use because of the side effects (Chen 1948). Chen presumed that the doses used in the experiments had been too high, causing nausea and overdose.

After the war, all German products, patents and trade names, including those for Polamidon, were requisitioned by the Allies as spoils of war. The I G Farbenindustrie factory in Hoechst was in a US occupation zone and therefore came under American management. The US Foreign Economic Management Department sent a 'Technical Industrial Intelligence Committee' team of four men (Kleiderer, Rice, Conquest and Williams) to investigate the wartime work at Hoechst. In 1945, the Kleiderer Report was published by the US Department of Commerce Intelligence. This documented, for the first time, the findings of Bockmühl and Ehrhart that Polamidon, despite having a different structure, closely mimicked the pharmacological action of morphine.

The formulae of all the analgesics developed by I G Farbenindustrie before and during the war were distributed around the world by the Allies. Because they were then freely available to many companies, drugs such as methadone have many different trade names around the world. As a result of this, the production of analgesics – which was now no longer commercially viable – practically stopped at Hoechst after the war. The new pethidine plant, by then half-finished, was instead dedicated to the production of penicillin. The I G Farbenindustrie empire was broken up by the Allies and the plant that had developed methadone became part of a new company called Hoechst A G.

Eli-Lilly and other American and UK pharmaceutical companies quickly began clinical trials and commercial production of the new drug, Polamidon. Although it has been widely asserted that one of the first trade names given to methadone – Dolophine – was a derivation of Adolf (and even that it was called Adolophine in Germany – the 'A' being dropped after the war), in fact the name Dolophine was created for the drug as a trade name after the war by the Eli-Lilly pharmaceutical company in America. It was probably derived from the Latin *dolor* meaning pain and the ending 'phine' is likely to have been an allusion to the morphine link.

Early use of methadone in general medical practice

In 1947, Isbell *et al.*, who had been experimenting extensively with methadone, published a review of their experimental work with humans and animals and their clinical work with medical patients (Isbell *et al.* 1947). They gave volunteers up to 200 mg 4 times daily, and found rapidly developing tolerance and euphoria. They had to reduce levels with patients on these high doses because of, among other things: '...signs of toxicity ... inflammation of the skin ... deep narcosis and ... a general clinical appearance of illness'. They also found that 'morphine addicts responded very positively'. They concluded that methadone had high addiction potential: 'We believe that unless the manufacture and use of methadon [methadone] are controlled, addiction to it will become a serious health problem'.

There were many early studies, all of which found methadone to be an effective analgesic. Bockmühl and Ehrhart were eventually able to submit for scientific publication the preliminary research results that they had given to Kleiderer on the 60 or so compounds they had discovered in the 'new class of spasmolytic and analgesic compounds' in July 1948. They were published in 1949.

The earliest accounts of methadone use in the UK include a study of its use as an obstetric analgesic at University College, London (Prescott and Ransome 1947). This study, however, was terminated because of respiratory depression in the newborn babies. Early advertisements claimed that Physeptone (Wellcome's trade name for methadone) carried 'little risk of addiction' and the consensus was that it was a better analgesic than morphine. It is therefore likely that the first people who became dependent on it had either been treated for pain or treated by doctors who thought it to be less dependence-forming than other opiates.

Although a weaker 2.5 mg in 5 ml linctus form is still used for treatment of chronic cough (usually those caused by malignant tumour), it is not generally used as an analgesic in the UK. In those countries where methadone is widely used as an analgesic, it has been chosen because of the less strict regulatory framework around the prescribing of methadone compared with diamorphine, which has a superior analgesic effect and fewer problems with accumulation of the drug in the system, rather than because of any greater efficacy of methadone.

The early years of methadone treatment for opiate addiction in the UK

The emergence of substitution treatment for opiate users, and of methadone as a mainstay of that response, was not an inevitability but rather due to a combination of social, medical, political and other historical events. These events have their roots in the First Opium Convention in the Hague in 1912, when Britain first agreed to the principle of adopting controls over opium, morphine and cocaine (Berridge 1999), and culminate in the Report of the Departmental Committee on Morphine and Heroin Addiction (Rolleston Committee), published in 1926. This report established the principle that all medical doctors could legitimately prescribe addictive drugs as part of the treatment of dependence where abstinence would be the long-term goal, and long-term prescribing a legitimate way of treating people who were unable to stop taking drugs in the shorter term. This was the beginning of 'The British System', a framework in which decisions about the prescribing of drugs of dependence were essentially a matter of individual clinical judgement by medical practitioners.

This pragmatic approach, in which the care of opiate users was entrusted to medical doctors, continued without serious review until the late 1950s. However the number of people being treated at any time was only a few hundred – and they were generally considered to be stable. When data were compiled for the first time in 1935, 700 'addicts' were counted. About one-sixth of these were medical practitioners. This size and pattern of addiction remained similar through the 1930s, 1940s and 1950s. In 1959 there were 454 known addicts of whom the majority (204) were addicted to morphine, 68 to heroin and 60 to methadone; 76% had become addicted following treatment for pain and 15% were health professionals (Spear 1969).

In 1955 the Home Office was aware of 21 methadone addicts; by 1960 the number had risen to 60. In 1968 the Home Office notification system was set up and, by the end of the year, 297 people had been notified as addicted to methadone. In 1969, as a result of the setting up of clinics, the number of people reported as using methadone had risen to 1687 (Edwards and Busch 1981).

In the UK in the early 1960s the number of opiate addicts increased and the pattern of use began to change: there were younger people and more people taking opiates for pleasure rather than as part of medical treatment. Heroin first overtook morphine as the most notified drug of addiction in 1962. Most of these 'new' addicts lived in London. All of the heroin was pharmaceutically pure and much of it was prescribed by a small number of general practitioners. There was concern that, contrary to the principles of the Rolleston report, some doctors were showing little, if any, inclination to 'make every effort for the cure of addiction'.

New evidence from the USA on methadone maintenance (1960s)

In the early 1960s in the USA, Dr Marie Nyswander and Dr Vincent Dole were finding that they could not stabilize opiate users on morphine without continually increasing the dose. They reviewed the medical literature in search of possible alternatives and pioneered the radical step of prescribing methadone which was effective orally, and seemed, from pain research and some detoxification experience, to be longer acting (they were not able to measure blood levels in those days). They soon found that, once they had reached an adequate treatment dose, they could maintain people on that dose for long periods of time. Within a year, Nyswander and Dole had coined the term 'methadone maintenance treatment' which was based on the belief that, once addicted, opiate addicts suffer from a metabolic disorder, similar in principle to disorders such as diabetes. They identified the need for large doses of methadone (80 mg to 150 mg) on the basis that they would establish a 'pharmacological blockade' against the effects of heroin, which would prevent addicts from experiencing euphoria if they took heroin.

Even though Nyswander and Dole viewed methadone treatment as a physical treatment for a physiological disorder, methadone maintenance was a combination of pharmacotherapy and intensive psycho-social rehabilitation. Most of the original work was done in the context of a residential setting; those who were treated as outpatients were required to take their methadone on site.

The gradual growth of methadone prescribing in the UK

These findings did not influence practice in the UK: the report of the Committee (known as the second Brain report) was published in 1965 and resulted in changes in policy and the law. These included a restriction of the right to prescribe heroin and other specified controlled drugs for the treatment of addiction, this being confined to doctors licensed by the Home Office. The legal requirement for doctors to notify addicts to the new Home Office Addicts Index was introduced, and by 1966 there were six times more notified heroin addicts than morphine addicts in the UK (Stimson and Oppenheimer 1982).

The report also recommended setting up specialist drug clinics to provide medical treatment of addiction, with the prescription of substitute drugs. They were designed to attract heroin users into contact with the service and to reduce the illicit market in drugs. It was hoped that they would be able to prevent crime associated with illicit drug use and help people give up drug use altogether. In 1968 the new drug clinics opened and began prescribing diamorphine and methadone (mostly in injectable form). These new services attracted a large number of opiate users into treatment and the number of notified addicts rose to 2881, of whom 2240 were addicted to heroin.

Doubts grow about the purpose of prescribing

During the 1970s the incidence of heroin use continued to rise. For the first time this included the use of a significant quantity of imported, illicit heroin. The clinics started to doubt the efficacy of prescribing the client's drug of choice as a way of producing change. In the search for something new and effective, clinic prescribing practice moved away from predominantly prescribing injectable heroin towards prescribing oral methadone, on the basis that it was more therapeutic to prescribe a non-injectable drug and its long half-life meant it could be taken once daily rather than every few hours. A landmark study from that time compared the effects of randomly allocating heroin users to either of these two treatments (Hartnoll *et al*. 1980). The study, carried out between 1971 and 1976, found that methadone treatment produced more polarized effects than heroin treatment. The methadone group were more likely to leave treatment but were also more likely to achieve abstinence. The heroin group were more likely to stay as they were. The researchers concluded that:

> The provision of heroin maintenance may be seen as maintaining the status quo, although ameliorating the problems of acquiring drugs ... by contrast the refusal to prescribe heroin (and offer oral methadone instead) may be seen as a more active policy of confrontation that is associated with greater change.

As the results of this study became known, the clinics were starting to deal with a new and different client group: large numbers of working-class heroin users who were smoking rather than injecting the relatively cheap heroin that had appeared on the market from the Middle East. In the light of the changing client group – who were not asking for injectable drugs – and the results of the study, the clinics redefined their role as one of promoting change, and increasingly moved towards the use of oral methadone.

Some clinics began to review the efficacy of methadone-maintenance prescribing. For example a small study carried out in 1975 by the Glasgow Drug Clinic found that new patients who did not receive a prescription for methadone improved as much as methadone-maintained patients, except in the area of crime (Paxton *et al*. 1978). Although weak scientifically, the publication of studies such as this in the late 1970s led to questioning the value of methadone-maintenance prescribing, or indeed any prescribing at all.

In the early 1980s there was a second period of dramatic increase in the prevalence of heroin use. The numbers of notified addicts, which had increased slowly through the 1970s from 509 in 1973 to 607 in 1976 and to 1110 in 1979, doubled from 1979 to 1982 and had doubled again by 1984. This great increase in the early 1980s differed from that of 20 years earlier in that it was not restricted to London: it occurred all over Britain and many of these new users smoked their heroin (known as 'chasing the dragon') rather than injected it. The increase in the number of opiate users meant that services had to expand and become more widely available. Prompted by this change, and the Advisory Council on the Misuse of Drugs (ACMD) Report on Treatment and Rehabilitation (Advisory Council on the Misuse of Drugs 1982), the Government responded with a funding initiative which saw the development of a non-statutory drug service and/or a community drug team in most health districts. Most of these new services got involved in methadone prescribing either by employing a clinical assistant or a consultant psychiatrist on a sessional basis, or through working with general practitioners.

The AIDS reappraisal: methadone moves back to centre stage

The recognition of the threat posed by HIV led to the 1988 report of the Advisory Council on the Misuse of Drugs entitled AIDS and Drug Misuse (Advisory Council on the Misuse of Drugs 1988). Its emphasis on prevention of the spread of HIV and a harm reduction approach led to the reversal of abstinence-orientated prescribing policy and legitimized longer-term prescribing to enable users to stop injecting. The funding for new drug services was devolved to area health authorities with little guidance on how it should be spent, other than the general stipulation that it be spent on developing drug services. This led to a diverse patchwork of service provision. In the UK, as in other countries that were pursuing a harm reduction approach, methadone became a central pillar of the prescribing response to opiate use.

Beyond the fear of the spread of AIDS ...

During the 1990s, as the threat of HIV appeared to recede, many practitioners, politicians and patients became disillusioned with methadone treatment. The possibility of getting people out of a cycle of drug-taking began to gather credence amongst all of these groups (despite the increased dangers of overdose and infection amongst detoxified heroin addicts) and the expectations of methadone treatment went beyond what could ever be expected of a pharmacological response to opiate dependence. At the same time, the levels of psycho-social support being offered to patients dropped in many cases, thus further decreasing their chances of achieving goals based on change. Media focus on issues such as accidental overdose and the sale of methadone to illicit markets served to increase disillusionment with the treatment. At the same time, new treatments such as levo-alpha-acetylmethadol (LAAM), buprenorphine and lofexidine were becoming available and services began to turn to these for a variety of reasons, not only because they have a legitimate place in the drug treatment armoury (Seivewright 2000) but also, sometimes, in the hope of achieving results that could not be achieved with methadone.

Conclusion

As the number of heroin users and treatment services grew in the UK, methadone – for a number of social, medical and political reasons – became the orthodox prescribing response. During the 1990s, optimistic expectations of drug treatment, combined with growing concern about the attendant risks of methadone treatment and the perception that public health goals (such as HIV prevention) could also be achieved by getting people off drugs, led many practitioners, politicians and patients to become disillusioned with methadone treatment despite evidence for its effectiveness. The political backlash against the failure of methadone to go beyond being a public health success to become a cure for opiate dependence has, to some extent, been reversed by the findings of the National Treatment Outcome Research Study (NTORS) in the UK (see Chapter 24), which has demonstrated the efficacy of the treatment against mental health and criminal justice objectives. With the agenda for responding to drug issues increasingly being set by the criminal justice system, it remains to be seen whether evidence for improvements in health and other areas of social functioning will regain ground in shaping the response to opiate dependence.

References

Advisory Council on the Misuse of Drugs (1988) *Treatment and Rehabilitation*. London: HMSO.

Advisory Council on the Misuse of Drugs (1982) *AIDS and Drug Misuse Part 1*. London: HMSO.

Bäumler, E. (1968) *A Century of Chemistry*. Dusseldorf: Econ Verlag.

Berridge, V. (1999) *Opium and the People: Opiate Use and Drug Control Policy in Nineteenth Century and Early Twentieth Century England*. London: Free Association.

Chen, K.K. (1948) Pharmacology of methadone and related compounds. *Annals of the New York Academy of Sciences,* 51: 83–94.

Edwards, G. & Busch, C. (eds) (1981) *Drug Problems in Britain: A review of 10 years*. London: Academic Press.

Isbell, H., Wikler, A. & Eddy, N. (1947) Tolerance and addiction liability of 6-dimethylamino-4-4-diphenyl-heptanon-3 (methadon). *Journal of the American Medical Association*, 135: 888–94.

Hartnoll, R.L., Mitcheson, M., Battersby, A., Brown, G., Ellis, M., Fleming, P. & Hedley, N. (1980) Evaluation of heroin maintenance in controlled trial. *Archives of General Psychiatry*, 37: 877–84.

Paxton, R., Mullin, P. & Beattie, J. (1978) The effects of methadone maintenance with opioid takers: a review and findings from one British city. *British Journal of Psychiatry,* 132: 473–81.

Payte, J.T. (1991) A brief history of methadone in the treatment of opiate dependence: a personal perspective. *Journal of Psychoactive Drugs,* 23: 103–7.

Prescott, F. & Ransome, S.G. (1947) Amidone (miadone) as an obstetric analgesic. *Lancet* 2: 501.

Preston, A. (1996) *The Methadone Briefing*. London: Institute for the Study of Drug Dependence.

Seivewright, N. (2000) *Community Treatment of Drug Misuse: More than methadone*. Cambridge: Cambridge University Press.

Spear, B. (1969) The growth of heroin addiction in the United Kingdom. *British Journal of Addiction,* 64: 245–55.

Stimson, G.V. & Oppenheimer, E. (1982) *Heroin Addiction Treatment and Control in Britain*. London: Tavistock.

3
Methadone prescribing in the United Kingdom: what can we learn from community pharmacy surveys?

Janie Sheridan

The UK context

In the UK, methadone forms the mainstay of substitute prescribing for opiate dependence, and from this point of view the UK is very much like most other countries. However, unlike many other countries, the UK has few restrictions on methadone prescribing – reflecting the freedom with which doctors are able to prescribe. This freedom means that doctors are able not only to prescribe methadone in any form (ampoules and tablets as well as the oral syrup), but also to refuse to prescribe methadone at all; many refuse to provide health care at all for this patient group (Deehan *et al.* 1997; Glanz and Taylor 1986), despite the General Medical Council statement that doctors should not discriminate on the basis of moral views about a person's lifestyle and the impact this may have had on the condition for which they are seeking treatment (Department of Health 1999).

Patients in the UK can gain access to medical treatment via the National Health Service (NHS) in which they see a doctor free of charge and pay a standard fee for each prescription unless they are exempt from payment (e.g. if they are under 16 years old, unemployed, over 60 years old). Additionally, some patients also choose to access treatment via the private health care system in which they pay the doctor for his/her time (and hence any consequent prescription) and also pay the pharmacist for the cost of the drugs and his/her professional fee.

Methadone can be prescribed by any medical practitioner (i.e. both hospital-based and general practitioner in the NHS or private sector) for the management of opiate dependence. There is currently no legal constraint on the dose, the dosage form or the frequency with which methadone may be supplied to the patient, although national and local guidelines and prescribing policies have been produced and are intended to guide the doctor's decisions. Thus, any doctor is able to prescribe methadone ampoules, methadone tablets or oral liquid formulations (almost exclusively the syrup formulation known as 'methadone mixture 1 mg/ml', although more concentrated forms are available, largely supplied to the patient at drug clinics with on-site supervision facilities). It is also the doctor who decides on the frequency with which the patient is required to attend the pharmacy for collection of methadone and whether or not dosing is to be supervised.

New guidelines may herald new regulations

The most recent Government guidance on treating drug users (Department of Health 1999) represents a move towards a more controlled and evidence-based approach to the management of opiate misuse, providing guidance on dosing during induction onto methadone, methadone maintenance doses and the management of methadone detoxification. These guidelines, along with the earlier 1991 version, and recommendations from a Government Task Force (Department of Health 1996) and the Advisory Council on the Misuse of Drugs (2000), have all advised that tablets should not be prescribed as they are liable to be abused by being crushed and injected. In the Guidelines and the Advisory Council report there are also strong recommendations for methadone to be prescribed as daily instalments, and for such instalments to be consumed under the supervision of a professional person (usually the community pharmacist) for new episodes of treatment – typically at least for the first few months.

This relatively informal situation may eventually change as the UK Government periodically considers alternatives such as the introduction of prescribing licences that could limit certain aspects of methadone prescribing, such as restricting some dosage forms (ampoules and tablets) to doctors with a special licence to prescribe these particular drugs in the treatment of addiction. Such licensing might, for example, be attached to a system of 'accreditation', requiring doctors who desire such a licence to be able to demonstrate they have undertaken appropriate training and that they are competent in prescribing to more complex cases. The challenge would be to identify a form of licensing which successfully introduced the desired changes without an unplanned effect of restricting the availability of some forms of prescribing (e.g. injectable methadone) even further than is currently the case, an issue which needs to be resolved by other means.

However, at present, the structure remains on the whole unregulated by government. Major variations exist in the systems for monitoring methadone prescribing. In Scotland, data on methadone prescribing are rigorously collected, whilst, in contrast, the prescribing of methadone is largely uncharted in England and Wales. It is not possible, for example, to state how many patients are, at any one time, in receipt of a methadone prescription. It is not even possible to make any more than the crudest of estimates. Nor is it possible to describe the mean daily dose or the frequency of instalment dispensing (the number of times a week the patient is required to collect their methadone from the dispenser). However, with regard to the different dosage forms of methadone, data are at least available from the Department of Health on the numbers of NHS prescriptions dispensed each year at community pharmacies (i.e. not including those dispensed at drug clinics) for methadone tablets, ampoules and oral mixture, although this will also include the relatively small numbers of prescriptions written for cough suppression and the management of analgesia (mainly in the terminally ill) (see Table 3.1).

These data show the steady increase in the number of prescriptions being written for methadone, an increase of 200% between 1990 and 2000. The data also show the relative stability of the proportions of methadone dosage forms, with oral mixture 1 mg/ml comprising approximately 80% and tablets and ampoules at around 10% each until 1996, and this despite recommendations against the prescribing of tablets (Department of Health 1996; 1999; Advisory Council on the Misuse of Drugs 2000). A small increase to around 90% in the proportion of mixture in 2000 is noted, with the proportions of prescriptions for tablets and ampoules falling off to around 5% each. It is possible that the majority of tablet prescriptions are for the management of analgesia, but national data collected through community pharmacies in 1995 indicate that tablet prescribing for opiate dependence comprised 11% of methadone prescriptions at that time (Strang et al. 1996). Furthermore, comparison of data for 1995 and 1997 for South East England, one year after the government's 'Task Force' report (Department of Health 1996), also indicated little change (Strang and Sheridan 1998a).

The first national survey in England and Wales – 1995

Owing to the lack of centralized audit of methadone prescribing to opiate dependent patients, an exploration of prescribing patterns first requires a review of published research literature. The most extensive report was published in 1996, based on data obtained from a national survey of community pharmacies in 1995. While the study was mainly concerned with exploring the involvement of community pharmacists in service provision for drug misusers (Sheridan et al. 1996), the researchers used the opportunity of this extensive contact with community pharmacists to collect data on the methadone prescriptions that they were dispensing at the time they completed the questionnaire, thus providing a national 'snapshot' of prescribing patterns. The study design used a random 1 in 4 sample of pharmacies in England and Wales, stratified by health authority. A questionnaire was mailed to 2652 pharmacies with three reminders, resulting in a 75% response rate. Through this survey, data were obtained on 3693 methadone prescriptions in respect of dosage form, daily dose, number of instalments per week, whether the prescription was from a hospital prescriber or a general practitioner, and whether the prescription was an NHS or private one. The data which follow are taken from the resulting paper by Strang et al. (1996), unless otherwise stated. Data for Wales alone are presented later.

The data comprise prescriptions which were being dispensed to patients on methadone maintenance and methadone reduction or detoxification at the time the pharmacist completed the questionnaire, and so represent a snapshot of

Table 3.1 Number of prescription items (thousands) for methadone hydrochloride dispensed in the community, by form type, 1990–2000 (England).

Dosage form	1990*	1991	1992	1993	1994	1995	1996	1997	1998	1999	2000
					Number of prescriptions (thousands)						
Injections	35.40	39.00	54.50	70.10	81.70	84.20	83.10	85.80	83.10	69.20	59.60
Mixtures	341.20	403.30	495.00	598.20	682.40	787.00	891.00	981.70	1022.80	1087.7	1144.4
Tablets	41.80	38.30	47.70	62.40	77.30	94.90	97.80	88.80	80.40	69.30	61.50
Linctuses	7.00	6.80	5.30	4.20	4.00	3.50	3.10	2.90	3.00	2.30	2.00
Other	0.00	3.10	4.70	0.20	0.70	1.40	1.00	4.10	3.50	2.80	2.30
Totals	425.40	490.50	607.00	735.10	846.00	970.90	1076.10	1163.20	1192.70	1225.3	1296.7

Sources: Department of Health (2001) Statistics Division 1E, Prescription Cost Analysis System, London

Note: *The data for 1990 are based on fees and cover prescriptions dispensed by community pharmacists and appliance contractors only. The data 1991 to 2000 are based on items and cover all prescriptions dispensed by community pharmacists and appliance contractors, dispensing doctors and personal administration.

prescribing patterns. The data are based on prescriptions and not patients. For reasons of confidentiality, pharmacists were not asked to identify patients or prescribers, and it is therefore possible that one patient may have been receiving a prescription for more than one methadone dosage form. The mean dose overall of 44.3 mg for the oral mixture is thus likely to be an underestimation of the mean methadone dose for those on methadone maintenance, since at least some of these patients will have been receiving methadone ampoules and oral mixture, leading to two separate entries to the dataset (one for ampoules, one for the oral mixture). Furthermore, maintenance dosing is not represented, as many of the prescriptions will have been for patients on reduction/detoxification programmes.

Of the 3693 prescriptions, 79.6% were for methadone oral mixture, 11.0% for tablets and 9.3% for ampoules. Daily instalments (defined as 5, 6 or 7 days per week as some pharmacies are not open at weekends) accounted for 36.6% of prescriptions, 37.2% for weekly or less frequent instalments, and the remainder were for 2, 3 or 4 times per week. There was little difference between the prescribing patterns of general practitioners and hospital prescribers with regard to dosage forms, and general practitioners tended to prescribe in less frequent instalments than their hospital colleagues (see Figure 3.1). GPs were, however, more likely to prescribe lower mean daily doses.

The vast majority of prescriptions were from NHS prescribers. However, there were 55 which were from private prescribers and they were distinctive. Private prescriptions were much more likely to be for methadone tablets and ampoules than were NHS prescriptions, and the private prescriptions never

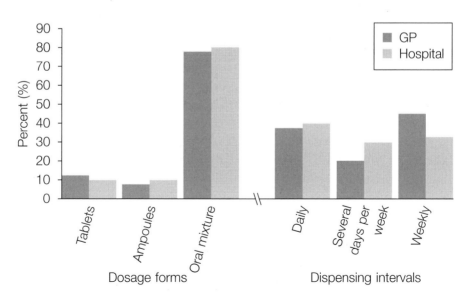

Figure 3.1 Dosage forms and dispensing intervals for GPs and hospital prescribers.

involved daily instalments, more typically being for weekly or less frequent pick-ups (see Figure 3.2). This may be as a result of a different patient population, it may be related to a concern for the potential increased cost to the patient who has to pay for each instalment, or it may represent a significant difference in the philosophy informing prescribing in the NHS compared with the private sector.

There were differences in the mean daily doses for the different dosage forms by type of prescription (NHS or private). For example, the mean daily doses for NHS and private prescriptions for oral methadone mixture were 44.3 mg and 55.2 mg respectively and for NHS and private tablet prescriptions were 51.9 mg and 82.5 mg, although the differences were not significant at the 0.05 level. However, for NHS and private ampoules prescriptions, the mean daily doses were 62.4 mg and 117.8 mg, and this difference was statistically significant at the 0.05 level.

Geographical variation in methadone prescribing patterns was also identified (Strang and Sheridan 1998b). When analysed by NHS region ($n = 15$ in England plus Wales), major variations were noted in the proportions of the different dosage forms, the frequency of instalments prescribed and the daily dose. For example, the proportion of prescriptions for daily instalment ranged from 15.6% to 65% (mean = 38.4%) and the mean daily dose per region ranged from 38.6 mg to 53.4 mg (mean 47.4 mg). The proportion of prescriptions for oral mixture ranged from 72.2% to 90.4% (mean 79.7%). It seems highly unlikely that such variation is a result of local prescribing protocols, and it is more likely to be a result of individual prescriber preferences.

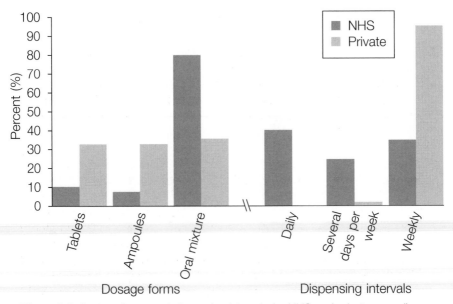

Figure 3.2 Dosage forms and dispensing intervals for NHS and private prescribers.

The second major survey – 1997 in the South East of England

The previous description of methadone prescribing patterns refers to data obtained through a national community pharmacy survey in 1995. One year after this survey was carried out, the Government made various recommendations about prescribing in their Treatment Effectiveness report (Department of Health 1996). Among the recommendations was the statement that the prescribing of tablet forms of methadone should cease and daily dispensing should be introduced to reduce the overdose risk and to limit the diversion of methadone to the illicit market. Also within the report was a recommendation for methadone maintenance doses to be within the range of 50–100 mg.

A second survey of community pharmacies, in the South East of England in 1997, created the opportunity to study the impact of this new Department of Health guidance, since methadone data had now been collected at two time-points – one year before and one year after the government report. Little change had occurred. Mean daily doses and the frequency of daily instalments remained largely unchanged, although there was a move from weekly dispensing to several days a week. While the proportion of methadone tablet prescriptions had fallen by 2.6%, when taking into account an overall rise in 20% of opiate addicts presenting for treatment (Home Office 1997) it is reasonable to assume that the actual number of tablet prescriptions had risen (Strang and Sheridan 1998a).

Prescribing in Wales – the Welsh component

Data for Wales have been separately extracted and studied from the national survey data (Sheridan and Strang 1998). Data on 89 methadone prescriptions were obtained: 73% were for methadone mixture, 17% for tablets and 10% for ampoules – a higher proportion of tablets than for England and Wales overall. The majority of prescriptions (65%) were from general practitioners.

Prescribing in Scotland – the 1995 national survey

A national survey of community pharmacy services for drug users was carried out by Matheson et al. (1999). A questionnaire, posted to all community pharmacies in Scotland received a 79% response rate after three mailshots. The questionnaire included a section in which responding pharmacists could describe the prescriptions they were currently dispensing for methadone.

Of the responding pharmacies, 54.6% dispensed methadone to 3387 methadone patients. The majority of prescriptions (74.6%) were from general practitioners, a higher proportion than in England and Wales. Two-thirds (65.6%) were for daily dispensing (with 32.9% for daily supervised methadone). However, there was considerable Health Board variation, for example, with daily dispensing ranging from 16.7% to 89.1% and supervised dispensing ranging from zero to 69.7% of the methadone prescriptions in the study.

Northern Ireland – national survey in 1999

A national survey of all 507 community pharmacies in Northern Ireland, based on the 1995 England and Wales survey (Sheridan *et al.* 1996), was carried out in 1999 (Fleming *et al.* 2001). A 67.5% response rate was obtained (n = 342). As part of this survey, pharmacists in Northern Ireland were asked to provide information about drugs they were dispensing for the management of drug misuse. Only 9.7% of pharmacies reported providing this service, compared with more than 50% in England and Wales (Sheridan *et al.* 1996) and 61% in Scotland (Matheson *et al.* 1999). Very few methadone prescriptions (n = 9) were recorded by pharmacists, the majority of these being for methadone tablets (n = 7). This low figure reflected the status of methadone prescribing in Northern Ireland, whereby methadone may only be prescribed from a specialist drug treatment agency.

Concluding remarks

The data presented here paint a picture of a 'non-system', or certainly one that is not regulated from the centre. There is considerable variation in pre-scribing practice between countries. This variation is also highly evident within the regions of England and Wales, which one might expect in an unregulated system. What might underlie the substantial diversity of mean daily doses noted in the NHS regions across the UK? There may be a greater level of maintenance prescribing than reducing doses in regions with a higher mean daily dose. Such a major difference in clinical practice probably reflects a difference in treatment philosophy, which is difficult to explain in the face of harm reduction strategies advocated to reduce the risk of HIV and other blood-borne viruses (maintaining someone in oral maintenance treat-ment has been shown to reduce the level of injecting). Again there is a lack of use of instalment prescribing facilities which are readily available to NHS prescribers through the use of specially provided 'instalment prescription forms', and with no extra cost to the patient. The use of instalment prescribing in many areas of Scotland is extremely high, leading one to presume that local guidance and treatment philosophy, motivated by a desire for high levels of compliance and low levels of diversion, can impact on local prescribing practices.

Current UK treatment plans presume the growth of the provision of this form of treatment and the increased diversity of contexts and locations. Our ability to steer developments healthily depends crucially on improved awareness of the puzzling variations in prescribing habits which have been described, as well as a more co-ordinated strategic approach to the chosen developments to achieve more effective and more available methadone prescribing.

References

Advisory Council on the Misuse of Drugs (2000) *Reducing Drug Related Deaths.* London: Home Office.

Deehan, A., Taylor, C. & Strang, J. (1997) The general practitioner, the drug misuser and the alcohol misuser: major differences in general practitioner activity, therapeutic commitment, and shared care proposals. *British Journal of General Practice*, 47: 705–9.

Department of Health (1999) *Drug Misuse and Dependence – Guidelines on Clinical Management.* London: The Stationery Office.

Department of Health (1996) *The Task Force to Review Services for Drug Misusers: Report of an Independent Review of Drug Treatment Services in England.* London: HMSO.

Fleming, G.F., McElnay, J.C., Hughes, C.H., Sheridan, J. & Strang, J. (2001) The role of the community pharmacist in drug abuse: a comparison of service provision between Northern Ireland and England/Wales. *Pharmacy World and Science*, 23: 13–16.

Glanz, A. & Taylor, C. (1986) Findings of a national survey of the role of general practitioners in the treatment of opiate misuse: extent of contact with opiate misusers. *British Medical Journal*, 293: 427–30.

Home Office (1997) *Statistics on the Misuse of Drugs: Addicts notified to the Home Office, United Kingdom, 1996.* London: HMSO.

Matheson, C., Bond, C. M. & Hickey, F. (1999) Prescribing and dispensing for drug misusers in primary care: current practice in Scotland. *Family Practice*, 16: 375–9.

Sheridan, J. & Strang, J. (1998) Community pharmacy in Wales: 1995 data on HIV prevention and drug misuse services. *Journal of Mental Health*, 7: 203–10.

Sheridan, J., Strang, J., Barber, N. & Glanz A. (1996) Role of community pharmacies in relation to HIV prevention and drug misuse: findings from the 1995 national survey in England and Wales. *British Medical Journal*, 313: 272–4.

Strang, J. & Sheridan, J. (1998a) Effect of government recommendations on methadone prescribing in South East England: comparison of 1995 and 1997 surveys. *British Medical Journal*, 317: 1489–90.

Strang, J. & Sheridan, J. (1998b) National and regional characteristics of methadone prescribing in England and Wales: local analyses of data from the 1995 national survey of community pharmacies. *Journal of Substance Misuse*, 3: 240–6.

Strang, J., Sheridan, J. & Barber, N. (1996) Prescribing injectable and oral methadone to opiate addicts: results from the 1995 national postal survey of community pharmacies in England and Wales. *British Medical Journal*, 313: 270–2.

Section B: Aspects of clinical practice and variations

4

Negotiating a script: the dynamics of staff/client relationships

Alan Quirk, Robert Lilly, Tim Rhodes and Gerry Stimson

> Studies are needed that closely examine how physicians and other staff members make decisions about clients' treatment. Treatment practices may vary from client to client or from one staff member to another. Such variance and the factors that account for it may be better understood in a study of clinical decision making (D'Aunno and Vaughn 1992).

Most research into methadone treatment has been outcomes based, focusing on determining the key treatment components or client characteristics that can be linked to successful outcomes. In contrast, little research has been conducted into the actual day-to-day delivery of methadone treatment, little is understood or known about the processes of treatment delivery and how these may influence outcome. This chapter aims to look inside the 'black box' of methadone treatment and describe what is involved in negotiating a 'script' (prescription), using data from our qualitative study of treatment process in the UK. The focus is on negotiation of methadone dose between staff and clients in National Health Service (NHS) specialist drug clinics, also known as Drug Dependency Units (DDUs). Such negotiation needs to be understood in its specific organizational, historical and policy context.

The 'British System' has, until recently, been uniquely characterized by the absence of a central co-ordinated policy. This has permitted more individual tailoring of the treatment response to the needs of the individual patient than is likely to be found elsewhere, and has left considerable room for manoeuvre in staff–client negotiation (for overviews see Strang 1989; Farrell et al. 1996; Royal College of Psychiatrists & Royal College of Physicians 2000). This was certainly the case in the years immediately after the DDUs were set up in the late-1960s, when 'bargaining' over treatment was first documented (Stimson and Oppenheimer 1982). Many specialist doctors of the time recognized their social control function and the difficult 'prescribing tightrope' they had to walk: to prescribe enough drugs so that patients did not turn to the illicit market for supplies, while not prescribing too much in case patients sold their supplies and fed that illicit market (Stimson and Oppenheimer 1982). Difficulties in decision-making about dosage were further compounded by the lack of experience staff had in dealing with this patient group, and the relatively heavy reliance on addicts' own reports of their drug-taking and dosages. Prescribing decisions were made no easier by the divergent aims of patients and staff – the former viewing the receipt of a regular and legal supply of drugs as their right, the latter seeing it as subject to the doctor's discretion (Stimson and Oppenheimer 1982; see also Bewley and Fleminger 1970).

Even today there are no formal limits on the maximum quantity of methadone that a doctor can prescribe with a single prescription, and centralized guidance on dosages and dose adjustments in maintenance treatment only recently emerged (Department of Health 1999). These clinical guidelines for doctors have recommendations on initial doses (in the region of 10–40 mg), dose increases (no more than 5–10 mg per day in the first seven days), daily maintenance doses (usually 60–120 mg, following careful dose induction and stabilization), and dose reductions in slow reduction regimes (5–10 mg per week or fortnight, until a stable dose is reached) (Department of Health 1999).[1] The guidelines also stress the importance of *patient agreement*, and thus the interactional dimensions of treatment, for successful outcomes in drug reduction regimes, noting that 'there is usually very little clinical improvement when a reduction regimen is carried out against the wishes of the patient' (Department of Health 1999). In addition, while guidance on how to negotiate dose decisions has been provided to both doctors (Martin *et al.* 1991) and patients (Preston 1999), there is scant research evidence on how this is currently done. Nonetheless, research focusing on dose and client characteristics has led to some interesting assertions regarding decision-making procedures. Metzger and Platt (1987) attributed certain client characteristics to the prescribing of higher doses, leading them to assert that this 'provides a basis for viewing the determination process as primarily interactional' and that 'it is imperative that dose determination procedure is better understood'. Yet as Roszell and Calsyn (1986) point out, 'even though clinicians seem to have hunches about which patients require higher doses there is little information on how these decisions are made'.

The research literature has shown dosage to be one of the key variables associated with client outcome. Higher doses have been found to be effective, particularly in relation to retention in treatment and reductions in heroin use (summarized in Ward *et al.* 1998). Increasing the methadone dose, as one of a variety of 'constructive responses' to client problems, has been found to increase the time clients are retained in treatment (Magura *et al.* 1998). However, dose is not the only factor to consider here. Among clients who occasionally 'topped up' their prescriptions with street heroin, the main reasons reported were availability and hedonism (Best *et al.* 1999). In other words, those who use opportunistically and/or for pleasure are unlikely to change their illicit use in response to a dose increase. By understanding such use in terms

---

[1] The extent to which doctors are following these new guidelines is unknown. Given the minimal impact of previous government recommendations on methadone prescribing (Strang and Sheridan 1998), some have called for this to be monitored (Royal College of Psychiatrists & Royal College of Physicians 2000).

of motivational and social factors, and not just as a response to physiological need, research has indicated the need for different clinical responses based on an assessment of its meaning to the client (Best *et al.* 1999).

The study

The findings come from our two-year, multi-method study of methadone treatment in London. Over an 18-month period in 1996–97, in-depth interviews were conducted with staff (*n* = 40) and clients (*n* = 45) recruited from four methadone prescribing agencies. These were supplemented by focus groups and participant observation in clinical settings. The agencies included two NHS DDUs, a private clinic and a general practitioner (GP) liaison project offering shared care to clients (see Lilly *et al.* 1999 for further description).

The aim of the research was to investigate how methadone treatment is delivered, and to elicit staff and clients' views about this. Our main focus was on the processes which influence how methadone prescribing decisions are made and the implications of these findings for understanding treatment delivery and outcome.

Negotiating the start dose

> When I actually see the patient there is no question of just telling him or her what the treatment will be, so that they can take it or leave it. It's always negotiation in that I have to listen to where they're at; what it is they think they want, work out whether I think that is appropriate and then discuss it with them; I will start knowing what I'm willing to accept and not willing to accept. (Psychiatrist, DDU).

After an initial assessment at the clinic, usually with a nurse, clients undertook a medical assessment with a doctor. Start dose was typically discussed during both encounters but was ultimately determined during the medical assessment. Clients had variable expectations regarding their start dose. Those with expectations, for example, based on previous experience of treatment, could be invited into a negotiated process: 'I was asked how much I wanted, if I wanted 70 or 80'. Staff said clients 'expect to barter, to kind of negotiate it'. One doctor said he would typically enter the assessment with a 'middle figure' in mind, offer 'a bit below' and 'work up' with the client until 'what you feel is right'.[2] Some clients were prone to start with unrealistic 'opening bids':

---

[2] Similar 'bargaining' was observed 25 years earlier by Stimson and Oppenheimer (1982). Doctors in the same NHS clinics in London were often reduced to using a simple rule of thumb: to 'divide what was asked for by two', as one doctor recalled, and prescribe the smaller amount.

> I asked for 120 [mls]. They naturally knocked me down, you know 'Sorry love, nice try'. (Client, DDU).

Staff emphasized that their foremost considerations in the start dose decision were caution and accountability. However, the decision was portrayed by some staff as bartering towards achieving a 'realistic decision' that may involve compromise. In this way, start dose becomes the outcome of a negotiated process where staff have to deal with client expectations within certain parameters (e.g. clinic policy). It was widely recognized, as in much prescribing, that setting the start dose was not an exact science, one doctor saying 'It's not quite out of a hat, you're sort of guided by certain things, but it's not that important'. Such inexactness left room for flexibility to accommodate clients' expectations and to avoid dose becoming a distraction.

Perceived importance of dose

Staff talked about some clients having 'fixed ideas' of the dose they wanted. However, staff also noted the importance of not getting 'bogged down' by dose, otherwise subsequent keyworking sessions can dissolve into game playing. Additionally, this can lead to confrontation:

> They're going to keep saying 'that's not enough, I'm going to withdraw'. They're not going to co-operate, your whole sessions are going to be that you're not giving them enough, until they get that amount. And then you give them that amount, then you can do the work. (Nurse, DDU).

This indicates how dose determination goes beyond considerations of pharmacological effectiveness – achieving favourable medical outcomes and behavioural change is a question of balancing medical and social dimensions of treatment because effective *relationships* are required. As we have already seen, client inclusion within the decision to set the start dose can aid the subsequent social interaction between staff and clients (discussed further in Lilly *et al.* 1999; 2000).

That noted, the relative importance of the pharmacological aspects of the start dose can vary according to the aims and level of structure of treatment packages. With clients on a short, structured reduction programme, the accuracy of the decision was seen to have a direct impact on the effectiveness and outcome:

> I think it's probably more important than in maintenance that we get the first dose right because they're only on it for two or three weeks and then they start reducing. And if you don't give them an opportunity to stabilise on a dose that actually covers them medically, then you really are setting them up to fail. (Nurse, DDU).

Control over change

Once the start dose had been set, dose decisions were typically negotiated on a local level between the keyworker and the client (for a detailed example, see Quirk *et al.* 2003).[3] While keyworkers consulted the doctor about changes in dose, especially regarding an increase, professional roles and levels of autonomy over decisions varied greatly within and between treatment agencies. Similarly, the nature and extent of client input into dose decisions varied considerably.

Rather than actual dose, the more pressing concern for many clients was how long the treatment episode would last and how much input and control they would have to change their treatment, especially dose reductions. For staff, a key skill in managing clients who were perceived to have unrealistic expectations was to reschedule their reductions. This would involve their 'putting the brakes' on change:

> I had a client recently, he's got some mental health problems and using as well. He wants to detox[ify] at a rate which I would consider is way too rapid and it's like 'No you're not stable, and to do this is an unrealistic option'. What you are trying to do is not put people in the situation where you are setting them up to fail. (Nurse, DDU).

Client perspectives on dose reductions were partly linked to their views of methadone (discussed further in this chapter). Some wanted to reduce and detoxify as soon as possible because of the perceived addictiveness of methadone. Others were reluctant to reduce, primarily because they feared difficult physiological and psychological effects of a dose change. It was common for the latter to be concerned about staff having unrealistic expectations about the pace of dose reductions:

> If they really push you and then you come off it too soon and then you go back onto drugs and you know your problem isn't solved. (Client, DDU).

Staff reported being well aware of such fears, and the challenge for them was helping clients to overcome this, especially when they 'have been on a dose for a long time'. This typically would involve careful negotiation:

> [My keyworker] will take into account what I've said to him, how I feel about it. I think we'll come to some compromise about it. If he feels that I'm not comfortable about reducing again, I think he'll probably say 'Okay then, fair enough', because he knows I've had trouble. (Client, DDU).

Yet other clients reported actively avoiding change and devising conversational strategies to achieve this:

---

[3] Previous research (Gossop *et al.* 1982) indicates how easily time-limited increases in dose, agreed in response to problems, can be negotiated upfront by staff and clients.

I knew the question [about reducing] would come up at some stage and I'd be waiting for it [in the keyworking session] – I'd have reasons made up why it would be better that I didn't. And I'd try to bring those reasons into the start of the conversation surreptitiously and try and get the conversation going in that direction. (Client, DDU).

Many meanings of methadone

What's different about methadone [to other medication] is that it's used by clients in so many different ways. Some clients see it definitely as medicine – even though they know it's an opiate, to them it's not, whereas obviously there are others who see it as a way of staying reasonably healthy and straight before getting another hit [of heroin]. (Nurse, DDU).

Methadone was found to have many meanings for clients and staff. It was variously perceived as 'boring', potentially 'dangerous' (especially at the start of a treatment episode), more 'addictive' than heroin, and occasionally 'pleasurable'. Furthermore, its perceived uses included to 'hold withdrawals', offer 'stability between hits', act as a 'medicine', provide 'capital' (via diversion onto the illicit market) and give people an 'opportunity for lifestyle change'. Such views were subject to change over the course of a treatment episode or treatment career, as indicated by the following quote:

I was really scared at first of taking methadone because I looked at methadone as being just like heroin except you're getting it from a doctor. Now I don't see it like that. Okay, methadone's addictive but it's a lot better than taking illegal drugs – it's not a drug as such, it's a cross-roads. It gives you the choice to carry on with life and it gets you normal. (Client, DDU).

Clients (and staff) will inevitably bring to their encounters such perceptions, which shape their *goals* in interaction. For example, clients who view methadone, or at least a part of their 'take-home' prescription, primarily as 'capital' – to be exchanged on the illicit market for money or drugs – are likely to be intent on maximizing their dose (Quirk *et al.* 2003). In contrast, those who see it as 'boring' are unlikely to aim for an increase (nor are staff likely to recommend it) in order to counter occasional hedonistic use of heroin.

Concern about methadone addiction

Interviews with both staff and clients indicated that there is growing concern about the long-term effects of methadone, particularly its addictive potential.[4] Again, such concerns are brought to medical encounters with staff and variously influence participants' actions and goals within them. First there were reports of clients withholding information at initial assessment in order to start on a lower dose than might have been the case:

> They may start off saying they use half a gram of heroin a day, which we'd convert [into the correct methadone dose]. It could turn out they're using much more than that, but they've been afraid to say – there's a rumour on the street about what methadone does to people, like it's more addictive [than heroin]. (Nurse, DDU).

Second, such concerns led some clients to request time-limited treatment or a reduction programme at initial assessment. On the other hand, it could make existing clients more fearful of detoxifying:

> I've heard methadone's supposed to be worse for withdrawing than heroin, it stays in your system. And most addicts fear that and put off coming off. (Client, DDU).

Such fears led to requests for dosage to be maintained among those who had no immediate intention of detoxifying:

> If I'm on 40 mls I can keep on going with my life. The question of reducing never arose again because I said to [my nurse-keyworker] 'Look just maintain [me and my partner] on what we're on' because we were managing. I did initially want to come off because methadone's a very insidious drug. It's worse than heroin for sure. I would dread coming off. (Client, DDU).

Alternatively, concerns about tolerance can lead to requests for dosage to be reduced in order to make detoxification easier in the long run:

> [Why did you want a reduction?] Because methadone is so much harder to come off than gear. I came off methadone once, about four years ago, and I didn't sleep one full night for six months. I want to come off it now because I know the detox is gonna slaughter me. I just wanna be clean now. (Client, DDU).

Staff were generally well aware of such concerns, and would seek to discuss them with clients when appropriate. But they also led some staff to regard shorter-acting drugs, such as diamorphine, as possibly more efficacious for clients undergoing detoxification. Indeed, both of the NHS DDUs involved in the research were increasingly using alternatives to methadone treatment

---

[4] Such concerns are well-founded in the sense that withdrawal symptoms of methadone take longer to subside than those of heroin (Department of Health 1999). In addition, our fieldwork coincided with the publication of scientific, specialist and mass media accounts of methadone problems, such as those relating to its toxicity (e.g. Newcombe 1996). These are likely to have fuelled clients' concerns. Further, they probably contributed more generally to the construction of methadone treatment in the UK as a social and policy problem (Quirk et al. 1998).

(e.g. lofexidine), in part as a response to meeting the needs of clients who were concerned about 'replacing one addiction with another'.

Contextual influences

> They wouldn't give me [a maintenance script] because I should imagine there's quite a lot of people trying to get into here. I've heard there's quite a big waiting list. My [reduction] script is not by choice, it's something I've really been forced into. (Client, DDU).

Our findings show that dose negotiation, and methadone decision-making more generally, is best understood in relation to the specific organizational context in which it is embedded. This is important because at the time of the fieldwork we found both of the DDUs to be undergoing organizational change, which was affecting staff–client interaction and limiting the scope for negotiation. The emergent picture was that the clinics were becoming 'stricter', more 'boundaried' and harder for clients to gain access to. This change in the nature of methadone treatment had been fuelled, in part, by a combination of organizational factors which had put pressure on the provision of 'open-ended' methadone maintenance. These included: growing demand for methadone maintenance, but limited resources to deal with it; lengthy waiting lists for non-priority cases; 'silting up' of the service with long-term maintenance clients; and detoxification had become a 'high risk' option (because it was difficult to get back into treatment in the event of relapse), making this an even more 'scary' option to clients.[5] At the same time, we saw evidence of changing attitudes among staff and some 'loss of faith' in HIV-oriented harm reduction approaches. Reasons for this included: emergent epidemiological evidence showing lower-than-predicted levels of HIV among injecting drug users in the UK; and the practical difficulties clinics were having in providing a genuinely 'low threshold' service at a time when demand for maintenance treatment outweighed supply, and when extra HIV funding for service expansion had become harder to justify (Quirk *et al*. 1998).

The key message here is that staff–client interaction does not occur in an institutional vacuum: contextual factors influence what staff and clients do in their encounters with one another, so need to be considered when investigating decision-making about dose.

Conclusions

Qualitative research asks different questions to those of outcomes studies and can give new insights into clinical practice (Fountain 2000). In this chapter

---

[5] These types of organizational pressures were forewarned by Strang in the late 1980s (Strang 1989).

we have described some of the negotiation that goes on between staff and clients in methadone treatment, as well as the organizational and contextual factors that influence this. Dingwall *et al.* (1998) argue the case for qualitative studies of this type. They note that clinical practice has two key aspects: first, a body of 'rules', as produced by evidence-based approaches founded on the randomized controlled trial (RCT), and second, a set of improvisational skills in fitting the general rules to the particular case. Having noted the need for professional work to decide which rules apply to which case, Dingwall and colleagues argue that qualitative research is able to *address the gap* between the findings of RCTs and similar research and the actual practice of decision-making in individual cases with individual patients. By investigating such improvisation and the organizational context in which it is embedded, as well as addressing topics of equity (fairness of access to services) and humanity (what happens to people when they get it), qualitative research has the potential to promote effectiveness. This is because, while evidence-based approaches increase the client's chance of getting the right treatment, for example, in terms of dose, more is needed to ensure that it is taken in a way that will reproduce the findings of RCTs without the special conditions that RCT design and management create (Dingwall *et al.* 1998). This chapter has attempted to take some steps in that direction, with the illustration of how open-ended methadone maintenance and retention rates can be pressured by organizational factors that are largely beyond the control of practitioners. Such factors need to be addressed in order to make evidence-based practice possible at the individual practitioner level.

Methadone has a wide range of often conflicting meanings to clients; these may go well beyond its official medical function of curbing opiate withdrawal and stabilizing patients. We have seen that such perceptions shape clients' goals in their interactions with staff and this complements previous findings about the variable functions of continued heroin use on top of a methadone prescription (Best *et al.* 1999). Further, it helps to explain the inconsistencies in the relationship between such use and methadone dose. It is evidently wrong to assume that continued heroin use is motivated by physiological factors alone. Future outcomes studies should, therefore, consider trying to capture issues of process such as clients' satisfaction with their level of input into treatment decisions and their perceptions of methadone and its functions. This will allow further exploration of the complex relationship between prescribed methadone dose and illicit drug use on top of it.

Finally, clients indicated that there are growing concerns about the perceived addictiveness of methadone. Methadone clients were found to constitute a comparatively 'wised up' patient group. However, those who were new to treatment seemed to be unaware of some of the risks associated with methadone, for example that it may prolong dependence and can be associated with changed patterns of alcohol use. While such issues were often discussed in intake assessments and relevant material was made available, there is a persuasive argument for eliciting formal informed consent from clients so that they are fully aware of the pros and cons of taking methadone.

Acknowledgements

The authors would like to thank the staff and clients of the agencies involved in the study, as well as Sarah Mars for her helpful comments on an earlier draft of this chapter.

References

Best, D., Gossop, M., Stewart, D., Marsden, J., Lehmann, P. & Strang, J. (1999) Continued heroin use during methadone treatment: relationships between frequency of use and reasons reported for heroin use. *Drug and Alcohol Dependence*, 53: 191–5.

Bewley, T.H. & Fleminger, R.S. (1970) Staff–patient problems in drug dependence treatment clinics. *Journal of Psycho-Somatic Research*, 14: 303–6.

Department of Health (1999) *Drug Misuse and Dependence – Guidelines on Clinical Management.* London: The Stationery Office.

Dingwall, R., Murphy, E., Watson, P., Greatbach, D. & Parker, S. (1998) Catching goldfish: quality in qualitative research. *Journal of Health Services Research and Policy*, 3: 167–73.

D'Aunno, T. & Vaughn, T.E. (1992) Variations in methadone treatment practices: results from a national study. *Journal of American Medical Association*, 267: 253–8.

Farrell, M., Sell, L., Neeleman, J., Gossop, M., Griffiths, P., Buning, E., Finch, E. & Strang, J. (1996) Methadone provision in the UK. *International Journal of Drug Policy*, 7: 239–44.

Fountain, J. (ed.) (2000) *Understanding and Responding to Drug Use: The Role of Qualitative Research.* Lisbon: European Monitoring Centre for Drugs and Drugs Addiction.

Gossop, M., Strang, J. & Connell, P.H. (1982) The response of out-patient opiate addicts to the provision of a temporary increase in their prescribed drugs. *British Journal of Psychiatry*, 141: 338–43.

Lilly, R., Quirk, A., Rhodes, T. & Stimson, G.V. (2000) Sociality in methadone treatment: understanding methadone treatment and service delivery as a social process. *Drugs: Education, Prevention and Policy*, 7: 163–78.

Lilly, R., Quirk, A., Rhodes, T. & Stimson, G.V. (1999) Juggling multiple roles: staff and client perceptions of keyworker roles and constraints on delivering counselling and support services in methadone treatment. *Addiction Research*, 7: 267–89.

Magura, S., Nwakeze, P.C. & Demsky, S. (1998) Pre- and in-treatment predictors of retention in methadone treatment using survival analysis. *Addiction*, 93: 51–60.

Martin, J., Payte, J.T. & Zweben, J.E. (1991) Methadone maintenance treatment: a primer for physicians. *Journal of Psychoactive Drugs,* 23: 165–76.

Metzger, D.S. & Platt, J.J. (1987) Methadone dose levels and client characteristics in heroin addicts. *International Journal of the Addictions*, 22: 187–94.

Newcombe, R. (1996) Staying alive: how safe is methadone? *Juice*, 1: 16–17.

Quirk, A., Rhodes, T. & Lilly, R. (2003) Combining ethnography with conversation analysis: the negotiation of methadone decisions. In: Rhodes T, ed. *Qualitative Methods in Drugs Research*. London: Sage.

Quirk, A., Lilly, R., Rhodes, T. & Stimson, G.V. (1998) *Opening the 'Black Box': A Study of Methadone Treatment Process in North Thames,* Final report. London: The Centre for Research on Drugs and Health Behaviour.

Preston, A. (1999) *The Methadone Handbook*, Fifth Edition. Dorchester: Exchange.

Roszell, D.K. & Calsyn, D.A. (1986) Methadone dosage: characteristics and clinical correlates. *International Journal of the Addictions*, 21: 1233–46.

Royal College of Psychiatrists & Royal College of Physicians Working Party (2000) *Drugs: Dilemmas and Choices.* London: Gaskell.

Stimson, G.V. & Oppenheimer, E. (1982) *Heroin Addiction: Treatment and Control in Britain,* London: Tavistock.

Strang, J. (1989) 'The British System': past, present and future. *International Review of Psychiatry,* 1: 109–20.

Strang, J. & Sheridan, J. (1998) Effect of government recommendations on methadone prescribing in south-east England: comparison of 1995 and 1997 surveys. *British Medical Journal*, 317: 1489–90.

Ward, J., Mattick, R.P. & Hall, W. (1998) The use of methadone during maintenance treatment: pharmacology, dosage and treatment outcome. In: Ward J, Mattick RP, Hall W, eds. *Methadone Maintenance Treatment and Other Opioid Replacement Therapies.* Amsterdam: Harwood.

5
Linking psychology and pharmacology

Duncan Raistrick

It is commonplace in the addiction field to hear talk of *methadone programmes* or *prescribing services,* as if the pharmacotherapy was of itself a treatment. This should never be the case. Pharmacotherapies are particularly useful for targeting discrete symptoms such as withdrawal or craving. In contrast psycho-social interventions are usually aimed at a much broader range of problems; it follows that judiciously combining the two is likely to produce the most robust and effective treatment package (Carroll 1997). The prescriber has a responsibility to ensure that any prescription is safe, can be justified in terms of efficacy, and is one element of a treatment plan which may in part or in whole be delivered by the prescriber.

Substitute treatment packages are typically delivered by more than one professional and, in the case of shared care, by more than one agency. Multi-professional and multi-agency working is difficult and will only be effective if those participating aspire to have complementary roles and be perceived by patients to be acting as one. This is a tall order, even where professionals share the same philosophies and have personal friendships. Kenyon *et al.* (2001) have identified some of the key elements that make for a successful shared care scheme – most notably a shared model of understanding to facilitate communication and shared protocols. It is often assumed that psychotherapies, or talking therapies generally, are safe and can be delivered by anyone without formal, professional training. This is incorrect – the example of false memory enhancement, particularly in cases of child sexual abuse (Andrews *et al.* 1999), is a reminder of the axiom: *first do no harm*. Addictions psychotherapy can do harm and so the competence of therapists is of paramount concern.

Interesting dynamics and tensions surround substitute prescribing. On the one hand there is a goal to reduce harm and reduce dependence on opiates at an individual level but, on the other hand, there is a goal to support social and public health policy objectives – the two may not be in harmony. In achieving the latter there is an implicit 'deal', namely *the state will give free drugs but you must agree to certain conditions*. The conditions are too often idiosyncratic to prescribers' interpretations of their responsibilities and need to be made more explicit through policy. This chapter sets aside these political issues and plays on the psychological interactions between the patient and their social context, the prescribed drug, the role of the therapist as treatment moderator, and the implications of specific psycho-social treatments.

The psychology of the drug effect

Methadone has a number of properties that are important elements of substitution therapy: it produces an opiate effect; it is cross-tolerant with other opiates and is able to suppress the emergence of withdrawal symptoms; it has a high affinity for opiate receptor sites and in high enough dose (usually considered to be 60–100 mg daily) is able to 'block' the effect of commonly misused opiates such as heroin. The so-called blocking effect occurs because methadone has a high affinity for opiate receptors and prevents other opiates having an action at the receptor sites for as long as methadone is active – typically 12–24 hours. In fact the block is only ever partial and less than that achieved with buprenorphine or naltrexone.

The key concept linking drug effect and behaviour is called *reinforcement.* In plain language reinforcement occurs because of a desired drug effect and means that the behaviour, drug-taking, is likely to be repeated. In the absence of a headache, taking aspirin has no effect and so people do not use aspirin for aspirin's sake. In contrast, heroin has a highly desired effect beyond analgesia and so people may use more heroin simply because they like its euphoriant effect. Reinforcement from a pleasant drug effect is called positive reinforcement; reinforcement from avoidance of something unpleasant, for example, withdrawal, is called negative reinforcement. The importance of the positive reinforcement effect of methadone is sometimes underestimated. Bickel *et al.* (1986) showed that, in a choice procedure paradigm, volunteer subjects were more likely to choose the higher available dose of methadone; subjects recognized and had a liking for the opiate effect even though they did not experience a high and did not experience withdrawal.

These pharmacokinetic properties of a substitute drug can readily be translated into psychological properties which can be manipulated, by choice of drug and prescribing regimen, to suit the particular purpose of the individual treatment. The psychoactive effect of methadone – positive reinforcement – is important to make acceptable the switch from more potent opiates such as heroin so that patients will engage and stay in treatment. The avoidance of withdrawal symptoms – negative reinforcement – lasts for about 24 hours and is equally important for creating a stable psychological state. Achieving receptor blockade may be necessary to prevent supplementation of the prescription by use of illicit heroin – in effect desensitization of heroin use. Methadone is itself an addictive drug, but less so than heroin because its effect is less potent and its long duration avoids the need for the regular 'topping up' which is characteristic of shorter-acting opiates.

Substituting heroin with methadone will reduce opiate dependence in the short term but longer term prescribing of methadone will lead to repeated learning of its own positive reinforcement potential, resulting in the reinstatement of higher levels of opiate dependence. Dependence should not be confused with the experience of withdrawal, which is more severe but of shorter duration for heroin.

There are alternatives to methadone and the differences in pharmacokinetics confer different psychological properties. Buprenorphine is a partial opiate agonist, meaning less positive reinforcement, and so it tends to be inferior to methadone on programme retention but has the benefits of being an effective antagonist at low doses and having less addictive potential so that it is easier to achieve abstinence (Walsh *et al.* 1994). It is probably best suited to those who have low to moderate dependence. LAAM (levo-alpha-acetylmethadol) is much longer acting than methadone but in other respects rather similar (Glanz *et al.* 1997). It is probably well-suited to people firmly engaged in long-term maintenance programmes. The dilemma of substitution therapy can be summarized in the statement that the more closely a prescription approximates to the route and drug of choice of the user then the more likely that they will stay in the treatment programme but the less likely that they will become drug free – this is no better illustrated than in the study by Hartnoll *et al.* (1980) of diamorphine versus methadone substitution. In this study, high dependence users were assigned either to injectable diamorphine or to oral methadone prescribing plus the standard psychosocial therapy of the day. In the diamorphine group, 74% were in treatment and 10% were abstinent after one year; for the methadone group the figures were 29% and 30% respectively. The picture for other outcome measures was quite mixed. It is not that one treatment is better than another, rather that different treatments deliver different outcomes.

Therapist characteristics

The way in which a therapist relates to patients, without delivering any specific treatment, is of critical importance. The concept of the 'therapeutic alliance' has become recognized as one of the most consistent predictors of outcome across different forms of psychotherapy. The therapeutic alliance can be thought of as having three key components: the personal therapeutic bond between patient and practitioner, agreement about the goals that are to be achieved and agreement about the method of achieving those goals. A therapeutic alliance is something that grows as therapy progresses and the timing of its measurement is therefore problematic. It would be logical routinely to measure therapeutic alliance at the end of treatment as a means of identifying those therapists who consistently had difficulty building an alliance. In a particularly lengthy treatment there could be advantage in taking repeated measures of therapeutic alliance to give early warning of a therapist in difficulty, although this would be impractical for many of the briefer therapies in use today.

A busy addiction clinic requires that therapists have the characteristics to build rapidly a positive therapeutic alliance. Much of the research in this area has been done outwith the addiction field or, if within the field, then it is not specifically related to substitute prescribing. For example, Cartwright (1980) proposed that effective therapists would score highly on what he called overall therapeutic attitude, which he formulated as being the sum of role legitimacy, role adequacy and self-esteem. The role legitimacy of those working in specialist agencies is self-evident but may not be so for generic workers; arguably addiction is the business of all caring professions and so it is important that substance misuse be included within the curriculum of all professional training courses, thereby marking the appropriateness of working with substance misuse problems. Role adequacy is a function of post basic training, gaining clinical experience, and having organizational support. Self-esteem is a more general concept; the important finding is that therapists with their own psychological problems tend to do less well than those without.

Matching therapists to patient characteristics is an attractive but usually impractical proposition: indeed, in so doing, patient choice and therapist improvement through a broadening of experience are likely to suffer. One important exception is where there is little chance of building a therapeutic alliance, for example, women who have experienced violence from men do better with all-women services (Jarvis 1992). A second exception might be where there is an unbridgeable gulf between cultures. The problem here is that there are just too many cultures; ethnic groups may have their overriding culture but within each group there are many sub-cultures based on such things as religion, wealth, education, leisure pursuits and so forth. The foremost concern of patients is that they have a competent therapist. Thereafter much can be done to facilitate building a therapeutic alliance through practising basic therapy skills.

If matching therapists and patients is impractical, then an alternative is for therapists to present themselves in as neutral a way as possible without taking away their individual flair and personality. Dress code is a good example: Wilson Jones and Keaney (2002) found that patients were most comfortable with staff dressed 'smart but casual' and they found spiky hair and body piercing intimidating. Another example is through interpersonal communication skills: attention to time keeping, collecting and greeting people in the waiting room, checking out the appropriate salutation, and being careful about body language. Perhaps more controversially, the general style of interacting with patients is something that can be learned. Motivational interviewing, that is a style of interviewing where the therapist's purpose is to elicit self-motivating statements, has become very popular in the addiction field. Some would argue that motivational interviewing is, of itself, a specific therapy; however, it may more usefully be seen as a therapist behaviour in that it can be applied to most, if not all, therapies commonly used in addictions. To separate therapist attribute effects from specific treatment effects is now seen as a challenge for psychotherapy research. For example, in Project MATCH (Project MATCH Research Group 1998) therapist characteristics were found to have modest and variable effects on outcome; however, in other studies of Motivational Enhancement Therapy, those therapists who scored high on 'need for nurturance' and low on 'need for aggression' delivered the best results.

What then is the impact of therapist behaviours in the clinic? Luborsky *et al.* (1985) studied the effectiveness of 27 addiction therapists trained to deliver one of three manual based, six-month treatments: counselling, behaviour therapy, and supportive expressive therapy. A total of 110 subjects were randomly allocated to the treatments. A raft of outcome measures were taken seven months after the start of treatment and an index of change, where 1.0 represents maximum change, across seven of the outcome measures was calculated. One therapist achieved large change, 0.74, four therapists were middle range achievers, 0.4–0.6, and four were small change achievers, less than 0.3. To take specific examples, on the outcome measure 'drug use' the best therapist achieved a 34% improvement and the worst therapist a 14% deterioration, and on the measure 'psychiatric status' the best achieved an 82% improvement and the worst a 1% deterioration when averaged across their whole caseloads. The therapist qualities associated with good outcome were labelled *interest in helping patients, therapist psychological health* and *psychological skill*. Therapists tended to drift from their assigned treatment regimens in inconsistent ways. For the more specific therapies, that is the supportive expressive and cognitive behavioural therapy, the purity of treatment delivery, the extent to which the therapist adhered exclusively to the intended treatment the better the outcome; in contrast the counselling intervention did better when borrowing from the other two modalities.

Similarly in a study of methadone dose as a determinant of outcome, Blaney and Craig (1999) found that most of the variation in outcome was attributable to therapists and not methadone dose. For example, on the measure of positive drug screens, the best therapist had 11% positive and the worst 60% positive. Programme retention was also found to be related to therapist differences rather than dosage differences. These variations in therapist performance are substantial and likely to confound outcome studies of specific treatments if the therapist variables are not controlled.

Psychotherapists from other disciplines show the same variability of performance. Lafferty *et al.* (1989) studied the differences between more and less effective trainee psychotherapists. Of the 30 trainees, 85% of the less effective therapists were identified by only three variables: empathy, patient involvement and therapist directiveness. Patients of the less effective therapists felt less well understood than did the patients of the more effective therapists, but the less effective therapists also overestimated their patients' involvement in therapy and overestimated their own contribution to the therapy process.

Measuring therapist competence is a formidable but not impossible task (Margison *et al.* 2000). Not least among the difficulties is the consistent finding that the most expert practitioner has an ability to use therapy manuals in novel ways in order to adapt to the particular therapeutic situation. Lifting and maintaining therapist competencies is a critical element in improving substitute prescribing programmes more generally, and it follows that therapist supervision including prescribers, assisted by video recording of therapy sessions, is now an essential part of clinical governance.

Specific treatments

Psychosocial treatments have always been part of substitute prescribing programmes. The task of evaluation has been made difficult by confusing terminology, and so the goals of each kind of service need to be understood by clinic staff, commissioners, users and the general public in order to secure continuing support. The key questions are: to what extent are psycho-social treatments necessary to maximize the benefits of substitute prescribing; and to what extent are psycho-social treatments necessary in order to move people on to achieve abstinence from opiates?

It has been known for a long time that the presence of positive social influences outweighs other factors in determining good outcome for substance misuse problems. Hunt and Azrin (1973) demonstrated that adding elements such as a buddying system, leisure skills, and employment assistance to standard treatments markedly improved outcome – they called this the Community Reinforcement Approach. Following the same principles in a methadone programme, Abbott *et al.* (1998) found that, when 180 subjects were randomized to standard treatment or Community Reinforcement Approach treatment, the latter was superior in terms of positive urinalysis and scores on the Addiction Severity Index. In a more pragmatic interpretation of the same need, Gallanter (1993) has described a style of therapy that utilizes existing social networks to support change in addictive behaviours; social network therapy lends itself to combining with other more established therapies.

If methadone alone is insufficient to deliver the best results from methadone programmes, then is there an optimum level of psycho-social input, or are the benefits 'dose' related (the more therapy the better the outcome)? McLellan *et al.* (1993) randomly allocated 92 subjects to three six-month treatment programmes where the minimum dose of methadone was 60 mg daily: i) minimum treatment was essentially prescribing only; ii) standard treatment was prescribing and structured counselling; and iii) enhanced treatment was prescribing, counselling and added psychiatric care, family therapy, and employment counselling. The clinical effectiveness was related to the amount of therapy; 'prescribing only' treatment performed so poorly that clinicians felt bound to transfer over two-thirds of subjects assigned to this modality to 'standard treatment'. In a further analysis of these data, the cost effectiveness ratio was established by comparing the total treatment costs against reductions in demand on welfare and criminal justice systems – standard treatment was found to be the most cost effective (Kraft *et al.* 1997). In order to investigate whether or not the dose response to therapy has a ceiling effect, Avents *et al.* (1999) randomized 308 subjects between the same enhanced treatment used by McLellan and a high intensity day treatment which included extensive skills training. There were no major differences between the results seen with the two intensities of treatment; however, those patients with no prior history of methadone treatment were more likely to stay in treatment and were more likely to be abstinent at follow-up if they received the lower intensity of intervention. The evidence here points to the conclusion that there is a minimum level of psycho-social therapy that is necessary within any methadone programme. More intensive therapy improves the clinical outcome but only when matched to assessed need and even then reaching a ceiling effect. As an example of targeted need, Avents *et al.* (1998) identified patients with social anxiety who had been referred for methadone treatment and offered anxiety management skills training; they found that those patients in the less intensive general treatment but with added anxiety treatment did better than those in the more intensive general treatment. An assessment of the significance of mental health problems and appropriate intervention should be built into any treatment package.

For organizational reasons it may be impractical to conduct a detailed individual needs assessment and provide a bespoke treatment programme. In these circumstances a more universal means of enhancing a methadone programme on the basis of *more problems more treatment* could be of value. Studies have shown that people can be persuaded to stop using drugs by giving them financial incentives. For example, Piotrowski *et al.* (1999) offered monetary contingencies for patients in methadone treatment and found that subjects allocated to the contingency condition had longer periods of abstinence and more drug-free urinalysis results than those without incentive. Financial incentives have little practical application in therapy but serve to make the point that if there is a sufficiently attractive alternative then people will give up the use of even powerfully addictive drugs such as heroin and cocaine. Unfortunately the changes in drug using behaviour stop when the financial incentives stop. In a more useful example of contingency management, Kidorff *et al.* (1998) set up a programme where continued prescribing of methadone was contingent upon patients securing employment, meaning paid or voluntary work or training, within two months of commencing treatment; those who did not achieve this goal were transferred to ever more intensive therapy until they succeeded; in the event of persistent failure, methadone was slowly tapered. Three-quarters of patients were able to secure and maintain employment, 78% of these continuing through the six-month follow-up; half were successful without referral to more intensive therapy.

Conclusions

Substitute prescribing programmes can be expected to deliver benefits across the major outcome domains, namely reducing illicit drug use, improving health, improving social circumstances, and reducing criminal activity. However, the specific reasons for prescribing and the intended outcomes need to be understood. Furthermore, the amount of benefit varies greatly according to how the treatment is delivered. In order to achieve the desired goals there is a need for an experienced prescriber, preferably working to a protocol, collaborating with a skilled therapist, preferably working to a manual. The amount of psycho-social intervention required to give maximum clinical effect depends on patient need – more than is needed might even be counterproductive. Aggregate cost effectiveness is probably best achieved from a standard treatment package, meaning structured therapy without enhancements. It has proved difficult to find pre-treatment factors that reliably predict outcome. For example Morral *et al.* (1999) found no useful pre-treatment predictors of outcome but did find that clean toxicology screens and attendance in counselling at two weeks correctly identified 80% of good outcome cases nine months later. It may well be productive to give priority to more intelligent programme monitoring in order to identify at an early stage either a therapist or patient in need of additional help and support.

References

Abbott, P.J., Weller, S.B., Delaney, H.D. & Moore, B.A. (1998) Community reinforcement approach in the treatment of opiate addicts. *American Journal of Drug & Alcohol Abuse*, 24: 17–30.

Andrews, B., Brewin, C.R., Ochera, J., Morton, J., Bekerian, D.A., Davies, G.M. & Mollon, P. (1999) Characteristics, context and consequences of memory recovery among adults in therapy. *British Journal of Psychiatry*, 175: 141–6.

Avents, S.K., Margolin, A., Sindelar, J.L., Rounsaville, B.J., Schottenfeld, R., Stine, S., Cooney, N.L., Rosenheck, R.A., Li, S. & Kosten, T.R. (1999) Day Treatment Versus Enhanced Standard Methadone Services for Opioid-Dependent Patients: A Comparison of Clinical Efficacy and Cost. *American Journal of Psychiatry*, 156: 27–33.

Avents, S.K., Margolin, A., Kosten, T.R., Rounsavillle, B.J. & Schottenfeld, R.

(1998) When is less treatment better? The role of social anxiety in matching methadone patients to psychosocial treatments. *Journal of Consulting and Clinical Psychology*, 66: 924–31.

Bickel, W.K., Higgins, S.T. & Stitzer, M.L. (1986) Choice of blind methadone dose increases by methadone maintenance patients. *Drug and Alcohol Dependence*, 18: 165–77.

Blaney, T. & Craig, R.J. (1999) Methadone Maintenance. *Journal of Substance Abuse Treatment*, 16: 221–8.

Carroll, K.M. (1997) Integrating psychotherapy and pharmacotherapy to improve drug abuse outcomes. *Addictive Behaviors*, 22: 233–45.

Cartwright, A.K.J. (1980) The attitudes of helping agents towards the alcoholic client: the influence of experience, support, training, and self-esteem. *British Journal of Addiction*, 75: 413–31.

Gallanter, M. (1993) *Network Therapy for Alcohol and Drug Abuse*. London: The Guildford Press.

Glanz, M., Klawansky, S., McAullife, W. & Chalmers, T. (1997) Methadone vs. L-alpha-acetylmethadol (LAAM) in the treatment of opiate addiction. A meta-analysis of the randomised controlled trials. *American Journal of Addictions*, 6: 339–49.

Hartnoll, R.L., Mitcheson, M.C., Battersby, A., Brown, G., Ellis, M., Fleming, P. & Hedley, N. (1980) Evaluation of heroin maintenance in controlled trial. *Archives of General Psychiatry*, 37: 877–84.

Hunt, G.M. & Azrin, N.H. (1973) A community-reinforcement approach to alcoholism. *Behaviour Research and Therapy*, 11: 91–104.

Jarvis, T.J. (1992) Implications of gender for alcohol treatment research: a quantitative and qualitative review. *British Journal of Addiction*, 87: 1249–61.

Kenyon, R.H., West, D., Raistrick, D.S. & Hatton, P. (2001) General Practitioner satisfaction with 'Shared Care' working. *Journal of Substance Use*, 6: 36–9.

Kidorff, M., Hollander, J.R., King, V.L. & Brooner, R.K. (1998) Increasing employment of opioid dependent outpatients: an intensive behavioural intervention. *Drug and Alcohol Dependence*, 50: 73–80.

Kraft, M.K., Hadley, T.R. & McLellan, A.T. (1997) Are supplementary services provided during methadone maintenance really cost-effective? *American Journal of Psychiatry*, 154: 1214–9.

Lafferty, P., Beutler, L.E. & Crago, M. (1989) Differences between more and less effective psychotherapists: a study of select therapist variables. *Journal of Consulting and Clinical Psychology*, 57: 76–80.

Luborsky, L., McLellan, A.T., Woody, G.E., O'Brien, C.P. & Auerbach, A. (1985) Therapist success and its determinants. *Archives of General Psychiatry*, 42: 602–11.

Margison, F.R., Barkham, M., Evans, C., McGrath, G., Mellor Clark, J., Audin, K. & Connell, J. (2000) Measurement and psychotherapy. Evidence-based practice and practice-based evidence. *British Journal of Psychiatry*, 177: 123–30.

McLellan, A.T., Arndt, I.O., Metzger, D.S., Woody, G.E. & O'Brien, C.P. (1993) The effects of psychosocial services in substance abuse treatment. *Journal of the American Medical Association*, 269: 1953–9.

Morral, A.R., Belding, M.A. & Iguchi, M.Y. (1999) Identifying methadone maintenance clients at risk for poor treatment response: pretreatment and early progress indicators. *Drug and Alcohol Dependence*, 55: 25–33.

Piotrowski, N.A., Tusel, D.J., Sees, K.L., Reilly, P.M., Banys, P., Meek, P. & Hall, S.M. (1999) Contingency contracting with monetary reinforcers for abstinence from multiple drugs in a methadone program. *Experimental and Clinical Psychopharmacology*, 7: 399–411.

Project MATCH Research Group (1998) Therapist effects in three treatments for alcohol problems. *Psychotherapy Research,* 8: 455–74.

Walsh, S.L., Preston, K.L., Stitzer, M.L., Cone, E.J. & Bigelow, G.E. (1994) Clinical pharmacology of buprenorphine: ceiling effects at high doses. *Clinical Pharmacology and Therapeutics,* 55: 569–80.

Wilson Jones, C.F. & Keaney, F. (2003) Guidelines for the millennium. How psychiatric patients would like their psychiatrists to dress. *Psychiatric Bulletin,* in press.

6
Assessment and outcome monitoring

John Marsden, Michael Gossop and Duncan Stewart

Patient assessment and treatment outcome monitoring arrangements for methadone prescribing services are explored in the context of a continuum of care approach for those people with opioid dependence who require agonist pharmacotherapy. An overview of the rationale and benefits of using a structured assessment and outcome monitoring approach is provided, with a description of the basic elements needed when deciding how to develop these arrangements.

Rationale for structured assessment and outcome monitoring

The evaluation literature on methadone prescribing indicates that treatment is generally effective in helping patients to reduce their heroin use and improve their personal and social functioning. However, methadone treatment services are not identical in their structure and operation, and outcome studies show that their level of effectiveness varies widely. Many service providers are interested in monitoring their own outcomes, reflecting organizational values. There has been some progress in this area in the UK but there are relatively few instances of fully integrated and sustained monitoring systems. There is an increasing expectation among UK health authorities, drug action teams and commissioning groups that service contracts will include a requirement for this information to be collected. Improvements in the resources and procedures that support outcome monitoring are at the forefront of priorities for many developed treatment systems and high quality service providers.

There are several benefits to be derived from collecting assessment and outcome information. First, many patients perceive that a structured approach to assessment and recording outcome reflects a service that is committed to providing the best care. The feedback of information describing the during-treatment changes to the patient (and his/her spouse/partner or carers) by clinical staff can be a powerful motivational influence to reinforce progress and assist in personal treatment goal setting. Secondly, clinical staff can monitor the characteristics and outcomes of their caseloads and identify areas of priority work. Thirdly, service managers can aggregate information across staff as an indicator of how well the agency is serving its patients. Fourthly, aggregate summaries of samples of cases across services can be provided to funding bodies and other government agencies to show the overall impact of treatment provision for a particular area.

This chapter is organized into three sections, beginning with conceptual issues and description of a framework. Examination of the key elements of structured assessment in the context of outcome monitoring and a summary of reliable structured assessment and outcome evaluation instruments follows. The chapter concludes with a discussion of some of the important implementation and operational issues that should be considered when establishing these arrangements.

Conceptual issues and framework

Treatment outcomes may be defined, technically, as the results of processes and can be positive or negative. Outcomes are therefore those subsequent conditions or events that can be established as plausible or likely effects of treatment processes. In the context of a methadone maintenance programme, for example, questions of outcome concern the retention of the patient, the reduction in heroin use and problem behaviours and whether desired treatment goals are achieved and maintained over time. The most logical and practical method of assessing treatment outcome is to use a parallel set of measures for intake assessment, at the completion of treatment and at one or more subsequent points during and/or following treatment. Seen in this way, outcome determination may be conceptualized as reassessment. This information can be used to improve the client assessment and care co-ordination process. Reassessing patients helps the treatment provider explore ways of improving their services, for example by identifying groups of patients who may not achieve the outcomes of the majority.

Identifying the various points in the system where information should be collected is not always straightforward. Drawing up a 'logic model' to represent the programme can be a helpful way of identifying the assessment information needed at various points in treatment. Logic models are essentially schematic diagrams that show how the programme is intended to operate and what it is expected to achieve (Rush and Ogborne 1991). When fully developed, logic models can lead naturally to the design of management information systems for the monitoring of services. A logic model can also be useful when inducting new staff and for communicating with funding bodies, board members, patients and others with an interest in the programme. The structure of a logic model is represented in Table 6.1 (see Marsden *et al.* 2000a for examples of logic models in the substance misuse service delivery field).

Table 6.1 Components of a methadone programme described by a logic model.

Elements	Description
Programme components	Activities which are directed to the attainment of specific goals
Implementation objectives	What a programme seeks to achieve
Short-term objectives	Changes that the programme seeks to induce in its target patients in the immediate or short term
Long-term objectives	Changes that the programme seeks to induce in its target patients in the longer term

In recent years, Integrated Care Pathways (ICP) have been developed in a variety of health care settings as a means of maximizing the efficient and effective use of resources and ensuring quality standards are met. ICPs are known by various names, including critical care pathways, treatment protocols, anticipated recovery pathways, treatment algorithms, care standards and benchmarks. All of these are designed to create professional consensus and standardize elements of care to improve efficiency, effectiveness and value for money. In practice, ICPs are locally developed structures that identify individual needs and the expected outcomes of treatment and care. ICPs are similar to logic models but resemble a detailed flow chart showing how patients move through the treatment programme. Importantly, ICPs can also show how patients can move from one treatment service to another in cases of continuing treatment need. For example, an ICP for a methadone programme might show how patients flow across the following stages: intake and methadone dose induction, stabilization/maintenance, reduction/withdrawal and community aftercare support. A special feature of ICPs is called variance tracking. Variance tracking involves monitoring departures from expected courses of treatment and examining the causes for these, thus improving the pathway of care. In this regard, ICP initiatives are similar to audit activities.

Outcome monitoring

A formal and structured approach – outcome monitoring – has been advocated as a useful means of assessing outcome as part of the day-to-day operation of treatment programmes. Coined by the US Institute of Medicine (1990), outcome monitoring is based on the following features: i) specification of the patients treated and their presenting problems; ii) specification of the treatment delivered (i.e. type, intensity and duration); iii) use of repeated parallel measures for pre-treatment problem assessment and outcome determination. The most logical and practical method of assessing treatment outcome is to gather a set of measures from a client at intake to a programme (baseline) and then collect the same measures again from the client at one or more points during and following treatment. In this way, outcome monitoring is conceptualized as reassessment and can be incorporated as part of routine clinical practice.

The elements of assessment

Comprehensive assessment is a prerequisite for effective treatment in methadone services. It may be preceded by screening (described in the next section) and will include the assessment of dependence, motivation and a selection of problem domains for the purpose of treatment planning, outcome monitoring and measurement.

Screening

Screening can be defined as the use of a rapid procedure designed to detect individuals who have a health disorder. In general medicine, this normally involves the identification of a risk factor, a marker of the condition, or some symptomatic early stage. A cost effective screening test should be simple, precise and validated. It should also be acceptable to the population being tested and it should link with further procedures for diagnostic assessment.

In the context of methadone treatment programmes, screening can be defined (McPherson and Hersch 2000) as an activity designed to determine whether an individual meets a set of criteria for a particular treatment, in other words, is he or she a 'case'? This involves detecting the presence of the signs and symptoms of primary opioid dependence. Screening is a critical procedure and ensures that opioid naïve individuals (i.e. those with no opioid tolerance) are not considered for substitution prescribing. Screening can involve either self-report or biological investigations or both (Wolff et al. 1999).

Screening in methadone programmes involves a combination of biological testing as part of procedures to confirm opioid tolerance and dependence, and interview to determine the precise nature and severity or problems. Several-substance focused screening instruments have been devised, but to date these have shortcomings that make their use in methadone programmes problematic. In conclusion of a review of screening procedures, a US Preventive Services Task Force was unable to recommend and support a single standardized self-report questionnaire (US Preventive Services Task Force 1998).

Comprehensive assessment

A comprehensive assessment for methadone treatment should commence with a characterization of a patient's personal details and situation. This can include: personal demographic details (gender, age, ethnic category, family relationships); location of current or most recent residence; local authority of residence; sources of income and weekly income received; accommodation details; number and age of dependents and whether residing with the patient; ability to self-care; financial status and debts. A treatment history should also be recorded including: age and details of first treatment; types of treatments received to date; whether currently in treatment, and history of completing or dropping out of treatment. The reason for presentation to current treatment should be recorded together with treatment readiness and motivation details, treatment goal preferences and current service contact.

A major goal of assessment is to make sense of the individual's drug use and to this end a functional analysis of drug use is proposed (see Kanfer and Phillips 1970). This involves a detailed analysis of the antecedents, context, expectations and consequences of an individual's drug use. Such an analysis contributes to the assessment of motivation and the system of rewards that is maintaining the drug use.

Since many people are heavy and problematic users of more than one drug, assessment should profile the harm arising from the range of substances used. Assessment of the route of drug administration is also of clinical importance, since intravenous drug use may lead to specific medical problems, including viral hepatitis, HIV, septicaemia, subcutaneous abscesses and endocarditis. Some patients are also heavy users of alcohol and this may not be recognized and properly treated if the focus of treatment is on the management of opiate problems. In addition to assessing the harm arising from drug use, the threat of HIV infection and other communicable diseases has made it important to assess certain drug use and sexual risk behaviours such as sharing injection equipment and unsafe sexual behaviour. An important task during assessment is the identification of barriers to change and the maintenance of change. These may include psychological problems, anxiety, negative mood states, psychiatric co-morbidity, social and relationship issues, living with a drug using or addicted sexual partner, and environmental issues, for example physical access to drugs. Comprehensive assessment packages have been developed in the UK (see Tober et al. 2000; http://www.lau.org.uk) and the USA (see Dennis 1998; http://www.chestnut.org/LI/gain/index.html).

Assessing dependence

Individuals experiencing problems with opioid drugs are not a single, unitary group and their problems are not all the same. However, one of the main problems likely to be associated with presentation for treatment is dependence. Although early definitions of dependence relied heavily on the central role played by tolerance and withdrawal, more recent formulations have placed greater emphasis on psychological aspects, including a subjective awareness of compulsion to use drugs, a diminished capacity to control drug use and salience of drug-seeking behaviour. The clinical diagnostic criteria for dependence adopted by both the World Health Organization (WHO) in the *International Classification of Diseases* (ICD-10) (World Health Organization 1992) and the American Psychiatric Association (APA) in the *Diagnostic and Statistical Manual of Mental Disorders* (DSM-IV) (American Psychiatric Association 1994) emphasize such psychological features over physiological aspects.

A number of standardized clinical rating scales have been used to assess drug dependence. The Severity of Dependence Scale is a short, easily administered scale measuring the degree of dependence experienced by users of different types of drugs (Gossop *et al.* 1995). The Leeds Dependence Questionnaire (LDQ) is a similar, but more comprehensive instrument, which enquires about 10 markers of dependence (Raistrick *et al.* 1994). The nature and extent of withdrawal symptoms are not included in these instruments and can be assessed by verbal report.

Although the dimension of dependence is important, many people experience health, social and legal problems as a result of opiate use, without being dependent. A diagnosis of substance 'abuse' in DSM-IV is made where there is evidence of recurrent drug use and social, interpersonal or legal problems. These drug-related problems can often be the main reason for drug users seeking help and are important measures of the need for treatment and its subsequent impact.

Table 6.2 Patient eligibility criteria for methadone treatment.

Patient meets criteria A–C and either D or E
A. Over the past six months, diagnostic criteria for substance dependence (with a physiological dependence specifier), are met for the opioid or amphetamine class (the latter as described by the conditions under the DH clinical guidelines).
and
B. The client expresses a preference for a substitute prescription or will accept an assessment for a community stabilization/maintenance programme.
and
C. The client is presently tolerant to opioids or amphetamines (having demonstrated this via objective verification) and abrupt cessation of use will lead to the onset of a characteristic withdrawal syndrome.
and either
D. There are reasonable grounds to assume that the client will be able to attend treatment and comply with the rules and regulations operating in the prescribing programme.
or
E. Owing to the nature of the client's substance dependence, he/she is not able to make an immediate commitment to abstinence and requires a period of stabilization/maintenance and monitoring based on appropriate substitution and other adjunctive pharmacotherapy, pending further assessment of treatment goals.

Once a patient has been diagnosed with opioid dependence, his/her eligibility for methadone prescribing needs to be established. This is an area in which there is substantial variability in practice. Table 6.2 presents a hypothetical example of a set of eligibility criteria that could be used.

Problem domains and the nature of outcome measures

In order to evaluate changes which result from treatment, measures are required which tap into broad domains of patients' functioning. The majority of variables suitable for the repeated assessment required for this purpose will be continuous, or scale measures, sensitive to recording change over time. Treatment outcome will need to measure status at intake, at treatment completion and at follow-up. Certain measures will be taken only on a single occasion pre- or post-treatment, for example, assessment of personal socio-demographic information, previous treatment experience, or client satisfaction with treatment provided.

Attenuation or cessation of drug, including alcohol, consumption is the obvious primary indicator of success for this treatment population. However, individuals entering treatment typically present with chronic and acute medical, psychological and social problems. Reflecting this, research has utilized a broad array of measures of patients' functioning with which to assess outcome, categorized in three problem domains: i) alcohol and drug use, dependence and adverse consequences; ii) physical and psychological health and iii) life functioning (psychological resources, interpersonal relationships, occupational functioning and criminality). Since the mid-1980s, the risk of exposure of substance users to the Human Immunodeficiency Virus (HIV) and other blood-borne infections, for example Hepatitis B and C viruses, has led to the important addition of a fourth domain concerning health risk behaviours. Measures of outcome from these four domains are described in the following section.

Substance use

It is recommended that service providers record the frequency of all substances used by a client during a recall period and the usual amount consumed (intensity) during a 24-hour 'using day' (Wells et al. 1988). These measures reflect the likelihood of harm to the user when substances are taken either with a high frequency and/or with a high intensity (that is, large amounts consumed on a single occasion). Alcohol consumption is usually measured by ethanol content, weight or fluid volume; measuring the content of illicit drugs doses is challenging and research has tended to focus on frequency rather than intensity measures because of concerns about the accuracy of self-report of drug concentrations and the size of drug doses. However, an estimate of the usual quantity consumed is a desirable additional clinical and research measure, not least because at follow-up an individual may have maintained the same frequency of use but have achieved a marked reduction in their level of consumption.

Physical and psychological health

A number of physical and psychological health problems and specific disorders may be linked to or concurrent with substance use (Wartenberg 1994; Rubin and Benzer 1997). The management of physical health problems and complications is a common service activity in many programmes. A high prevalence of anxiety and depressive disorders of a transient and chronic nature has been reported amongst substance users in treatment (e.g. Rounsaville *et al.* 1982).

Health risk behaviour

Injecting drug users may be exposed to blood-borne infections through the direct sharing of infected needles/syringes, and potentially through the indirect sharing of certain items used in the injection procedure. At the population level, HIV is mainly transmitted through sexual intercourse. Since many substance users are sexually active, the assessment of penetrative sexual risk behaviour is also important.

Personal and social functioning

In this broad domain, three important problem areas are usually assessed. First, relationship conflicts and problems: most treatment programmes aim to promote improved relations between a client and his/her sexual partner, family and friends and conflict in these areas has been shown to be an important negative predictor of outcome (Moos *et al.* 1988). Secondly, employment issues: although the ability of a treatment programme to secure a job for a client may be very limited, full-time employment has been found to be a major predictor of retention in treatment and good outcome (Simpson *et al.*1986). Many services will seek to support a client to improve employment opportunities and securing or maintaining a job is consistently recognized to be an important goal (French *et al.* 1992). A third area concerns criminal activity. For some individuals crime is instrumental for funding drug use. The reduction in criminal involvement is seen as an important public safety benefit of treatment as well as being an individual gain in social functioning; the number of property crimes, particularly shoplifting which is the most frequently reported property crime, drugs distribution, and other crimes are usually recorded for the purpose of outcome evaluation.

Multi-dimensional outcome instruments

Choice of suitable outcome questionnaires should be guided by certain principles; they should:

- be relevant to the target population and treatment programme
- be relevant to the drugs strategy and capable of direct reporting against national targets and priorities
- be suitable for face-to-face interviewing with a client or self-completion by the client
- have established psychometric properties (validity and reliability)
- be sensitive to change over time
- make administration time brief
- ensure that the client and other non-professional audiences are able to understand the meaning of scores and reporting.

Instruments based on the domains described in the previous section have been developed in the USA (Addiction Severity Index (ASI) McLellan *et al.* 1995), Australia (Opiate Treatment Index (OTI) Darke *et al.* 1992), and the UK (Maudsley Addiction Profile (MAP) Marsden *et al.* 1998). Also in the UK, RESULT has been developed as a comprehensive data management system incorporating the key outcome monitoring domains already described (www.lau.org.uk; Tober *et al.* 2000). The ASI is a structured interview containing seven dimensions across medical, employment, legal, family, psychological status, alcohol use and drug use and is capable of yielding a single composite score. It was originally developed by McLellan and his colleagues as a generic instrument to evaluate treatment outcome of both problem drinkers and drug users and is now in its fifth edition. Drug-use items record lifetime use and frequency of use during the past 30 days. The ASI is amongst the most widely used outcome monitoring instruments and has been translated into nine languages, and a number of versions for particular target populations (e.g. adolescent drug users) have been produced. A shortened version (the ASI-*Lite*) has also been developed (http://www. densonline.org/ASIlite_CF.pdf).

The OTI contains measures from six domains: drug use, HIV risk-taking behaviour, social functioning, criminality, health status and psychological adjustment. Drug use is recorded by the client on the last three days' use for each of 11 classes of drugs: heroin, other opiates (including illicit methadone), amphetamines, cocaine, tranquillizers, alcohol, cannabis, barbiturates, hallucinogens, inhalants and tobacco. The MAP is a brief (12-minute) multi-dimensional treatment outcome research instrument developed in London also validated in three countries in continental Europe (Marsden *et al.* 1998, 2000b; http://www.ntors.org.uk/map.pdf). RESULT is a modular system including agency activity and costs linked to brief self-completion and therapist completed outcome measures (http://www.lau.org.uk).

Activity reporting and outcome monitoring

Reporting on the outputs of a methadone programme (the activities and work undertaken by the service) and the outcomes of the programme (the measurable benefit of the service), are critical activities. In England and Wales, for example, a National Drug Treatment Monitoring System (NDTMS) has been established to record patient treatment episodes and is a statutory reporting requirement for specialist methadone programmes (http://www.dtmu.org.uk/guidance.pdf). In the European Union, the Pompidou Group and the European Monitoring Centre for Drugs and Drug Addiction (EMCDDA) Treatment Demand Indicator Project have developed a Treatment Demand Indicator (TDI) to generate consistent and comparable information on patients seeking treatment. A panel of experts has developed a basic set of treatment contact, socio-demographic and drug-related information about the characteristics of people presenting to treatment services. The TDI is offered as a core set of information from which member states can gather additional information as required (http://www.emcdda.org). All services should record a basic set of information about patient referral, assessment and treatment activity of the programme for a specified reporting period (for example annually). This information should include the number of people who are referred for assessment, the number who are referred to another service, the number who complete assessment and the number commencing treatment.

While the basic information above can be gathered on all patients who are assessed and treated by a programme, it is more challenging to agree on the scope of outcome monitoring activities. Clearly one does not want to deploy scarce resources to implement a continuous research study in a treatment programme. These tasks can be relatively easily undertaken by formal evaluation studies in which a battery of information is gathered by research staff on a sample of patients for analysis. However, the collection of even a basic set of information with which to characterize patients and their treatment outcomes has been a challenge for many agencies. The UK NDTMS requires the following reasons for discharge to be recorded:

- treatment completed, drug free
- treatment completed
- treatment withdrawn/breach of contract
- no appropriate treatment available
- referred on
- dropped out/left
- moved away
- prison
- died.

At the most basic level, services should be able to record this departure status information and duration of treatment for all patients. This provides a lot of information with which to characterize the impact of treatment. Some agencies will also be able to gather a basic set of during-treatment outcome information as part of the day-to-day operation of the service and regular review of patients' progress (see Tober *et al.* 2000). A structured assessment instrument can be administered at one or more points during treatment as part of care management; for methadone services assessment, during treatment at three monthly intervals for the first year is recommended.

Conclusions

There are benefits for patients, programme staff, management and funding agencies in using a structured approach to assessment and treatment planning that incorporates routine outcome monitoring. Individual outcomes, comparisons between patients with different characteristics and the relative efficacy of different treatments are among these benefits. Two central obstacles remain: where treatment modalities have different objectives, the need to specify measurable objectives in order to determine whether such objectives are achieved may result in different outcome measures which are not comparable. The lack of consensus about the best instruments to employ may have its roots in a difference of view regarding treatment goal.

It is not only the outcome, but also the process of treatment which is important in its evaluation. It may be that there are specific components of the methadone programme which are influential in outcome and those that are less so. Monitoring the delivery of treatment will form the basis of evidence for capitalizing on effective components and discarding those which are not relevant to the outcome. An example would be the information derived from monitoring dose and duration of methadone treatment with the simultaneous monitoring of compliance. The recording of basic information for programme monitoring is best approached as part of patient care management. Outcome monitoring does not need to be an elaborate or costly activity. A basic characterization of treatment should be provided for all patients, and monitoring activities of increasing sophistication can be incorporated according to the resources and the needs of each treatment agency.

References

American Psychiatric Association (1994) *Diagnostic and Statistical Manual of Mental Disorders* (4th edition). Washington DC: APA.

Darke, S., Hall, W., Wodak, A., Heather, N. & Ward, J. (1992) Development and validation of a multi-dimensional instrument for assessing outcome of treatment among opiate users: the Opiate Treatment Index. *British Journal of Addiction*, 87: 733–42.

Dennis, M.L. (1998) *Global Appraisal of Individual Needs (GAIN) manual: Administration, Scoring and Interpretation.* Bloomington Il: Lighthouse Publications.

French, M.T., Dennis, M., Mcdougal, G.L., Karuntzos, G.T. & Hubbard, R.L. (1992) Training and employment programs in methadone treatment: Client needs and desires. *Journal of Substance Abuse Treatment,* 9: 293–303.

Gossop, M., Darke, S., Griffiths, P., Powis, B., Hall, W. & Strang, J. (1995) The Severity of Dependence Scale (SDS) in English and Australian samples of heroin, cocaine and amphetamine users. *Addiction*, 90: 607–61.

Institute of Medicine (1990) *Broadening the Base of Treatment for Alcohol Problems. Report of a study by a committee of the Institute of Medicine.* Washington DC: National Academy Press.

Kanfer, F. & Phillips, J. (1970) *Learning Foundations of Behaviour Therapy.* Chichester: Wiley.

Marsden, J., Ogborne, A., Farrell, M. & Rush, B. (2000a) *Psychoactive Substance Use Disorders: Guidelines for the evaluation of treatment services and systems.* Geneva: World Health Organization.

Marsden, J., Nizzoli, U., Corbelli, C., Margaren, H., Torres, M., Prada de Castro, J., Stewart, D. & Gossop, M. (2000b) New European instruments for treatment outcome research: reliability of the Maudsley Addiction Profile and Treatment Perceptions Questionnaire in Italy, Spain and Portugal. *European Addiction Research*, 217: 115–22.

Marsden, J., Gossop, M., Stewart, D., Best, D., Farrell, F., Lehmann, P., Edwards, C. & Strang, J. (1998) The Maudsley Addiction Profile (MAP): a brief instrument for assessing treatment outcome. *Addiction*, 93: 1857–68.

McLellan, A.T., Kushner, H., Metzger, D., Peters, R., Smith, I., Grisson, G., Pettinati, H. & Argeriou, M. (1995) The fifth edition of the Addiction Severity Index. *Journal of Substance Abuse Treatment*, 9: 199–213.

McPherson, T.L. & Hersch, R.K. (2000) Brief substance use screening instruments for primary care settings: a review. *Journal of Substance Abuse Treatment*, 18: 193–202.

Moos, R.H., Fenn, C. & Billings, A. (1988) Life stressors and social resources: an integrated assessment approach. *Social Science and Medicine*, 27: 999–1002.

Raistrick, D., Bradshaw, J., Tober, G., Wiener, J., Allison, J. & Healey, C. (1994) Development of the Leeds Dependence Questionnaire (LDQ): a questionnaire to measure alcohol and opiate dependence in the context of a treatment evaluation package. *Addiction,* 89: 563–72.

Rounsaville, B.J., Weissman, M.M., Kleber, H.K. & Wilber, C. (1982) Heterogeneity of psychiatric diagnosis in treated opiate addicts. *Archives of General Psychiatry*, 39: 161–6.

Rubin, J.M. & Benzer, D.G. (1997) Treatment of co-morbid medical complications. In: Miller NS, Gold MS, Smith DE, eds. *Manual of Therapeutics for Addictions.* New York: Wiley-Liss.

Rush, B.R. & Ogborne, A. (1991) Program logic models: expanding their role and structure for planning and evaluation. *Canadian Journal of Program Evaluation*, 6: 95–106.

Simpson, D.D., Joe, G.W. & Lehman, W.E.K. (1986) *Addiction Careers: Summary of Studies Based on the DARP 12-year Follow-up.* NIDA Treatment Research Report, DHHS Publication No. (AMD) 86–1420. Rockville MD: National Institute of Drug Abuse.

Tober, G., Brearley, R., Kenyon, R., Raistrick, D. & Morley, S. (2000) Measuring outcomes in a health service addiction clinic. *Addiction Research*, 8: 169–82.

US Preventive Services Task Force (1998) *Report of the US Preventive Services Task Force.* (2nd edition). US Department of Health and Human Services.

Wartenberg, A.A. (1994) Management of common medical problems. In: Miller NS, Gold MS, Smith DE, eds. *Manual of Therapeutics for Addictions.* Chevy Chase MD, American Society of Addiction Medicine.

Wells, E.A., Hawkins, J.D. & Catalano, R.F. (1988) Choosing drug use measures for treatment outcome studies. I. The influence of measurement approach on treatment results. *The International Journal of the Addictions,* 23: 851–73.

Wolff, K., Farrell, M., Marsden, J., Monteiro, M.G., Ali, R., Welch, S. & Strang, J. (1999) A review of biological indicators of illicit drug use: practical considerations and clinical usefulness. *Addiction,* 94: 1279–98.

World Health Organization (1992) *International Statistical Classification of Diseases and Related Health Problems* (10th edition). Geneva: World Health Organization.

7

Plasma methadone monitoring: an aid to dose assessment, monitoring compliance and exploration of drug interactions

Kim Wolff

Methadone measurements

Although clinical pharmacology is a well-established discipline, its influence on addiction treatment services has been minimal. Dose control has been the traditional paradigm for defining efficacy, safety and dose response in methadone programmes and substitution therapy for drug dependence. The majority of clinicians use absolute quantity of methadone to gauge patient management, most adopting the approach of prescribing an initial small dose with subsequent titration to an acceptable level. Dosage alterations during treatment are similarly construed. Although safe, these procedures are rather limited, unscientific and often insensitive to the individual patient's needs (Wolff *et al*. 1997).

Therapeutic drug monitoring is the science that combines measurement of serum (blood, plasma) drug concentrations with clinical pharmacokinetics. Rarely can the concentration of a drug at the site of action be measured directly; instead the concentration is measured at an alternative site – the plasma. Plasma measurements are thus based on the premise that therapeutic benefit is well correlated with a specific drug concentration (usually a narrow range) achieved after fixed dosing with a pharmacological agent.

In much the same way (although for different reasons) that a wide range of daily doses are required of the oral anticoagulant warfarin to produce a similar prothrombin time, doses of methadone required to prevent the onset of opioid withdrawal symptom complaints also vary. Sources of variability in drug response typically include the patient's age, weight, type and degree of severity of the disease, the patient's genetic makeup, other drugs concurrently administered and environmental factors (Rowland and Tozer 1995).

For the majority of patients, knowledge of a drug's therapeutic plasma concentration range and pharmacokinetics would lead to more rapid establishment of a safe and efficacious dosage regimen. Methadone is no exception and plasma drug monitoring has the potential advantage of being beneficial to those involved in the prescription of methadone. Plasma measurements would allow more flexible individualized dosage schedules, reveal unrecognized under- or over-dosage and detect poor compliance with methadone dosing. There are also indirect benefits associated with plasma methadone monitoring such as the documentation of drug–drug interactions to warn clinicians of the possibility of toxicity (plasma level too high) or the possibility of side effects from concomitant drug administration. Similarly documentation of drug–drug interactions could monitor the effect of endogenous factors (concomitant diseases, pregnancy, gender and size), and exogenous factors (nutritional habits, smoking and lifestyle) and finally, indicate when there is little point in persisting with a particular treatment programme. However, plasma methadone measurements have not been widely utilized for methadone treatment programmes (Ward *et al.* 1992).

An aid to dose assessment

The usual procedure for assessing opioid users at clinics that prescribe methadone involves interviewing techniques (extensively reliant on the accuracy of self-report) and examination of results from urinalysis for drugs of abuse. Such screening procedures are able to provide meaningful information regarding recent drug use and are important clinical tools. Efficacy of prescribing with methadone involves additional observer report systems. These systems usually measure subjective and objective signs of opioid withdrawal symptoms and while circumventing self-report bias, they nevertheless remain insensitive, detect only gross changes and are difficult for the inexperienced to interpret.

Although urine drug screening is the predominant tool for assessing opioid users receiving treatment, a drug may be detected in any body fluid or tissue; indeed, methadone has been detected in hair, saliva, sweat, meconium and seminal fluid (Wolff and Strang 1999). In the clinical framework of substance misuse, the information required usually concerns whether or not an illicit compound has been consumed within the last 24–72 hours. The best biological tool for this purpose is urine, which is collected easily in large volumes and usually contains metabolites as well as the parent drug. Screening urine for illicit drugs will satisfactorily enable an initial diagnosis of substance misuse, gauge illicit drug use during a treatment programme and is a useful adjunct to a full drug history. However, urinalysis cannot usefully provide clinical information about efficacy or compliance with methadone prescribing.

Although urine samples can be collected fairly easily, there remains the problem of interpreting the results for clinical use. The main problem is that the picture in urine is often complex; unchanged methadone in urine only represents 2–5% of the total dose, the rest being excreted as metabolites. Furthermore, methadone excretion into urine is pH dependent, so that when urine is acidified for example, the amount of unchanged drug detected in urine is significantly increased. Clinical interpretation in such circumstances is thus affected by inter- and intra-individual variation in values for urinary pH.

There have been recent reports that advocate the quantitative measurement of methadone and its primary metabolite EDDP (2-ethylidene-1.5-dimethyl-3.3-diphenylpyrrolidine) in urine in order to confirm consumption of methadone in the context of treatment evaluation. EDDP is the non-pharmacologically active primary metabolite of methadone accounting for 17–57% of the dose excreted in urine (Anggard et al. 1975). Its presence in urine is a useful guide for practitioners to be able to confirm that methadone has been ingested. However, there is large variation in the ratio of EDDP: methadone, which suggests that the use of this procedure for monitoring compliance would be difficult. Such an approach remains an experimental option but some of the issues raised may have applicability in analysing the relationship between self-report and drug use (Kell 1994; 1995).

Stabilization of patients on to methadone involves achieving a steady-state condition. This is thought to occur at a rate of five to seven times the elimination half-life, for methadone approximately seven to twelve days. During this time there is some accumulation of methadone in tissues. Even if the same dose of methadone were given daily, however, the peak plasma methadone concentration on the first day of dosing would be lower than peak concentrations at steady-state (Figure 7.1).

One important consideration during dosage induction is the pharmacokinetic characteristics of methadone at the onset of treatment. In a study of opioid addicts about to commence dosing with methadone, it was found that the clearance of methadone was significantly lower in opioid addicts at the start of treatment (mean elimination half-life 128 hours) than in those who

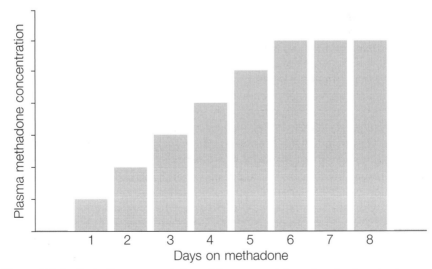

Figure 7.1 An illustrative representation of the accumulation of methadone in plasma with fixed, constant daily dosing.

had reached steady-state (mean elimination half-life 48 hours). Because the half-life of the drug is extremely long relative to the dosing interval at the onset of treatment, the degree of accumulation is large in some individuals during the first few days of treatment (Rostami-Hodjegan *et al.* 1999; Wolff *et al*. 2000), with fatal consequences in some instances (Caplehorn 1998).

Monitoring compliance

Methadone would seem ideal for plasma monitoring because once-daily administration is convenient and has the potential to promote patient compliance. Lack of compliance is a major problem in pharmacotherapy. The most frequent pattern of non-compliance is the occasional omitted dose or failure to take several consecutive doses. The impact of a missed dose is particularly important in methadone treatment for two key reasons. Firstly, omitting a single daily dose produces a lower trough (minimum) concentration of methadone at the end of the dosage interval than the usual steady-state concentration, which may then cause the onset of initial withdrawal symptoms. Secondly, missed doses of methadone may incur loss of tolerance. Department of Health Guidelines (Department of Health 1999) recommend reassessment following omission of maintenance doses of methadone.

One of the major benefits of plasma methadone measurements is the ability to monitor compliance. Studies of treatment response to methadone maintenance have shown that patients who comply with the recommended course of treatment have longer lasting post-treatment benefits. Thus, it is discouraging for many practitioners that opioid addicts are frequently non- or poorly compliant and subsequently resume substance use. Barring the difficulty of blood collection in some sections of this population, it seems that methadone treatment is one area where there is growing evidence that quantitative measurements of methadone could be a useful clinical tool. For example, it is highly desirable to know if a patient is taking all their medication (at the correct time and in the correct amount) and to find out whether the patient is using extra methadone (obtained illicitly or by 'double-scripting') or is not taking part of their prescription, perhaps selling the surplus to other users. Neither urinalysis drug screening or hair analysis will provide answers to these questions. These procedures are largely qualitative and results only indicate whether or not a patient has taken the drug under study; they give no meaningful information on quantities taken or circulating blood levels.

Poor, or insufficient compliance is of considerable importance for the relationship between plasma concentration and methadone dose. When compliance is good, the relationship between plasma concentration and methadone dose is highly correlated and plasma methadone concentrations can be used effectively to validate dosing regimens, as well as to assess compliance (Wolff and Hay 1994). There is a linear relationship between plasma concentration and methadone dose for those patients who have reached a condition of steady-state and thus there is a window within which patients prescribed a fixed daily dose should fall.

Pharmacokinetics

Methadone is an unusual opioid in that it is orally effective and is well absorbed from the gastro–intestinal tract, particularly the small intestine. The fraction of the oral dose that reaches the blood stream is very high (bioavailability = 70–95%) compared with other opioids such as morphine (oral bioavailability = 40–50%). However, methadone is highly lipophilic and so is sequestered into the tissues with continued dosing. It is also highly bound to plasma proteins (mainly alpha-1-acid glycoprotein) so that the free (unbound) pharmacologically active fraction of the drug is very small, ranging from 6% to 14%. Hence plasma methadone levels in the general circulation are usually quite low. After oral administration it takes about four hours in opioid addicts for the methadone concentration in blood to reach a peak (range 1–6 hours).

Unlike most other opioids, methadone is also a very long-acting drug whose action is prolonged because there is little significant first-pass-effect (rate of extraction from the liver ER = 0.089) as observed with morphine (ER = 0.7). The half-life most commonly ascribed to methadone is conveniently about 24 hours. However, in truth the elimination kinetics of the drug are highly complex and subject to wide variation between patients depending on a number of key factors, some of which have yet to be fully characterized. Figure 7.2 shows the variability in half-life values for a cohort of patients prescribed methadone.

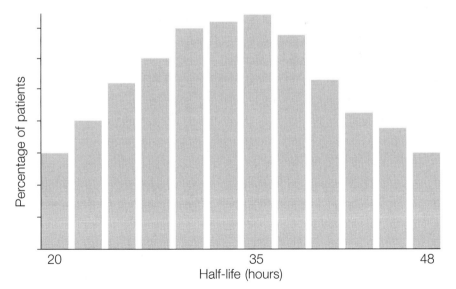

Figure 7.2 Illustrative representation of the terminal elimination half-life for methadone (in hours) showing steady-state variability conditions have been reached.

Several studies have investigated the possibility of an optimal methadone blood level for methadone treatment. However, it must be stressed that significant inter-individual variability may occur among individuals in both the efficacy and toxicity response curves, leading to differences among individuals in the location and the range of the therapeutic window. Hence efficacy should be monitored on an individual basis and should centre on maintenance of a trough blood level that sustains the patient for the whole dosing interval and prevents the onset of withdrawal symptom complaints.

For the same reasons there does not appear to be a unique fatal dose of methadone – nor plasma concentration above which, if the individual were untreated, death would occur. This is because it is possible for addicts to tolerate different quantities of methadone depending on the degree of previous exposure to opioid drugs. Consequently blood concentrations that cause toxicity in some are safe and effective in others. There is much uncertainty regarding a patient's tolerance and difficulty remains in determining objectively the degree of tolerance in someone presenting for treatment; the rate at which tolerance to methadone is developed or lost is not certain. Nevertheless a lethal dose for a non-tolerant adult could be as little as 30 mg (less if taken with alcohol or benzodiazepines). In children, if untreated, as little as 10 mg can be fatal. Most opioid addicts have experienced an overdose and many have witnessed it in others. Variability in purity, uncertain effects following combination drug use (especially benzodiazepines, alcohol and opioids) and generalized poor health make the opioid addict population a vulnerable group from both intentional and accidental overdose. Poly-drug users who embark on a methadone maintenance programme are also at risk of pharmacokinetic interactions occurring between methadone and other drugs.

The signs of opioid overdose are:

(1) in an adult, respiratory arrest with a pulse
(2) pinpoint pupils unreactive to light
(3) snoring, giving way to shallow respirations (rate <8/min)
(4) bradycardic and hypotensive, peripherally shut down in later stage
(5) varying degree of reduced consciousness/coma.

Exploration of drug interactions

Co-administration of other prescribed drugs is common practice for the addict population in treatment and can present clinical problems. Although the response produced by each drug may be known and thus predictable, that produced by the combination may be less certain. In some circumstances where patients self-administer either prescribed or illicit drugs the response may be unpredictable and potentially problematic. Drug–drug interactions are thought to be graded, and changes in the action of a drug vary continuously in relation to the plasma concentration of the interacting drug(s) and hence with time. Indeed, given in sufficiently high doses, almost any drug can interact with another. Thus the incidence of drug interactions is likely to be very high on occasions when there is the use of substances in excess of recommended dosing regimens, binge style consumption and poly-substance use. Methadone dosing and maintenance therapy have traditionally been solely based on observations of the effects produced. However, control on a dosage basis alone often proves difficult. Therapeutic control is achieved more readily and accurately when plasma drug concentration data and the kinetics of the drug are known (Rowland and Tozer 1995).

Drug interactions often involve a change in pharmacokinetics. Some drugs inhibit metabolizing enzymes and slow elimination. Drugs that inhibit activity of certain cytochrome P450 liver enzymes (CYP3A4) have the potential to increase the concentration of methadone in blood. However, individuals will respond differently to combinations of drugs. The time frame over which inhibitors exert their maximum effect is generally in the order of days, and therefore should not incur significant adverse effects. Theoretically, complete inhibition of CYP3A4 could halve methadone clearance with significant repercussions for the drug's pharmacological effects. For instance, serotonin re-uptake inhibitors such as sertraline variously inhibit isoenzymes responsible for the metabolism of methadone. Hamilton *et al.* (2000) recommend that clinicians should consider monitoring serum methadone levels when treating depressed or anxious methadone patients with second generation antidepressants.

Inhibition of methadone clearance is most probable with strong liver enzyme inhibitors like erythromycin and diazepam. The transient increase in plasma methadone levels and the positive subjective opiate-like effects that occur are likely to be the reason in the latter case that benzodiazepines are commonly consumed by those prescribed methadone. Sedation and nausea are the most common clinical indications of toxicity, although at the onset of methadone treatment there may also be the risk of the onset of respiratory depression.

Ciprofloxacin caused profound sedation, confusion and respiratory depression in a patient who had been previously stable on methadone for six years (Herrlin *et al.* 2000). Co-administration of the following drugs with methadone may cause adverse (though transient) effects in some susceptible patients:

(1) calcium channel antagonists: verapamil, nifedipine, diltiazem
(2) protease inhibitors used in the treatment of HIV infection, e.g. ritonavir, zidovudine
(3) antidepressants: desipramine (raised plasma levels of desipramine)
(4) antibiotics: erythromycin
(5) histamine H_2-antagonists: cimetidine and ranitidine
(6) antibacterials: clotrimazole, ketoconazole
(7) hormones: progesterone, ethinyloestradiol

(8) selective serotonin re-uptake inhibitors (SSRIs) e.g. sertraline, fluvoxamine, fluoxetine
(9) miscellaneous: isoniazid, disulfiram, allopurinol, cyclosporin, quinidine, bromocriptine.

Other drugs stimulate drug metabolizing enzymes (induction) and hasten drug loss from the body. Those that induce activity of the liver enzyme CYP3A4 may decrease the plasma level of methadone and precipitate the onset of withdrawal symptoms. For instance, doubling the activity of the enzyme CYP3A4 could increase the clearance of methadone by up to 50%. The time frame over which inducers exert their maximum effect is two to three weeks. In order to prevent treatment failure, dosages of methadone may need to be increased as a result of co-medication with a strong enzyme inducer. This should not be attempted until after the onset of withdrawal symptoms and should be undertaken in an incremental fashion. Moreover, methadone dosing for patients already on medications that inhibit or induce CYP3A4 should err towards caution.

A pertinent clinical example is co-medication with the anti-tuberculous drug rifampicin, which causes the onset of significant withdrawal symptoms in individuals prescribed methadone. It is therefore important to monitor plasma methadone levels before the onset of treatment with rifampicin in order that doses of methadone may be subsequently titrated to the correct level. It is also advisable to monitor compliance with rifampicin dosing and carefully to educate patients so that they know what to expect, otherwise the onset of unexpected withdrawal symptoms may initiate use of illicit substances or methadone obtained illegally. Potent enzyme inducers include:

(1) anti-epileptics: carbamazepine, phenobarbitone, phenytoin
(2) anti-tuberculous drugs: rifampicin, rifabutin – confounded by isoniazid
(3) steroids: dexamethasone
(4) diuretics: spironolactone
(5) non-nucleoside reverse transcriptase inhibitors: nevirapine, efavirenz
(6) nucleoside reverse transcriptase inhibitors: abacavir
(7) protease inhibitor: amprenavir
(8) anxiolytics: barbiturates like quinalbarbitone, amylobarbitone

Frequency of monitoring is a function of the presumed change in factors that govern the therapeutic response. For example, the plasma concentration of methadone in a long-term maintenance patient, whose state of health and illicit drug use remains stable, may need to be monitored only a few times a year; more frequent monitoring may be indicated if the patient's drug-using behaviour deteriorates, withdrawal symptom complaints are frequent and when therapy with other drugs is altered. For instance, weekly or more frequent monitoring may be needed for optimal use of methadone in HIV positive patients about to commence combination therapy or when a course of anti-tuberculosis therapy is required, because these drugs are known to alter the metabolism of methadone in a clinically significant way. Figure 7.3 presents an aide-memoire for the purpose of alerting the clinician to those conditions that may prompt plasma methadone monitoring, and their interpretations are listed in Table 7.1.

Table 7.1 Indications for plasma methadone monitoring.

Decision to request plasma measurement	Interpretation
Assessment of compliance with methadone – monitor take-home medication – monitor prescription of ampoules – suspect multiple prescriptions	**Sub-therapeutic concentrations** – not taking all dose **Higher than expected concentrations** – consuming extra methadone
Change in dosage regimen	**Sub-therapeutic concentrations**
Dose reduction	Steady-state may not have been achieved Dose reduction is too quick
Detoxification	
Withdrawal symptom complaints	
Change in clinical state of patient e.g. pregnancy	**Sub-therapeutic concentrations** In third trimester may be reduction in drug concentration with possibility of the onset of opioid withdrawal
Chronic liver disease (acute viral hepatitis)	**Toxic concentrations** Severe liver damage can prevent the normal clearance of methadone and cause nausea, sedation
Induction of methadone	**Sub-therapeutic concentrations** Enzyme inducing drugs (rifampicin, phenobarbitone, phenytoin, carbamazepine) will cause the onset of opioid withdrawal symptoms
Inhibition of methadone	**Toxic concentrations** Enzyme inhibiting drugs (protease inhibitors – ritonavir, isoniazid, possibly cimetidine) may cause nausea, sedation

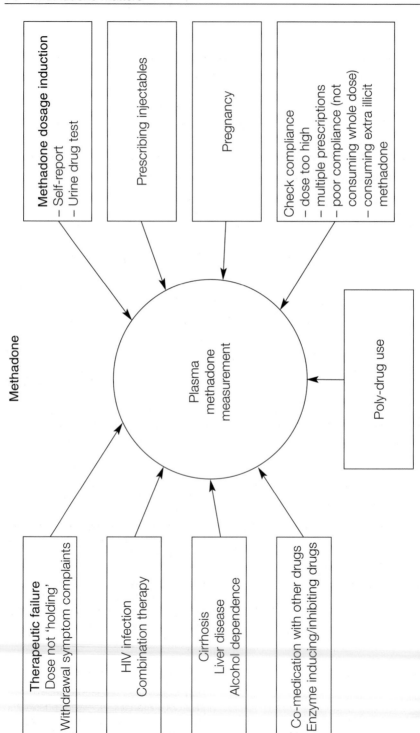

Figure 7.3 The potential uses for plasma methadone measurements.

Conclusion

The rational design of safe and efficacious dosage regimens is essential for the success of methadone maintenance programmes. Methadone dosage regimens are designed to prevent the onset of opioid withdrawal symptoms for the duration of the dosing interval. This objective may be achieved by various modalities. Evidence exists that response is often better correlated with plasma concentration than with dose administered. Accordingly it would seem prudent to apply pharmacokinetic principles to methadone maintenance treatment.

References

Anggard, E., Gunne, L.M., Holmstrand, J., McMahon, R.E., Sandberg, C.G. & Sullivan, H.R. (1975) Disposition of methadone in methadone maintenance. *Clinical Pharmacology & Therapeutics*, 17: 258–66.

Caplehorn, J.R.M. (1998) Deaths in the first two weeks of maintenance treatment in NSW in 1994: identifying cases of iatrogenic methadone toxicity. *Drug and Alcohol Review*, 17: 9–17.

Department of Health, The Scottish Office Department of Health, Welsh Office, Department of Health and Social Services, Northen Ireland (1999) *Drug Misuse and Dependence – Guidelines on Clinical Management.* London: HMSO.

Hamilton, S.P., Numes, E.V., Janal, M. & Weber, L. (2000) The effect of sertraline on methadone plasma levels in methadone maintenance patients. *American Journal on Addictions*, 9: 63–9.

Herrlin, K., Segerdahl, M., Gustafsson, L.L. & Kalso, E. (2000) Methadone, ciprofloxacin and adverse drug reactions. *Lancet,* 356: 2069–70.

Kell, M.J. (1995) Utilisation of plasma and urine concentration measurements to limit narcotics use in methadone maintenance patients: II Generation of plasma concentration time curves. *Journal of Addictive Disease,* 14: 85–108.

Kell, M.J. (1994) Utilisation of plasma and urine methadone concentrations to optimise treatment in maintenance clinics: I. Measurement techniques for a clinical setting. *Journal of Addictive Diseases*, 13: 5–25.

Rostami-Hodjegan, A., Wolff, K., Hay, A.W.M., Raistrick, D. & Tucker, G.T. (1999) Population pharmacokinetics of methadone in opiate users: characterisation of time-dependent changes. *British Journal of Clinical Pharmacology,* 48: 43–52.

Rowland, M. & Tozer, T.N. (eds) (1995) *Clinical Pharmacokinetics: concepts and applications* (3rd edition) Philadelphia and London: Lea and Febiger.

Ward, J., Mattick, R. & Hall, W. (1992) *Key Issues in Methadone Maintenance Treatment.* Australia: University of New South Wales Press.

Wolff, K. & Strang, J. (1999) Therapeutic drug monitoring for methadone: scanning the horizon. *European Addiction Research,* 5: 36–42.

Wolff, K. & Hay, A.W.M. (1994) Plasma methadone monitoring with methadone maintenance treatment. *Drug Alcohol Dependence*, 36: 69.

Wolff, K., Rostami-Hodjegan, A., Hay, A.W.M., Raistrick, D.S., Tucker, G. (2000) Population-based pharmacokinetic approach for methadone monitoring of opiate addicts: potential clinical utility. *Addiction,* 95: 1771–83.

Wolff, K., Rostami-Hodjegan, A., Shires, S., Hay, A.W.M., Feely, M., Calver, R., Raistrick, D. & Tucker, G.T. (1997) The pharmacokinetics of methadone in healthy subjects and opiate users. *British Journal of Clinical Pharmacology*, 44: 325–34.

8
Withdrawal from methadone and methadone for withdrawal

Nicholas Seivewright and Olawale Lagundoye

When given as an outright 'maintenance' treatment, methadone is highly effective in reducing many indicators of illicit drug misuse. It is inevitably controversial, as doubts as to the principle of such prescribing will never completely go away, but it is clear that methadone can routinely reduce other opiate use, injecting, psychological distress and social complications such as crime in opiate-dependent individuals. Such evidence has been presented in reviews and meta-analyses (e.g. Bertschy 1995; Marsch 1998), while differences in approach, which relate to whether methadone is viewed as a direct treatment that normalizes the behaviour of an addict or as a 'substitute' enabling largely secondary benefits through removing individuals from illicit drug-taking, have also been the subject of investigation (Seivewright 2000a).

Unfortunately as soon as methadone is used in ways other than ongoing maintenance, the evidence for effectiveness weakens greatly. This applies to both the areas covered in this chapter, namely withdrawing from established methadone treatment and using methadone as a detoxification drug. Indeed there are observers who look upon non-maintenance or otherwise 'flexible' methadone treatment with some dismay, as flying in the face of so much solid evidence. Arguably we should pay more attention to a warning that followed the early studies of the drug, that 'each withdrawal [from methadone] is an experiment with the life of a patient' (Dole 1973).

Indisputably, however, many things have changed since that time, most importantly in this context the actual usage of heroin. This drug has become hugely available in the UK and elsewhere, and many relatively mildly dependent users present to services when traditional high dose methadone maintenance would be quite inappropriate. Of course at the lowest levels of heroin usage methadone would be avoided anyway, with recourse instead to other detoxification treatments such as lofexidine, but that still leaves a very large middle range of patients who may require methadone initially, with no suggestion that this need be lifelong. This is partly the territory of this brief review, in which we will critically examine the common clinical situations relating to shorter term methadone treatment.

Withdrawal situations

Methadone may, in different circumstances, be either the drug that is being withdrawn from, or the one used to detoxify from another opiate. The distinction is not absolute, as it is very common in UK community treatment to encounter the hybrid situation whereby a heroin user is given methadone in relatively high dose for an initial stabilization period, and then in a reducing course lasting weeks, months or even longer, the process therefore including both elements. The term 'methadone detox' can consequently be rather ambiguous, but here we will endeavour to be clear about which withdrawal situations are being discussed at each point; ironically, it is the common clinical process of a slow detoxification which has been investigated least in terms of formal studies.

The move away from outright maintenance

We should briefly consider the main forces that have been at work in the move away from methadone maintenance programmes. The modern use of methadone can be seen as a classic exercise in pragmatism, taking account of some very basic matters: the level of heroin use, patients' views, medico–legal and service considerations. With reference to heroin use, the sheer availability of impure, smokeable heroin means that a wide range of individuals will present to services, not simply the committed 'hardcore' injectors who used to be typical. Methadone treatment has generally needed to become more 'lightweight' in response to this, with inevitably more prospects for full detoxification.

In all areas of clinical practice, patients' own views are increasingly considered. Despite the stereotypical view that drug misusers try to obtain as much in the way of medication as possible from their doctors, it is actually quite rare to meet a patient in a UK clinic who definitely wants to be on methadone forever. Many see that the routine of going to a pharmacy for methadone virtually every day can be a truly stultifying process.

With regards to medico–legal considerations, we should be wary of forcing individuals to take a very addictive drug for longer then they intend to. The unfortunate precedent here is the extensive prescribing of benzodiazepines for psychological problems, which has resulted in a highly litigious situation. There are admittedly similarities and differences between the two scenarios, while the risks of using methadone in relatively mildly dependent individuals raise the prospect of alternative treatments (see next section).

Finally, in terms of service considerations, if most methadone patients receive long-term treatment, any service providing this will rapidly become overburdened, as new cases are taken on and very few leave. This is exactly what has happened in many parts of the UK, especially in services that operate along undemanding 'harm reduction' lines, with a reluctance to discharge individuals for breaches of treatment contract. Some prescribing can be passed on from specialist services to primary care, but not usually at a rate sufficient to ease the congestion, and in order at least to give more people a chance, time limits are sometimes placed on methadone treatment.

There has also been the recommendation within HIV prevention policies that methadone should be available, in effect, to attract users into services to receive other advice (Stimson 1996), with methadone being given to many individuals who are not definite maintenance candidates. We repeat that it is possible to view these general changes in methadone usage as fundamentally misguided, but in summarizing the withdrawal treatments we now need to leave the major controversies on the 'evidence base' aside. We will, however, consider briefly some properties of the drug which are relevant to its use in detoxification.

Properties of methadone

Some methadone users complain bitterly about prolonged symptoms they experience on stopping or reducing the drug, typically citing severe muscle or joint aching, insomnia and general weakness (Rosenbaum and Murphy 1984). Even during a relatively short course of treatment, marked symptoms appear to build up, and the widespread opinion that methadone is more difficult to come off than heroin seems to relate to methadone's long duration of action and receptor-binding properties. Some clinics routinely use a shorter-acting opioid such as dihydrocodeine or even diamorphine itself in the withdrawal process, but whether it is a problem per se to use a long-acting drug for detoxification is debatable; in benzodiazepine dependence, for instance, this is positively recommended.

An aspect that is often ignored is inter-individual variability in the pharmacokinetics of methadone as discussed in Chapter 7. The elimination half-life is usually considered to be about 24 hours but the range is fairly wide, affected by hepatic, renal and other factors (Garrido and Troconiz 1999). Also, methadone is known to be highly plasma-protein bound with the free form active, and there are further differences among individuals in the plasma concentration of the main protein involved. It is currently recommended that all initial methadone treatment is carried out on the basis of supervised (therefore nearly always once-daily) consumption in a pharmacy (Department of Health 1999), but complaints by some patients that their methadone does not 'hold' them for a full day may often be legitimate. Although the relationships are not direct, this may be a particular problem towards the end of a detoxification, when dosages are low and also auto-induction of enzymes can have occurred (Rostami-Hodjegan et al. 1999).

Withdrawal from methadone

One reason for the controversy surrounding methadone treatment is that attempts to come off the drug often appear unsuccessful. Some early studies showed single-figure percentages for completion of withdrawal, although these tended to be in services where there had been a policy change away from maintenance treatment, and therefore the patients had not chosen to detoxify at the time. In general provision, there are always some individuals who do elect to detoxify even if they are entitled to ongoing maintenance, a situation studied by Eklund et al. (1994); outcomes included an untoward number of deaths, inability to tolerate abstinence from methadone in half of those who attempted it, some cases of switching to alcohol misuse after detoxification, but the best quality of life in those who managed to become free of all substance dependence. It is not known whether current 'flexible' UK policies have led to general improvements in successful withdrawal from methadone, but there has been interest in various methods, with some reasonable results reported.

Most withdrawal treatment takes place in the community, but some individuals are admitted, especially if there are adverse social circumstances or if specialized methods are to be used. Strang et al. (1997) found that acceptability was higher and outcomes better at various stages if opiate detoxification occurred in a specialist addiction unit rather than a general psychiatric ward, and such units are better placed to develop new treatment regimens. A recent focus of interest has been accelerated detoxification, in which withdrawal is stimulated by an opiate antagonist and completed under heavy sedation. Using such a technique in heroin and methadone addicts, Beaini et al. (2000) found almost universal completion of detoxification, high tolerability, and a subsequent confirmed abstinence rate of 34% at three months which appeared to compare well with other methods.

Withdrawal regimens from methadone involving alternative medications can be carried out in hospital or the community. In the latter situation there may be concerns as to the tolerability of withdrawing from very high dose methadone, and it is common to bring the methadone dosage down gradually before switching to an alternative at, say, 20–50 mg. The mixed agonist–antagonist buprenorphine may prove useful in withdrawal from such amounts but particular care is required in the transfer, a situation investigated in a UK clinic by Law et al. (1997). Lofexidine is another option that is widely used, and has been recently studied in 5- and 10-day regimens in inpatients (Bearn et al. 1998) and in the community (Carnwath and Hardman 1998). In the latter study of individuals who were taking up to 40 mg of methadone daily or other opiate equivalent, 58% completed detoxification with lofexidine or clonidine and were abstinent one month later.

Methadone for withdrawal

A series of studies of methadone detoxification was undertaken in the 1980s at the Maudsley Hospital, mainly involving inpatients and much shorter courses than are typically used in the community. Findings included a peaking of withdrawal symptoms towards the end of detoxification with persistent symptoms afterwards (Gossop *et al.* 1987), similar severity of symptoms in ten and 21-day courses (Gossop *et al.* 1989), but worse symptoms in ten days in patients being withdrawn from methadone rather than heroin (Gossop *et al.* 1991). Completion of methadone detoxification was higher in inpatients than outpatients (Gossop *et al.* 1986), while the option of outpatients being able to choose their rate of reduction conferred no advantage (Dawe *et al.* 1991), perhaps contrary to what many clinicians believe.

A much larger cohort study of drug misusers in UK treatment, the National Treatment Outcome Research Study (NTORS), is currently underway, with one of the investigated modalities being outpatient methadone reduction programmes. This work is described in Chapters 22 and 24 and in general has shown improvements across treatment groups with respect to drug use, health and criminality. Just how long supposed detoxification courses have become, however, was illustrated by the finding that at one year the group designated as methadone reduction had not reduced their drugs to levels significantly below the maintenance group, having also started at similar dosages (Gossop *et al.* 2000).

In practice, a methadone detoxification often progresses fairly satisfactorily up to a certain point, before troublesome symptoms then emerge and a relapse into drug use occurs. This is typically around the 30–40 mg per day mark, and therefore if clinicians decide to continue the withdrawal process with treatments such as lofexidine or buprenorphine, the situation is analogous to that discussed above. The evidence from the NTORS study suggests that plans for detoxification are, however, often delayed or abandoned, and various personal and social factors, in addition to physical symptoms, may affect that situation. One such consideration is personality disorder, which appears to exert a generally adverse influence on detoxification attempts, but not to the same degree on maintenance treatment (Seivewright and Daly 1997).

Ending a failing treatment

If methadone withdrawal prescribing is prolonged, then, as in outright maintenance, decisions are needed regarding what is acceptable in terms of additional drug use and other problems in progress. This is a neglected area in advisory literature, given that methadone is undoubtedly a much easier treatment to start than to stop, when dependence on the drug and also a sense of entitlement have been established. As an illustration, the UK guidelines on managing drug misuse (Department of Health 1999) are 130 pages long but contain just half a page on terminating a failing treatment, stating generally that 'if a patient fails to make progress towards agreed and reasonable goals, the doctor may have to consider ending that particular treatment'. There is a recommendation that referral to other services could be made, while a specific point is that 'due notice should be given of a reduction regime'. This is clearly the territory of treatment contracts, which as a rule should be unequivocally in place at the start of methadone treatment, rather than introduced at a later stage.

Alternatives to methadone

In opiate misuse treatment in general there are many situations in which pharmacological and other alternatives to methadone are used from the outset (Seivewright 2000b; c). Here we provide a little more detail on two medications that we have discussed in terms of withdrawing from methadone.

Lofexidine

This is an alpha-2 adrenergic receptor agonist, which partly through negative feedback mechanisms reduces the features of opiate withdrawal that are due to noradrenergic over-activity. Lofexidine is an analogue of clonidine and lacks the latter drug's hypotensive and sedative side effects, and so can be used safely in community detoxification. It is undoubtedly effective in withdrawal symptom relief (Strang *et al.* 1999), and has been widely taken up by drug services in the UK as the standard non-opioid detoxification method. This medication is also used in settings, such as prisons, where it is desirable to avoid prescribing opioids. Additional medication may be required alongside lofexidine for relief of particular symptoms such as insomnia, stomach cramps or diarrhoea.

Buprenorphine

This is potentially another important treatment as it may offer some distinct advantages over methadone in substitution therapy, particularly in detoxification. These advantages relate to buprenorphine's profile as a mixed opiate agonist and antagonist.

Buprenorphine appears to be genuinely less addictive than methadone, with the relevant evidence drawn in from studies of the withdrawal features from discontinuation of long-term treatment with the two drugs, and of symptoms which occur during detoxification courses (Bickel and Amass 1995). In practice, as indicated above, clinicians have come to expect that a detoxification using methadone will become problematic at some stage in terms of emerging symptoms; it would therefore be extremely welcome if this were to occur less with buprenorphine. Other significant benefits are: it seems impossible to over-dose fatally through respiratory depression on buprenorphine alone; there is less reinforcing interaction with other euphoriant drugs; and transfer to naltrexone after detoxification can be quicker than with methadone, possibly as little as 1–2 days (Rosen and Kosten 1995).

Buprenorphine for this indication was introduced in the UK in 1999 with the strong recommendation that consumption of the sublingual tablets should be supervised in pharmacies, as there is a history of injected abuse of the medication as a separate analgesic product (Temgesic).

Relapse prevention

Relapse rates after detoxification from opiates by any method are high, and an assertive approach is required to avoid this. Relevant counselling can be provided, while the pharmacological treatment indicated is the oral opiate antagonist, naltrexone (Farren 1997).

Naltrexone may be used in precipitated withdrawal under sedation, but the main licensed use in the UK is after detoxification, to 'block' the effect of opi-ates. An opiate-free period of about 6–10 days is usually required before the first dose can be given, to avoid withdrawal symptoms occurring, but after that if 50 mg is consumed per day, any opiates subsequently taken are ren-dered ineffective, the treatment therefore operating as a strong disincentive to such use. Compliance is critical and can be enhanced by the involvement of a 'third person'.

Conclusions

Methadone, a medication extremely familiar to drug misuse clinicians, dom-inates the activity within many treatment services. Its benefits are striking, in terms of psychological and social stability and improvements in physical health. Unfortunately it is also highly addictive, which is a particular problem when the time arrives to come off the drug or when it is used as a detoxifi-cation treatment.

Many individuals undoubtedly manage to withdraw from methadone suc-cessfully, especially if they have particularly high motivation to do so at the time. A variety of methods can be used, with no clear evidence for benefit of one over another. There is increasing interest in regimens which can sub-stantially shorten the detoxification process, in view of the protracted withdrawal features which can otherwise occur.

The most questionable aspect of the current usage of methadone is the widespread prescribing to individuals with relatively mild dependence on heroin. Usually this is intended to be on a detoxification basis, but there is often a drift into a semi-maintenance situation with unclear treatment aims. In responding to large numbers of heroin users and attempting to fulfil objectives in HIV prevention, clinicians have reached for methadone as the simplest way of reducing individuals' other drug use, probably without enough consideration of the longer-term implications. While many kinds of factors contribute to difficulties in completing detoxification, methadone is far from being an ideal drug for this purpose, and alternatives such as buprenorphine could offer some advantages. After any detoxification, the matter of avoiding relapse should be assertively addressed.

References

Beaini, A., Johnson, T., Langstaff, P., Carr, M., Crossfield, J. & Sweeny, R. (2000) A compressed opiate detoxification regime with naltrexone maintenance: patient tolerance, risk assessment and abstinence rates. *Addiction Biology*, 5: 451–62.

Bearn, J., Gossop, M. & Strang, J. (1998) Accelerated lofexidine treatment regimen compared with conventional lofexidine and methadone treatment for inpatient opiate detoxification. *Drug and Alcohol Dependence*, 50: 227–32.

Bertschy, G. (1995) Methadone maintenance treatment: an update. *European Archives of Psychiatry and Clinical Neuroscience*, 245: 114–24.

Bickel, W.K. & Amass, L. (1995) Buprenorphine treatment of opioid dependence: a review. *Experimental and Clinical Psychopharmacology*, 3: 477–89.

Carnwath, T. & Hardman, J. (1998) Randomised double-blind comparison of lofexidine and clonidine in the outpatient treatment of opiate withdrawal. *Drug and Alcohol Dependence*, 50: 251–4.

Dawe, S., Griffiths, P., Gossop, M. & Strang, J. (1991) Should opiate addicts be involved in controlling their own detoxification? A comparison of fixed versus negotiable schedules. *British Journal of Addiction*, 86: 977–82.

Department of Health (1999) *Drug Misuse and Dependence – Guidelines on Clinical Management*. London: The Stationery Office.

Dole, V. (1973) Detoxification of methadone patients and public policy. *Journal of the American Medical Association*, 226: 747–52.

Eklund, C., Melin, L., Hiltunen, & Borg, S. (1994) Detoxification from methadone maintenance treatment in Sweden: long-term outcome and effects on quality of life and life situation. *The International Journal of the Addictions*, 29: 627–45.

Farren, C. K. (1997) The use of naltrexone, an opiate antagonist, in the treatment of opiate addiction. *Irish Journal of Psychological Medicine*, 14: 26–31.

Garrido, M.J. & Troconiz, I.F. (1999) Methadone: a review of its pharmacokinetic/pharmacodynamic properties. *Journal of Pharmacological and Toxicological Methods*, 42: 61–6.

Gossop. M., Marsden, J., Stewart, D. & Rolfe, A. (2000) Patterns of improvement after methadone treatment: One year follow-up results from the National Treatment Outcome Research Study (NTORS). *Drug and Alcohol Dependence*, 60: 275–86.

Gossop, M., Battersby, M. & Strang, J. (1991) Self-detoxification by opiate addicts: a preliminary investigation. *British Journal of Psychiatry,* 159: 208–12.

Gossop, M., Griffiths, P., Bradley, M. & Strang, J. (1989) Opiate withdrawal symptoms in response to a 10-day and 21-day methadone withdrawal programmes. *British Journal of Psychiatry,* 154: 360–3.

Gossop, M., Bradley, M. & Philips, G. (1987) An investigation of withdrawal symptoms shown by opiate addicts during and subsequent to a 21-day inpatient methadone detoxification. *Addictive Behaviors,* 12: 1–6.

Gossop, M., Johns, A. & Green, L. (1986) Opiate withdrawal: inpatient versus outpatient programmes and preferred versus random assignment to treatment. *British Medical Journal,* 293: 103–4.

Law, F.D., Bailey, J.E., Allen, D.S., Melichar, J.K., Myles, J.S., Mitcheson, M.C., Lewis, J.W. & Nutt, D.J. (1997) The feasibility of abrupt methadone-buprenorphine transfer in British opiate addicts in an outpatient setting. *Addiction Biology,* 2: 191–200.

Marsch, L.A. (1998) The efficacy of methadone maintenance interventions in reducing illicit opiate use, HIV risk behaviour and criminality: a meta-analysis. *Addiction*, 93: 515–32.

Rosen, M. & Kosten, T.R. (1995) Detoxification and induction onto naltrexone. In: Cowan A, Lewis JW, eds. *Buprenorphine: Combatting Drug Abuse with a Unique Opioid.* New York: Wiley-Liss 289–305.

Rosenbaum, M. & Murphy, S. (1984) Always a junkie? the arduous task of getting off methadone maintenance. *Journal of Drug Issues*, 14: 527–52.

Rostami-Hodjegan, A., Wolff, K., Hay, A., Raistrick, D., Calvert, R. & Tucker, G. (1999) Population pharmacokinetics of methadone in opiate users: characterisation of time-dependent changes. *British Journal of Clinical Pharmacology*, 48: 43–52.

Seivewright, N. (2000a) Methadone maintenance: a medical treatment for social reasons? In: Seivewright N, ed. *Community Treatment of Drug Misuse: More than Methadone.* Cambridge: Cambridge University Press.

Seivewright, N. (2000b) More than methadone? The case for other substitute drugs, In: Seivewright N, ed. *Community Treatment of Drug Misuse: More than Methadone* Cambridge: Cambridge University Press.

Seivewright, N. (2000c) Achieving detoxification and abstinence. In: Seivewright N, ed. *Community Treatment of Drug Misuse: More than Methadone.* Cambridge: Cambridge University Press.

Seivewright, N. & Daly, C. (1997) Personality disorder and drug use: a review. *Drug and Alcohol Review,* 16: 235–50.

Stimson, G.V. (1996) Has the United Kingdom averted an epidemic of HIV-infection among drug injectors? *Addiction,* 91: 1085–8.

Strang, J., Bearn, J. & Gossop, M. (1999) Lofexidine for opiate detoxification: Review of recent randomised and open controlled trials. *The American Journal on Addictions,* 8: 337–48.

Strang, J., Marks, I., Dawe, S., Powell, J., Gossop, M., Richards, D. & Gray, J. (1997) Type of hospital setting and treatment outcome with heroin addicts. Results from a randomised trial. *British Journal of Psychiatry*, 171: 335–9.

Section C: The special case of injectables

9
Injectable methadone: a peculiar British practice

John Strang and Janie Sheridan

Injectable methadone maintenance for the treatment of opiate addicts is an almost exclusively UK practice. Apart from a handful of patients in Australia and New Zealand (less than half a dozen) and other small numbers of patients in Switzerland or the Netherlands who may have recently been started on injectable methadone ampoules on an experimental basis, no other country includes injectable methadone as one of the options for treatment of opiate addiction. Even within the UK, this prescribing practice is almost entirely restricted to certain parts of England. Although no precise data are available about the extent of prescribing of injectable methadone ampoules in the UK, a snapshot was taken through the 1995 national survey of community pharmacists (see later section), at which time approximately 10% of the methadone prescriptions were for the ampoule form.

The methadone in methadone ampoules is pharmacologically the same as the methadone in various oral forms prescribed in the UK and many other countries worldwide. In virtually all other respects, the injectable ampoules are so different that they might better be considered separately, as if they were an altogether different drug. These differences include the clear 'hit' or 'rush' which results from intravenous methadone (in contrast to oral methadone). This chapter consists of a bringing-together of evidence about the different characteristics of injectable methadone (for the user experience) and the different ways in which it is prescribed and dispensed. The limited number of studies of this form of treatment will then be summarized. Clinical issues with regard to prescribing injectable methadone are considered separately in Chapter 10 and the different position of injectable methadone ampoules in the illicit market in the UK is covered in Chapter 15. Finally, consideration will be given to the options for development of clinical treatment and public policy with regard to injectable methadone, alongside recognition of the need to establish a more legitimate evidence base for this unusual clinical practice.

The history of injectable methadone prescribing in the UK

Injectable methadone was first prescribed in the UK in the mid-1960s by independent and private doctors such as Lady Frankau, who prescribed intravenous methadone along with heroin and other drugs to some of the heroin addicts whom she was treating (for further background information, see Spear 1994). However, it was in the years following the opening of the new drug clinics in 1968 that injectable methadone came to be prescribed more widely. During the first five years of their operation, there was a gradual reduction in the total amounts of heroin prescribed by the clinics, with an increase (broadly equivalent) in the amount of injectable methadone being prescribed so that, for the first time in 1973, substantially more injectable methadone was being prescribed than injectable heroin (Mitcheson 1994). Thereafter the amounts of injectable methadone being prescribed continued to exceed the amounts of heroin in the years that followed and increasingly so in later years.

The amounts of oral methadone were substantially lower than injectable methadone during the first decade of operation of the clinics and it was not until 1978 that, for the first time, quantities of oral methadone prescribed reached the same level as injectable methadone; since then the amounts of oral methadone have grown to exceed substantially the amounts of injectable methadone. There has also, since that time, been a marked reduction in the proportion of methadone prescriptions that have been for injectable methadone ampoules. Probably the best data source for tracking this change over a long period of time is the NHS prescription data set, which provides evidence of the great increase in the extent of methadone prescribing (see Chapter 3) and also enables tracking of the proportion of these methadone prescriptions that are in injectable form.[1] These data are displayed in Figure 9.1; during the first half of the 1980s the position of injectable methadone steadily reduced so that, from a position of making up at least one-third of all methadone prescriptions, its proportion had dropped to only 10% by the mid-1980s. Thereafter, there seems to have been a gradual increase back up to 15%, which may possibly have been a reaction to awareness about the new HIV risk and a particular concern to draw opiate addicts into treatment. However, this increase was not sustained and the proportion of methadone prescriptions given out as ampoules stayed between 8% and 10% through most of the 1990s until the last few years, when it seems to have reduced still further as a proportion, down to the 1999 level of 5.6% and a level of less than 5% for the year 2000.

---

[1] Several important limitations of this data set need to be made clear at the outset. The data cover only NHS prescriptions (i.e. they do not include private prescriptions) dispensed from community pharmacies and there is no filter or link to diagnosis (i.e. they include methadone prescriptions for other possible indications such as pain relief). Nevertheless unpublished information collected by commercial organizations studying GPs prescribing patterns consistently indicates that virtually all methadone prescribed is in the context of the treatment of addiction, with other indications probably comprising only a few per cent of all methadone prescriptions.

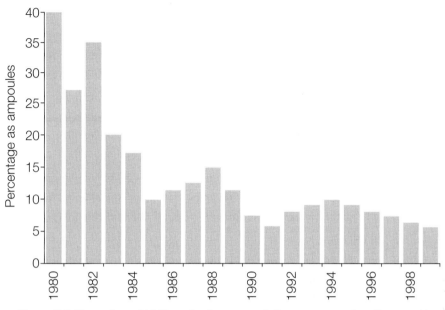

Figure 9.1 Proportion of NHS methadone prescriptions as ampoules dispensed by community pharmacists (England 1980–1999) (Derived from data kindly supplied by the Statistics Department, Department of Health).

A distinctively different effect

Much confusion is caused by the mistaken presumption that the effects of injectable methadone will be broadly the same as the more widely studied and understood effects of oral methadone. Since methadone has internationally almost always been considered in its oral form, reports of its effects are often presented as if the drug did not even exist in its injectable form.

When it was first introduced more widely into the UK, the methadone ampoules were often viewed by heroin addicts with disdain – perhaps partly because of their association with oral methadone and certainly because their introduction was associated with an attempt to transfer the addict away from injectable heroin. However, as injectable ampoules tended to be used more widely, they soon assumed a position (in treatment and on the illicit market), which was broadly comparable to injectable heroin. As Mitcheson (1994) described in his account of this period, initial customer reaction '…. was that they were only good for rinsing out one's works', but 'this rapidly gave way to a general realisation that intravenous methadone was a rapid-acting drug with euphoriant properties', after which 'the price of 10 mg units of injectable methadone and injectable heroin rapidly achieved parity'. At roughly the same time, a research study of heroin users in London found that they considered the hedonistic appeal of injectable heroin and injectable methadone to be broadly comparable (Blumberg *et al.* 1974).

Mitcheson's account relates to the clinics in London. A similar picture seems to have been occurring at a national level. Stimson and Oppenheimer (1982) report data collected by earlier researchers on the amounts of heroin and methadone prescribed to addicts attending NHS hospitals in England and Wales. The amounts of methadone ampoules were shown to increase steadily until they exceeded the amounts of heroin for the first time (and thereafter) in 1973, with a later increase in the amounts of oral methadone (described as 'linctus and tablets') which eventually exceeded the amount of injectable methadone in 1978 (the last year for which they presented data).

When prescribing injectable opiates in clinical practice in the UK, a typical experience was described by Strang *et al.* (1994): 'the committed injector seeking a prescribed supply of injectable drugs would usually be quite amenable to moves between heroin and methadone in injectable form – in sharp contrast to the determined opposition which may be encountered to suggestions of moving from injectable methadone to its oral form'. A particularly graphic verbatim quote from an addict (receiving one of the rare injectable prescriptions in Amsterdam) illustrates this point: 'I have been taking it for half a year now, it's far out; they can take anything from me, my beer, my wife – so long as they keep their hands off my injectable methadone' (Kools 1992).

The extent of recent prescribing of injectable methadone

(1) The 1995 Community Pharmacy Survey

In 1995, a national survey of community pharmacists was commissioned to explore the scope for increasing their involvement in provision of services to drug misusers (Sheridan *et al.* 1996). It was, at the same time, possible to construct a national picture with unprecedented detail, of the prescriptions which doctors issued in the treatment of drug misuse and addiction. The particular strength of this approach was that there was much less likelihood of distortion of the data from non-response bias. If an attempt had been made to obtain this information from the prescribing doctors themselves, it would not only have been dogged by the much higher non-response rate which is characteristic of doctors, but there would also have been more grounds for concern that the non-responder might be prescribing in a very different manner from the responder sample. By looking at these data through the keyhole of the community pharmacy, the likelihood of any such non-response bias was greatly reduced.

Self-completion questionnaires were sent to a random one in four sample of all community pharmacies in England and Wales, and repeat mailshots were sent on three subsequent occasions to non-responders. At the end of four postal mailshots, a highly respectable 75% response rate had been secured. Embedded within these self-completion questionnaires was a section within which information was gathered about all prescriptions currently

Table 9.1 Example of grid response by community pharmacist to drug prescription enquiry in community pharmacy survey (1995).

Dispensing controlled drugs

If you have **6 or less** clients, please enter details of their treatment. Where a client has more than one item (e.g. two dosage forms of same drug, or more than one drug) please bracket together.

Drug name	Form	Strength (mg)	Daily dose (mg)	Supervised consumption? Tick if 'Yes'	Private	NHS	GP	Hospital or clinic	Number of dispensings per week as stated on prescription
					Please tick one			Please tick one	
Methadone	Mixture	1mg/1ml	50		✓		✓		1
Methadone	Mixture	1mg/1ml	45	✓		✓		✓	6
Methadone	Amps	10mg	50			✓		✓	6
Codeine	Tabs	30mg	240			✓	✓		1
Buprenorphine	Tabs	2mg	8			✓	✓		3
Methadone	Amps	50mg	250	✓			✓	✓	1

If more space is required, please telephone … for supplementary sheet.

being dispensed to drug misusers by the community pharmacy using a grid recording system as shown in Table 9.1. With this method, information was obtained on nearly 4000 prescriptions that were being dispensed from pharmacies at that time (mid-1995), of which 3693 were prescriptions for methadone – and it is these 3693 methadone prescriptions that form the basis of the data presented at the time (Strang *et al.* 1996) in the next section[2] and in Figure 9.2.

The injectable methadone ampoules comprised 9% of these prescriptions, while methadone was most commonly prescribed as the oral liquid (e.g. methadone mixture: 1 mg per ml) – 80% of all of the prescriptions. The remainder (11%) was for tablets. These prescriptions had emanated from doctors working in both the specialist and generalist settings. Nearly half of the prescriptions (42%) had been issued by general practitioners, whilst the other half (58%) had been issued by hospital doctors. The average daily dose of methadone was 44.3 mg, although there was a wide range of daily doses (range 2–200 mg daily). A wide range of dispensing arrangements was also evident. Whilst a third of the prescriptions (37%) were being dispensed on a daily basis (which was defined operationally as a separate pick-up on 5, 6 or 7 days per week), another third (37%) were being dispensed on a weekly basis (a figure which included a small number of prescriptions for fortnightly or even monthly pick-up). Further details of the main data from this survey are contained in Chapter 3, and in the associated publications about the methadone data (Strang *et al.* 1996; Strang and Sheridan 1998a; b).

Was the prescribing of injectable methadone different?

The next step was to search for distinctive features of the prescriptions for injectable methadone in an attempt to gain a better understanding of the way in which this different form of methadone was being prescribed. With roughly half of the prescriptions having been issued from general practice and half from hospital settings, the opportunity existed to look for some prescribing evidence of effective triage, with specialist services perhaps having

---

[2] In order to understand properly the data presented on methadone prescriptions, the reader needs to be aware of the manner in which the data were collected and stored. If a single patient was simultaneously receiving more than one form of methadone (e.g. ampoules and syrup), then these appear as two separate entries; hence, whilst the data presented in this chapter are an accurate report of the methadone ampoule prescribing data, it needs to be borne in mind that the actual methadone dose of individual patients will often have been greater than the doses reported if a patient receiving injectable methadone ampoules was also receiving an oral form. For presentation of the data on the oral liquid methadone, which comprised 80% of all prescriptions, the potential distortion of the actual mean daily dose could only be small, since it could only affect a small proportion of the prescriptions: however, for the smaller number of prescriptions for methadone ampoules the extent of the distortion would depend on the proportion who were also receiving oral methadone, which, from examination of our data alone, could be anywhere between none and all.

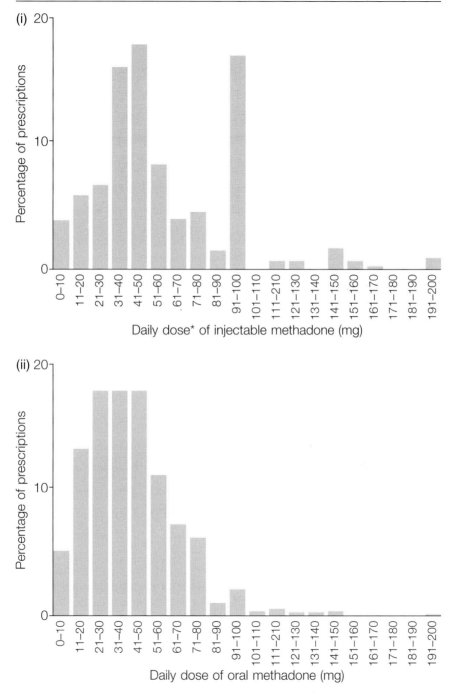

Figure 9.2 Distribution of daily doses on prescriptions of (i) methadone ampoules, and (ii) oral syrup methadone.
*Two further values of less than 1% for 230 mg and 250 mg are not displayed.

assumed responsibility for more difficult patients (for whom there might be evidence of the need for a greater proportion on injectable methadone, for example). Thus, if more complicated patients and more complicated treatments were correctly finding their way through to specialist services then one would expect to see a much higher proportion of patients on injectable methadone in the patient populations being seen in specialist clinics, just as one might expect to see other specialist services within the National Health Service having particular concentrations of more difficult patients and more complicated treatments. However, there was only modest evidence of any such difference in the likelihood of prescribing injectable methadone, with 8% of prescriptions from general practitioners being for methadone ampoules compared with 10% for hospital doctors. It is of course possible that some of these patients receiving injectable methadone from general practitioners may have been receiving a treatment that was either initiated by, or recommended from, a specialist clinic who subsequently asked the general practitioner to continue with the prescription for methadone ampoules – but no data were collected in this survey to allow this to be considered further; it is possible to consider this question further in the later study by Beaumont (2001), which is summarized later in this chapter.

Private prescriptions were markedly different. Private prescribing to addicts was mostly a London phenomenon, and comprised only 2% of all prescriptions. These private prescriptions were distinctive for the much larger proportion (33%) which were for injectable ampoules, with a further 33% being for tablets (comparative figures of 9% and 11% respectively for NHS practice). Doses were also significantly higher – most strikingly for injectable ampoules where the average private prescription was at a mean daily dose of 118 mg (compared with the equivalent NHS figure of 62 mg).

Regional variations in methadone prescriptions were pronounced. Since a large data set of methadone prescriptions had now been collected from across the whole of England and Wales, the types of prescriptions could be studied for local differences between the regional health authority areas (each region containing a catchment population of typically 2–4 million). Major variation was seen in the distribution of different forms of methadone (i.e. the proportion of prescriptions for either the oral liquid form, the tablets, or the ampoules).

Across all regions the most commonly prescribed form of methadone was the oral liquid form (e.g. methadone mixture 1 mg per ml). However this ranged from a low of 68% in one region to a high of 90% in two of the other regions. Marked differences also existed in the extent to which injectable methadone was prescribed – only 4% of prescriptions in three of the regions, with a high of 23% in one region (Strang and Sheridan 1998a).

(2) The 1997 Community Pharmacy Survey

In 1997, a repeat survey of community pharmacists was commissioned for the South East of England to allow the study of barriers to greater involvement of community pharmacists (Sheridan *et al.* 1999). This created the opportunity to repeat the collection of data on methadone prescriptions, thereby enabling us to look at any evidence of change in the intervening two years. The striking overall conclusion was that there was very little change, despite significant national policy initiatives in the intervening periods (Strang and Sheridan 1998b).

Let us look at these 1997 data from the South East of England in more detail. For the 1997 survey, a 50% sample of community pharmacists was surveyed and during the first mailshot, the same information was gathered about current methadone prescriptions. It was thus possible to compare these new 1997 data with the South East fraction of the national survey in 1995 (Strang and Sheridan 1998b). This comparison was of considerable interest as it represented the comparison of two surveys which bracketed the Department of Health Task Force Report (Department of Health 1996) and could hence reasonably be regarded as 'before and after' snapshots of methadone prescribing. With regard to injectable prescribing, there was very little difference between the two surveys: by 1997 there had been a very small reduction in the proportion of the prescriptions for injectable methadone ampoules – from 9.8% of all methadone prescriptions in 1995 to 8.1% in 1997. However, even this apparent reduction in the extent of pre-scribing injectable methadone had occurred against a backdrop of an annual increase of approximately 20% per annum in the extent of all methadone prescribing (Home Office 1997). This would indicate that the true number of injectable methadone prescriptions had probably not reduced and may even have increased over the intervening years, although not by as large an extent as the number of oral methadone prescriptions.

It is also possible to look at the 1997 data to establish whether there is the same evidence of regional variation as was seen with the 1995 data – sum-marized above. The picture is generally similar. It is also possible to apply this examination at a more local level – the level of the local health authority. At this level, the proportion of methadone prescriptions for ampoules varied substantially. Across the 15 local health authorities in South East England, injectable methadone comprised less than 5% of methadone prescriptions for three of the health authorities whilst it comprised more than 15% of methadone prescriptions for three of the health authorities, including one in which it comprised 23%.

(3) The National Survey of General Practitioners Prescribing Injectable Methadone

The third study in this section is the 1999 survey undertaken by Beaumont (2001). Beaumont surveyed all 105 health authorities in England and Wales and established, via the pharmaceutical advisers, that three-quarters of these health authorities contained at least one practice from which injectable methadone was being prescribed. The responses indicated that there were a total of 407 practices in these 75 health authorities, from which at least one general practitioner had been prescribing injectable methadone during the six-month period in question. Further data were then sought from the relevant practices in 57 of these health authorities (who complied with the requests to circulate further questionnaires) and responses were received from 149 of the surveyed sample of 324 practices: 42 of these returned questionnaires indicated that no injectable methadone had been prescribed, thus leaving 107 practices that had been correctly identified as currently or recently prescribing injectable methadone.

Fuller data were obtained from 93 of the doctors working in these practices. Sixty per cent of these doctors were prescribing injectable methadone to only one patient, although 10 of the practitioners were prescribing it to 5 or more patients. These 93 general practitioners were, between them, treating 211 patients with injectable methadone and they were also treating a further 2003 patients with oral methadone – i.e. the patients on injectable methadone comprised 9.5% of the 2214 patients receiving methadone treatment from these 93 doctors.

The most strongly endorsed reasons for prescribing injectable methadone were that the patient was 'already on injectable treatment from a specialist drug service' (scored as the 'most likely' or 'likely' reason by 79% of the practitioners), that 'injectable treatment was requested after assessment by the local drugs agency' (78%) or that there were 'serious health and social problems and can't stop injecting' (70%) whereas the 'failure of oral methadone' was identified as the most likely or likely reason by only 48%. Within the practice of these doctors there was also evidence of considerable diversity with, for example, more than half 'always or usually' requiring their patients to collect their methadone ampoules on a daily basis from a local pharmacy, whilst 20% of the practitioners reported that they rarely invoked these pick-up arrangements.

Other research studies of injectable methadone prescribing

The most important observation to make is that there has been surprisingly little clinical research on injectable methadone prescribing. Most of the limited amount of published material comprises reports from clinicians describing their recent practice. This includes reports from clinicians working in specialist drug clinics (Gossop et al. 1982; Strang et al. 1990; Battersby et al. 1992) and also from those working in primary care (Martin et al. 1998; Ford and Ryrie 1999) and a substantial observational report of injectable opiate prescribing from Sell et al. (2001).

What research evidence do we have if we restrict ourselves to randomized clinical trials, or at least recognizable clinical research trial design? The answer is – very little. However, two clinical research studies of injectable methadone prescribing have recently been reported and warrant fuller scrutiny. The Sell *et al.* (2001) report will also be examined. The first (Metrebian *et al.* 1998) was the observational, self-selection study of injectable heroin versus injectable methadone prescribing. The second (Strang *et al.* 2000) reported the feasibility and six-month outcome of the randomized trial of supervised injectable versus oral methadone mainte-nance. These two studies will now be considered more fully in the next two paragraphs.

The Metrebian *et al.* (1998) study was undertaken in a large West London drug clinic, and involved the prescribing of either injectable heroin or injectable methadone to an opiate addict treatment population who had pre-viously tried and failed with oral methadone treatment and who were unable or unwilling to cease injecting. The investigators studied 58 patients who were taken on by the clinic for injectable maintenance with either injectable heroin (diamorphine) or injectable methadone. This patient group represented a chronic addict population (median age 38 years) with long-standing histories (had been injecting heroin for a median duration of 19.5 years). Each patient was given the choice of injectable heroin or injectable methadone: two-thirds (64%) chose heroin whilst the remainder (36%) chose injectable methadone. Retention in treatment was reported as 86%, 69% and 57% of the study samples still being in treatment at 3 months, 6 months and 9 months after starting treatment. Major improvements in health and social domains were found amongst both groups of patients, with these changes already evident by the first assessment after the start of treatment. However, no consistent picture of major changes thereafter was seen with the study population with, for example, an increase in illicit drug injecting between the 3-month and 6-month follow-ups, in contrast to a reduction in HIV risk behaviour, illicit drug injecting and sexual risk behaviour between 6 and 12 months. The investigators noted the substantial proportion (more than one-third) who chose injectable methadone in preference to heroin, and also noted the improvements across all domains seen in the patients who remained in treatment. However, they also drew attention to the persistence, although typically at substantially reduced levels, of both illicit drug use and criminal activity.

The Strang *et al.* (2000) study was undertaken in a South London catch-ment area drug treatment clinic, to test the acceptability of a new supervised injecting facility within the clinic and also to examine the acceptability of ran-domization between supervised injectable and oral methadone maintenance (for the purposes of a randomized treatment trial). Forty opiate addicts par-ticipated in the study. Both the supervised injectable and oral methadone treatment were generally acceptable to the study participants, and there was a reassuringly high level of agreement to enter the randomization (after an explanation to the patients that they would be receiving active treatment in both arms of the randomization). Retention within both treatments was good and indeed was higher than that seen in the Metrebian *et al.* study (see pre-ceding paragraph), for which there had been no requirement of daily attendance and supervised injecting. On this basis the investigators concluded that the supervised injectable clinic was a treatment modality that should be explored more fully. Substantial benefits were found to be associated with the supervised injectable methadone maintenance at the time of the 6 month follow-up, with the average number of days (per month) of illicit heroin use having reduced from 22.2 to 7.6 and the average number of days (per month) of illicit injecting being reduced from 25.7 to 10.8. Other measures of well-being, such as the patients' physical and psychological health status and the extent of involvement in criminal activity, also showed improvements. However, similar results were seen in patients randomized to oral methadone maintenance, for whom the average number of days per month of illicit drug use and illicit injecting also reduced – from 22.4 to 8.7 (for reduction in illicit heroin use) and from 20.1 to 11.9 (for reduction in illicit injecting).

The investigators felt able to draw several conclusions that have a direct bearing on future research study of injectable methadone prescribing. First, the new, supervised injecting clinic seemed broadly acceptable to the patient population and was associated with acceptable retention rates in treatment. Secondly, the use of a randomized study design (with active treatment in both arms) was generally acceptable to most of the target group of potential study participants. Thirdly, it is essential for the outcomes with the less studied treatment (i.e. injectable methadone maintenance) to be compared with outcomes from oral methadone maintenance treatment applied to the same study population, in order to gauge the extent to which any observed benefits can legitimately be attributed to the injectable methadone treatment itself.

The Sell et al. (2001) study was an audit of 125 patients receiving prescriptions for injectable opiates from the regional drug services in Manchester. The great majority of patients on injectable opiate prescriptions were receiving injectable methadone (86%) with most of the remainder receiving injectable heroin (13%), and five of these were also receiving injectable methadone. Most (87%) were injecting their methadone ampoules intravenously, with all but one of the remainder injecting them intramuscularly. A third were receiving no medication other than the injectable methadone, whilst two-thirds were additionally receiving oral methadone in syrup or tablet form. They were generally an older chronic addict population who had been injecting heroin for an average of 16 years. Many no longer had easy venous access so that, for example, 41% had injected in their groin during the past month, including many who injected only in their groin. Finally, Sell and her colleagues uncovered an interesting difference between the opinions expressed by the patients about the drug they would ideally choose compared with the drug they believed best for their treatment. Half of the sample (50%) reported that, if they could choose their drug, they would choose heroin, with 31% reporting that they would choose methadone ampoules; but these figures changed when the respondents were asked which drug they believed was best for their treatment, with the proportion selecting heroin dropping to 34%, and 46% selecting the methadone ampoules.

Conclusion

The single most important conclusion is that injectable methadone treatment is a world apart from oral methadone treatment. Whilst the drug itself is obviously the same, the differences far exceed the similarities. The issues underlying discussion of injectable methadone prescribing sit more comfortably alongside the heroin prescribing debate, and it is disappointing that this heroin debate (e.g. Bammer *et al*. 1999) has given so little attention to injectable methadone prescribing, especially since the latter is so much more widespread – at least in the UK.

Many specialist clinicians in the UK (with experience of prescribing injectable and oral methadone treatment) are of the opinion that injectable methadone treatment is a legitimate tool in the armamentarium. However, most consider it a more difficult form of treatment to manage, and one which should only be prescribed by those doctors with a greater level of expertise in the addictions field, perhaps only by the specialized generalist or the specialist described in the recent Department of Health guidelines (Department of Health 1999). This was the conclusion with regard to the prescribing of injectable heroin found by Sell *et al*. (1997) in her survey of doctors holding special Home Office licences for the prescribing of heroin to addicts, and it is likely that much the same conclusion would have been elicited if the survey had also covered injectable methadone prescribing (not covered in this survey since no equivalent licence is required).

If injectable methadone prescribing is to be seen as typically more specialist in nature and requiring more essential monitoring, then it will require greater organization and clarity of purpose, since at present there is no evidence of any such differentiation between generalist and specialist prescribing (Strang *et al*. 1996). Indeed the marked regional variation in the extent of injectable methadone prescribing (Strang and Sheridan 1998a; Beaumount 2001) is unlikely to be due to some regional difference in the nature of the patients; it is much more likely to be associated with local organizational differences or the different personal views of individual physicians, which result in a postcode prescribing lottery with regard to injectable methadone prescribing. As Sarfraz and Alcorn (1999) have argued, it is essential that there is a clearer evidence-based prescribing policy in order to address the serious practical, ethical and legal implications of injectable methadone prescribing.

The 'British System' is a strange and wonderful animal. One of its great strengths (and reasons for its international fame) is the lack of tight definition and regulation of the system (or non-system) which allows both innovation and eccentricity, and crucially allows the clinician to consider the fullest range of options in selecting the most appropriate package of treatment for each individual patient. On the other hand, the British System can be seen as a rudderless ship being tossed this way and that by the tides and winds of fashion and panic, with a lack of any steering influence from research evidence (into which no investment is made), resulting in an unhealthy reliance on policy-by-committee or policy-by-default (Strang and Gossop 1994). Should the peculiarly British inclusion of injectable methadone maintenance as one of the treatment options be regarded as an example of the riches and benefits that can result from the absence of regulatory constriction, or should it be seen as evidence of lack of clear purpose, ignorance of the evidence base and consequent therapeutic anarchy? The answer is probably 'yes' to both.

The challenge before us is to find ways of reaping the benefits of this more controversial treatment without exposing ourselves and our patients to excessive harm from its inappropriate or careless application. In the absence of an accepted system and with evidence of great individual and geographical variation in clinical practice, criteria for suitability for injectable maintenance are now urgently required, alongside funding for an adequate system of triage and a new funded capacity to address the special heath care needs of the important minority of patients for whom injectable maintenance may be an essential part of their optimal care. Without such organisational and funding commitment, the current pattern of arbitrary clinical responses and postcode prescribing of injectable methadone is destined to continue, with resulting harm to patients, disillusionment amongst clinicians, and damage to the international standing of the peculiar British System.

References

Bammer, G., Dobler-Mikola, A., Fleming, P., Strang, J. & Uchtenhagen, A. (1999) The heroin prescribing debate: integrating science and politics. *Science*, 284: 1277–8.

Battersby, M., Farrell, M., Gossop, M., Robson, P. & Strang, J. (1992) 'Horse Trading': prescribing injectable opiates to opiate addicts – a descriptive study. *Drug and Alcohol Review*, 11: 35–42.

Beaumont, B. (2001) Survey of injectable methadone prescribing in general practice in England and Wales. *International Journal of Drug Policy*, 12: 91–101.

Blumberg, H.H., Cohen, S.D., Dronfield, B.F., Mordecai, E.A., Roberts, J.C. & Hawks, D. (1974) British opiate users: I: people approaching London drug treatment centres. *International Journal of the Addictions*, 9: 1–23.

Department of Health (1999) *Drug Misuse and Dependence – Guidelines on Clinical Management*. London: The Stationery Office.

Department of Health (1996) *Task Force Review of Services for Drug Misusers: Report of an Independent Review of Drug Treatment Services in England*. London: HM Stationery Office.

Ford, C. & Ryrie, I. (1999) Prescribing injectable methadone in general practice. *International Journal of Drug Policy*, 10: 39–45.

Gossop, M., Strang, J. & Connell, P. (1982) The response of out-patient opiate addicts to the provision of a temporary increase in their prescribed drugs. *British Journal of Psychiatry*, 141: 338–43.

Home Office (1997) *Statistics on the Misuse of Drugs: Addicts notified to the Home Office, United Kingdom, 1996*. (Home Office Statistical Bulletin). London: Home Office.

Kools, J.-P. (1992) Injectable methadone: policy for supplying methadone. *Mainline: Drugs, Health and the Street*, Special edition: 5.

Martin, E., Canavan, A. & Butler, R. (1998) A decade of caring for drug users entirely within general practice. *Journal of Substance Abuse Treatment*, 13: 521–31.

Metrebian, N., Shanahan, W., Wells, B. & Stimson, G.V. (1998) Feasibility of prescribing injectable heroin and methadone to opiate dependent drug users: associated health gains and harm reductions. *Medical Journal of Australia*, 168: 596–600.

Mitcheson, M. (1994) Drug clinics in the 1970s. In: Strang J, Gossop M, eds. *Heroin Addiction and Drug Policy: the British System*. London: Oxford University Press; 178–91.

Sarfraz, A. & Alcorn, R. (1999) Injectable methadone prescribing in the United Kingdom: current practice and future policy guidelines. *Substance Use and Misuse,* 34: 1709–21.

Sell, L., Segar, G. & Merrill, J. (2001) One hundred and twenty-five prescriptions for injectable opiates in the North West of England. *Drug and Alcohol Review*, 20: 57–66.

Sell, L., Farrell, M. & Robson, P. (1997) Prescription of diamorphine, dipipanone and cocaine in England and Wales. *Drug and Alcohol Review*, 16: 221–6.

Sheridan, J., Strang, J. & Lovell, S. (1999) Central and local guidance on services for drug misusers: do they influence current practice? Results from a survey of community pharmacists in South East England. *International Journal of Pharmacy Practice*, 7: 100–6.

Sheridan, J., Strang, J., Barber, N. & Glanz, A. (1996) Role of community pharmacies in relation to HIV prevention and drug misuse: Findings from the 1995 national survey in England and Wales. *British Medical Journal*, 313: 272–4.

Spear, H.B. (1994) The early years of the 'British System' in practice. In: Strang J, Gossop M, eds. *Heroin Addiction and Drug Policy: the British System*, London: Oxford University Press; 3–28.

Stimson, G.V. & Oppenheimer, E. (1982) *Heroin Addiction: Treatment and Control in Britain.* London: Tavistock.

Strang, J. & Gossop, M. (1994) The 'British System': visionary anticipation or masterly inactivity? In: Strang J, Gossop M, eds. *Heroin Addiction and Drug Policy: the British System*, London: Oxford University Press; 342–51.

Strang, J. & Sheridan, J. (1998a) National and regional characteristics of methadone prescribing in England and Wales: Local analyses of data from the 1995 national survey of community pharmacies. *Journal of Substance Misuse*, 3: 240–6.

Strang, J. & Sheridan, J. (1998b) Effect of government recommendations on methadone prescribing in South East England: comparison of 1995 and 1997 surveys. *British Medical Journal*, 317: 1489–90.

Strang, J., Marsden, J., Cummins, M., Farrell, M., Finch, E., Gossop, M., Stewart, D. & Welch, S. (2000) Randomised trial of supervised injectable versus oral methadone maintenance: report of feasibility and 6 month outcome. *Addiction,* 95: 1631–45.

Strang, J., Sheridan, J. & Barber, N. (1996) Prescribing injectable and oral methadone to opiate addicts: results from the 1995 national survey of community pharmacies in England and Wales. *British Medical Journal*, 313: 270–2.

Strang, J., Ruben, S., Farrell, M. & Gossop, M. (1994) Prescribing heroin and other injectable drugs. In: Strang J, Gossop M, eds. *Heroin Addiction and Drug Policy: the British System*, London: Oxford University Press; 192–206.

Strang, J., Johns, A. & Gossop, M. (1990) Social and drug taking behaviour of 'maintained' opiate addicts. *British Journal of Addiction,* 85: 771–4.

10
Prescribing injectable methadone: to whom and for what purpose?

Louise Sell

The UK is almost unique worldwide in using injectable methadone for opiate maintenance treatment. Treatment with methadone, whether oral or injectable, is not regulated by statute. Guidelines issued in 1999 by the Department of Health (DOH) state that injectable methadone may be an appropriate treatment for a minority of opiate-dependent individuals. They were able however to give little guidance about who these individuals are or how their treatment should be provided (Department of Health 1999). Despite the lack of detailed clinical guidelines, injectable methadone is used for a sizeable proportion of patients' opiate maintenance treatment in England and Wales. Nine per cent of the methadone dispensed in 1995 in England and Wales was injectable methadone (Strang *et al*. 1996). The answer to the question 'To whom and for what purpose?' is essentially decided by clinicians and treatment teams taking a view as to what is correct for their treatment population. This chapter discusses the clinical practice of prescribing injectable methadone maintenance, drawing from both clinical and research settings.

Why injectable methadone?

To understand why injectable methadone maintenance is used, we start by considering harm minimization treatment philosophy (Strang 1992). This takes as its starting point the view that it is more important to reduce the harm (initially HIV infection, but more recently encompassing other physical and even non-physical harm) accruing from drug use, than to stop drug use completely. At the individual level, injectable methadone may be prescribed in order to improve individual treatment outcome, while at the population level injectable prescriptions may attract greater numbers of heroin addicts into treatment. Injectable methadone may be particularly useful for treating three groups: those who are not attracted into treatment where only methadone mixture is available, those who are not retained in treatment with methadone mixture and those who continue to inject heroin regularly despite oral methadone treatment. Injectable methadone is prescribed with the intention that it will improve the outcome of treatment. Improvement may be achieved in the following domains: a reduction or cessation of injecting, a reduction in the use of other drugs and alcohol, a reduction in the risk of transmission of blood-borne viruses, a reduction in drug-related crime, facilitation of job seeking and employment and other socially productive behaviours and improved family relationships.

The use of injectable methadone extends the application of harm minimization strategies into increasingly difficult territory. In addition to the known benefits, the provision of oral methadone carries risks, including that of diversion and overdose (see Chapter 14), therefore any methadone maintenance treatment (oral or injectable) must be offered after considering the likely risks and benefits of doing so. Injectable methadone is prescribed in order to achieve benefit which is unlikely with oral methadone alone. However, the risks are arguably greater in the case of injectable methadone. Injecting of the prescribed drug may itself be associated with injection-related damage; injectable methadone has a higher street value than oral methadone and may be sold on illicitly, increasing supplies of diverted drugs. Most clinicians therefore take the view that injectable methadone should be offered only when the complications arising from injecting drug use are severe and when there is evidence that alternative treatments with fewer disadvantages themselves have not proven effective.

From majority to minority

National Health Service Drug Clinics, set up from the late 1960s onwards, originally prescribed more injectable than oral methadone. Indeed, the initial practice was to prescribe for patients the drug which they were already taking, and for the majority this was diamorphine. Injectable methadone was prescribed to a few patients who were already taking it, and thereafter increasingly to heroin addicts. The initial response of patients treated in this way was not positive, and it has been reported that methadone ampoules were used to flush out equipment used to inject heroin. However, the ampoules did acquire a value in the illicit drug market by the end of 1969, indicating an appreciation of their heroin-like properties (Mitcheson 1994). At this time the practice of prescribing injectable opiates was the standard method of opiate maintenance. Thus the answer to the question 'to whom?' would have been 'to most opiate addicts in medical treatment'. As the prevailing practice in the drug treatment field changed, the population of opiate addicts on injectable maintenance became a smaller proportion of all addicts in treatment: during the 1970s the volume of diamorphine prescribed fell steadily, that of oral methadone rose, that of injectable methadone peaked in 1975 and fell significantly by 1980. Prescribing injectable methadone became distinguishable from the general treatment of opiate addicts. It was carried out in specific settings and with specific intent, i.e. in clinics where the responsible doctor agreed with its role within the management of opiate dependence. Following Health Service reorganization the opinion of local treatment commissioners about the effectiveness of this treatment became a further factor determining availability. Prescribing injectable methadone has provoked international interest. However, the lack of prospective research or detailed guidelines has also been cause for comment. Zador (2001) has questioned whether injectable opiate treatment is good clinical practice, and found the evidence with which to answer the question wanting. She argues cogently for audit and governance of the large amount of clinical activity which currently goes unevaluated.

By whom

To understand the prescribing of injectable methadone, we should also pay attention to the question of who provides this treatment. The 1991 Department of Health Guidelines included the prescribing of injectable drugs as an example of a complicated intervention, 'best tackled by doctors with the relevant specialised training expertise and back up' (Department of Health 1991). This point of view is repeated in the 1999 Guidelines, which state that individuals prescribing injectable formulations should have appropriate training and experience (Department of Health 1999). There is not currently a specific curriculum for such training; trainee specialists (usually psychiatrists) who have a placement with an individual who prescribes injectable maintenance have access to training, but those who do not have this opportunity will not have such training.

Injectable methadone prescribing is a significant activity in the private sector. Of the methadone prescribed in private practice, 30% is the injectable form, compared with 9% of that prescribed in NHS practice (Strang *et al*.1996).

The studies

A number of studies which include patients on injectable methadone have been reported from clinics in the UK. These reports contain valuable information about the patients for whom this treatment has been provided and the clinics' treatment aims or philosophy. Some studies are of patients already in treatment, while others are of services set up or altered for the purpose of the study. Table 10.1 shows some characteristics of these patients, their treatment history and treatment in the study. Medication may be dispensed with a range of frequencies, and this information is included in the table. Unless otherwise stated, medication is dispensed from a hospital or community pharmacy and is consumed elsewhere.

An early report of injectable opiate treatment was a descriptive study of 40 opiate-dependent patients at the drug dependence clinic at the Maudsley

Table 10.1 UK studies of injectable methadone: patient characteristics, study selection criteria, treatment aims and study treatment.

Study	Age (yrs)	Gender	Length of opiate history	Selection criteria	Aim of treatment	Assessment methods	Dose	Pick-up (days/week)
Battersby et al. 1992 n = 40	Mean 35.4 Range 24–60	Female n = 13 32.5%	15.7 (4–43) Mean length of opiate use	Request injectables Previous injectables Long injecting history No abstinence Needle fixation Chaotic poly-drug use Physical complications	Engagement in treatment Transition to stop injecting and drug use Harm reduction and health promotion	2–3 interviews Physical examination Urine test Test dose	70.25 mg Mean, methadone equivalent Oral+inj methadone 31 Inj heroin 4 Inj methadone 4	
Metrebian et al. 1998 n = 58	38 yrs median (24–29)	Female n = 16 28%	19.5 yrs median (4–30) injecting heroin	Age at least 21 Opiate-dependent Unable/unwilling to stop injecting Previous treatment at least 80 mg oral methadone Drug-related problems	Reduce illicit drug use Reduce HIV-risk behaviour Improve physical and psychological function Transition to oral methadone and abstinence	Tolerance testing Opiate treatment Index (OTI)	21 (36%) methadone 148.18 mg/day (SD45.1, 100–200) 37 (64%) heroin, dose 181.43 mg/day (SD22.2, 120–200)	Five initially, then at least 1
Ford C, Ryrie I 1999 n = 35	35 yrs mean (27–54)	Female n = 15 42.9%	16 yrs mean Opiate use	Previous limited success of oral/detoxification Serious health/social problem unwillingness of specialist services to prescribe; 'insufficient' prescribing Advocacy by non-stat. agency	Harm reduction; physical, crime, social Cessation injecting ultimately	Questionnaire & semi-structured interview Urine test 23/35 (65.7%)	124 mg mean (50–250)	6 n = 15 2–5 n = 12 1 n = 5
Strang et al. 2000 n = 40	32.0 mean	Female n = 3 7.9%		Aged at least 23-yrs Illicit injecting for the last 3-yrs At least one previous opiate substitution treatment Venous access on arms No current serious physical psychiatric co-morbidity Not pregnant	Determine acceptability and clinical feasibility of supervised on-site injectable MMT Assess retention of patients and treatment outcomes over first six months of treatment	Physical examination Urinalysis Maudsley Addiction Profile (MAP)	96.9 mg mean injectable methadone 79.6 mg mean oral methadone	5
Sell L, Segar G, Merrill J. 2001 n = 125	36.0 mean (21–49)	Female n = 22 17.6%	16.5 yrs mean (4–30) opiate using	Committed injector Lack of benefit of oral methadone Able to engage in treatment	Manage patients referred by other teams Improve individual treatment outcome Harm minimization	Interview Urinalysis	88 mg mean inj methadone, n = 107 216 mg mean inj diamorphine n = 16	6 n = 34 5 n = 5 3 n = 39 2 n = 17 1 n = 32

hospital in London (Battersby *et al.* 1992). Patients were managed using individual treatment contracts. Metrebian *et al.* (1998) published a pilot study into the feasibility of prescribing injectable heroin and methadone to opiate-dependent drug users. The study was conducted at a West London drug treatment clinic which already offered injectable prescriptions. Ford and Ryrie (1999) reported on the provision of injectable methadone in three London general practices. This study described the cohort of patients currently in treatment and included information about patients' perceptions of treatment. A randomized trial (feasibility study) of supervised injectable versus oral methadone maintenance was carried out at the Maudsley Hospital in South-East London (Strang *et al.* 2000). Patients were randomized to oral or injectable treatment. This study required patients to take their methadone in a supervised setting with two staff members who prepared the injection and helped the patient to find a suitable site. If a patient was unable to inject intravenously, they did so intramuscularly or took an oral dose. We have reported (Sell *et al.* 2001) on 125 patients treated with injectable opiate maintenance at a regional clinic which takes referrals from Greater Manchester and Lancashire in North West England. These patients had been referred by community drug teams following lack of progress with other forms of treatment, or had been referred having had injectable treatment elsewhere.

The characteristics of opiate-dependent patients who have been treated with injectable methadone maintenance (shown in Table 10.1) reveal these patients to be older and to have long injecting histories. In our clinic, patients have typically started to inject opiates in their late teens; most had first used heroin by injection, although many had injected amphetamine before heroin. Their mean and median ages show them to be considerably older than patients entering treatment in the National Treatment Outcome Research Study (NTORS) where the average age was 29, range 16 to 50 (Gossop *et al.* 1998). The mean or median duration of heroin/opiate use reported by the patients in these studies varied from 15.7 years to 19.5 years, all considerably longer than that reported by the patients presenting to services in the NTORS, who had an average opiate using history of 8.8 years.

There is no consistent proportion of female patients in the studies reported. The selection criteria include an indication that patients are likely to remain dependent and continue injecting in the absence of injectable treatment, that they should have tried alternative treatments and that they should have problems as a result of injecting. Interestingly, the selection criteria also make reference to the influence of other treatment services; some patients in the Battersby *et al.* (1992) trial had previously been prescribed injectables by another service, while the Ford and Ryrie (1999) study makes reference to treating patients who had *not* been offered injectable treatment by another service. The studies reported varying aims, including aims for individual patient outcomes and aims to be achieved at a population level. Of interest is the intended use of an injectable drug to help a person to stop injecting. In theory a prescription for an injectable drug can be planned as a transition to oral treatment en route to abstinence. Treatment regimens often include both oral and injectable methadone with this in mind. The transition rarely happens quickly and this is discussed further below. Assessment methods seek to confirm the history of opiate dependence and injecting. Mean methadone doses vary, ranging from 70.25 mg to 148 mg daily. Medication is usually dispensed at frequent intervals and in the Strang *et al.* (2000) study was provided on site with supervision. In the other studies, community pharmacy dispensing occurred as infrequently as once weekly, with the highest frequency at once daily except Sunday. In the 1995 pharmacy survey of community pharmacies, methadone was being prescribed for dispensing at the following frequencies: 5–7 times weekly, 35.7%; 2–4 times weekly, 33.6%, once weekly or less, 30.6% (Strang *et al.* 1996).

Minimizing the harm from injecting – how far do we go?

Physical problems resulting from injecting drug use may be a pertinent reason to consider prescribing injectable substitutes. The risky activity which one hopes to reduce by prescribing injectable opiates is illustrated by the fact that in our clinic, 113 out of 121 patients studied, or 90.4%, had previously crushed tablets for injection; only 13 out of 121 or 10.7% had done so in the past month. Events during treatment reported by Battersby (1992) include osteomyelitis of the cervical spine, injecting methadone linctus into the femoral vein and using the inguinal area to inject prescribed injectable methadone. Physical complications occurring during treatment can present a dilemma. Doctors who prescribe injectable methadone as a harm minimization strategy need to decide where the limit is drawn, beyond which, whatever the problem arising from injecting drug use, the patient must find a solution which does not involve injectable prescribing. Few doctors would want to continue prescribing injectable methadone for a patient who had had a deep vein thrombosis while injecting prescribed drugs, but the risk of further medical problems may remain higher without the prescribed drug than with it.

The question of where patients inject can be an even thornier issue. Venous access and current practice by patients in treatment at our unit are described in Table 10.2. Many doctors require patients who are receiving injectable methadone to be able to inject the drug into an arm vein, and indeed to do so. However, many patients who are long-term injectors and therefore suitable for treatment no longer have patent arm veins. Other doctors find the practice of patients injecting their prescribed methadone into their femoral vein acceptable. Few, if any, would knowingly prescribe to a person who was injecting in their neck veins. Practitioners draw the line as to what is acceptable harm minimization in different places.

Table 10.2 Venous access and injecting sites used in patients at Drugs North West (*n* = 121).

Site	Remains patent	Used in past month
Intravenous – arms	59 (48.8%)	33 (27.5%)
Intravenous – hands	59 (48.8%)	26 (21.5%)
Intravenous – legs	83 (68.6%)	26 (21.5%)
Intravenous – femoral	112 (92.6%)	49 (40.5%)
Intramuscular	N/A	12 (9.9%)

Clinical indications

Although injectable methadone has been prescribed in England and Wales for decades, evidence of effectiveness is only now being tested. Clinical indications are arrived at as a result of applying harm minimization principles and also by individual assessment and monitoring. Some clinicians reach the conclusion that injectable methadone (or other injectable opiates) should not be used. However, for those who reach the conclusion that injectable methadone does have a role in the management of injecting opiate dependence, Sarfraz and Alcorn (1999) have suggested helpful clinical guidance, including patient eligibility criteria (see box).

Clinical guidance suggested by Sarfraz and Alcorn (1999)

(1) Objective evidence of:
   • opiate dependence
   • injecting for several years
   • current intravenous opiate use.
(2) Previous unsuccessful treatment including detoxification, oral methadone maintenance or residential rehabilitation. Most clinicians would require previous unsuccessful treatment with oral methadone at adequate dosage.
(3) Unwillingness or inability to stop injecting.
(4) No evidence of severe mental health problems (affective disorder, psychotic illness, cognitive impairment) which may reduce compliance or increase risk to self or others.
(5) No use of alcohol or other psychoactive drugs in amounts that would severely affect physical or cognitive state.
(6) No medical contra-indications to intravenous administration including anti-coagulant treatment, deep vein thrombosis, subacute bacterial endocarditis, pregnancy.
(7) Demonstrated ability to co-operate with the service including reliable attendance, examination, and urinalysis.

In addition, the patient's assessment should identify problems that are likely to be resolved if injecting and illicit use cease, and include a method of measuring progress. Treatment with injectable methadone will usually be stopped if there are medical complications, although this can be a difficult decision as discussed above. Further situations in which injectable treatment will stop include poor compliance, evidence that the medication is being diverted, the obtaining of supplies from another prescriber, and violent or illicit activity on clinic premises.

Treatment – for how long?

Treatment with methadone ampoules is very rarely a short-term treatment option. Patients may often present requesting the ampoules as a transitional measure and this approach can be attractive to clinicians. However, in practice once patients have commenced methadone ampoules, and especially if they significantly reduce their illicit drug use or make other progress, it becomes difficult to change the treatment. In our clinic, with a mean current age of 36 years, our patients had first been prescribed injectable methadone at a mean age of 29.5 years. The mean length of the current treatment episode was 3.5 years with a range from 3 months to 14 years. Some patients had first been prescribed injectable opiates elsewhere, while others had had treatment breaks for a number of reasons. Figure 10.1 shows the time since injectable treatment was initiated. Of those whose treatment was initiated 5 years ago or less, 9 were initiated 1 year ago, 11 were initiated 2 years ago, 15 were initiated 3 years ago, 12 were initiated 4 years ago and 8 were initiated 5 years ago. Only 24 patients (20%) had voluntarily reverted back to oral methadone they were first started on injectable treatment (Sell *et al.* 2001). Where relapse occurs during the treatment

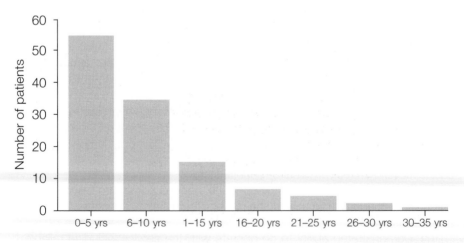

Figure 10.1 Time from initiation of injectable prescription to the present in Drugs North West 1997 cohort.

planning stage when the intention to limit the duration of treatment is stated, the treatment plan is renegotiated, often resulting in long-term treatment. It is important for both patients and treatment providers to be aware of this.

There are several ways of considering the tendency for treatment with injectable methadone to be long-term treatment. It reflects the practice of pre-scribing oral methadone on a maintenance, and therefore long-term, basis, which is an effective practice (Farrell *et al.* 1994). Maintenance treatment in the context of injectable treatment allows the patient to decide when to change from injectable treatment, according to constraints that vary from clinic to clinic. Patients are often very reluctant to consider a change from injectable to oral methadone. Those who are not doing particularly well value their methadone ampoules as part of their ongoing drug use. Those who have stopped using illicit heroin become very fearful of the consequences of relapse. Patients and clinicians can be wary of risking newly found 'stability'. Achieving an injectable prescription can take much of the urgency out of a patient's motivation to change. With many of the immediate day-to-day prob-lems of injectable drug procurement removed, making further change is often put on hold. Patients may find it less pressing to take action to avert longer term and less obvious consequences of continued injecting. For example, once a person no longer experiences abscesses as a result of injecting street heroin, the long-term risk of venous thrombosis may not concern them enough to motivate further change. The provision of a legal and sterile injectable drug may become part of a stable and socially productive lifestyle. Change may not be precipitated until there is a further event. Retention in treatment is clearly a benefit, given the evidence that this is an important mediating factor in achieving a good outcome in opiate-dependence treat-ment. Clinicians need to be aware that, for this patient group, transition to oral methadone without relapse to injecting street opiates happens slowly if at all.

There are situations in which the prescriber needs to make a unilateral decision that injectable methadone treatment will stop on safety grounds. However, when the decision is made in collaboration with the patient, there are options other than a simple switch. Many patients are treated with a combination of oral and injectable methadone and the proportions of these can gradually shift in favour of oral methadone. This can be done on each day; alternatively the number of days each week on which a patient receives injectable methadone can gradually be reduced. Some patients request detoxification from injectable methadone, either as an inpatient or as an out-patient. However, it is usually advisable to make the transition to oral treatment before attempting to become opiate free.

Injectable methadone or diamorphine?

Just as there is no evidence about the effectiveness of injectable opiate pre-scribing per se, there is no evidence of any difference in effectiveness between injectable methadone and injectable diamorphine. It may be argued that if one is going to prescribe an injectable drug then one may as well prescribe heroin, the drug which has actually been used and which is likely to remain the drug of choice. Patients may continue to desire the specific euphoric effects of heroin. This may limit the effectiveness of treatment as people continue to use street heroin, or may result in chronic dissatisfaction and tension between the patient and doctor. Patients report that injectable diamorphine is easier to inject, being reconstituted from dry powder into a small volume which is not irritating, while many report venous irritation and scarring when using methadone ampoules. This issue is worthy of further study. Methadone needs to be injected once daily and a patient is likely to achieve more effective suppression of withdrawal symptoms than would occur with short-acting drug alone. Once-daily administration reduces the intrusive effect of frequently repeated drug administration on a person's lifestyle. Some patients specifically prefer the effect of methadone. For service providers and purchasers it cannot go unnoticed that injectable methadone is typically four times less expensive in terms of drug costs than injectable diamorphine (Brewer 1995). When patients are prescribed injectable methadone it remains possible to monitor their use of street heroin with standard laboratory or bench-top analysis of urine. Some laboratories are able to differentiate between licit and illicit origins of heroin, but this is not universal. It may be that injectable methadone is prescribed in part precisely because it is not heroin. Policy makers and doctors may reject the notion of simply replacing a drug of abuse with 'like for like', but do not experience the same taboo about methadone.

Patient opinion

Patient opinion about injectable methadone has been expressed in strong terms. The prescription of injectable methadone in England and Wales varies from region to region, resulting in different expectations of prescribing for opiate dependence. In the study by Metrebian et al. (1998), patients who were eligible chose treatment with injectable diamorphine or injectable methadone; 21 out of 58 (36%) chose the latter. In our study we asked patients whether, given the choice they would continue on their current treatment or prefer an alternative. None of those on injectable diamorphine wished for an alternative, but 48 out of 107 (44.9%) who were prescribed injectable methadone wished for an alternative, usually diamorphine (Sell et al. 2001). Reasons advanced by our patients about why they would choose methadone ampoules include the fact that since methadone is long acting, it is only necessary to inject once daily. Many report that it has allowed them to resume a socially productive life, be it work, study or family. Conversely, those who dislike it often report that it is difficult to inject; the volume may be too large or the injection painful if the formulation is more concentrated.

Many indicate a strong preference for the euphoric effects of heroin.

Leigh and Leigh (2000) have commented on the use of methadone ampoules. They have expressed concern about the use of methadone ampoules outside the terms of their product data sheet and have described first-hand accounts of non-healing skin lesions arising as a result of methadone ampoules. They advance the opinion that patients should be better informed about possible side effects of methadone ampoules. The case for injectable diamorphine is advanced, but it is also suggested that when methadone ampoules are used, the dose should be higher.

Conclusions

Prescribing injectable methadone is a small but significant part of the UK response to opiate dependence. It was part of the treatment developed at the new NHS clinics set up in the late 1960s, and more recently has found a place within harm minimization philosophy. The clinical practicalities of prescribing injectable methadone emphasize the dilemmas inherent in opiate replacement therapy. Resolving the individual risk benefit analysis for each patient is crucial in deciding on treatment. This balance may change over time, and long-term management decisions can become more difficult. The potential for long-term injection-related damage, despite treatment, should be born in mind. There is a substantial body of clinical experience with this form of treatment and helpful suggested guidelines. Whether offering this treatment does indeed improve patient outcome remains an unanswered question, although welcome research is beginning in this area. A robust answer to the question needs to consider whether the provision of treatments that are readily accepted by patients may in fact prolong drug using over the life span and increase harm overall. Prospective audit and research into the extent of injection-related harm during treatment is also warranted given the long-term nature of treatment. Provision of injectable methadone is patchy; the question remains whether it should be a routinely available option or whether its demise is indicated.

References

Battersby, M., Farrell, M., Gossop, M., Robson, P. & Strang, J. (1992) 'Horse trading': prescribing injectable opiates to opiate addicts, a descriptive study. *Drug and Alcohol Review*, 11: 35–42.

Brewer, C. (1995) Recent developments in maintenance prescribing and monitoring in the United Kingdom. *Bulletin of the New York Academy of Medicine*, 72: 359–70.

Department of Health (1999) *Drug Misuse and Dependence – Guidelines on Clinical Management*. London: HMSO.

Department of Health, Scottish Office Home and Health Department Welsh Office (1991) *Drug Misuse and Dependence – Guidelines on Clinical Management*. London: HMSO.

Farrell, M., Ward, J. & Mattick, R. (1994) Methadone maintenance treatment in opiate dependence: a review. *British Medical Journal*, 309: 997–1001.

Ford, C. & Ryrie, I. (1999) Prescribing injectable methadone in general practice. *International Journal Of Drug Policy*, 10: 39–45.

Gossop, M., Marsden, J. & Stewart, D. (1998) Substance use, health and social problems of service users at 54 drug treatment agencies. Intake data from the National Treatment Outcome Research Study. *British Journal of Psychiatry*, 173: 166–71.

Leigh, J. & Leigh, J. (2000) Never mind the heroin, it's meth amps that screw you up. *Monkey,* 2: 4–5.

Metrebian, N., Shanahan, B., Wells, B. & Stimson, G. (1998) Feasibility of prescribing injectable heroin and methadone to opiate-dependent drug users: associated health gains and harm reductions. *The Medical Journal of Australia*, 168: 596–600.

Mitcheson, M. (1994) Drug clinics in the 1970s, In: Strang J, Gossop M, eds. *Heroin Addiction and Drug Policy, The British System.* London: Oxford University Press.

Sarfraz, A. & Alcorn R. J. (1999) Injectable methadone prescribing in the United Kingdom – current practice and future policy guidelines. *Substance Use and Misuse*, 34: 1709–21.

Sell, L. A., Segar, G. & Merrill, J. (2001) One hundred and twenty-five patients prescribed injectable opiates in the North-West of England. *Drug and Alcohol Review*, 20: 57–66.

Strang, J. (1992) Harm reduction for drug misusers: exploring the dimensions of harm, their measurement, and strategies for reductions. *AIDS and Public Policy Journal,* 7: 145–52.

Strang, J., Marsden, J., Cummins, M., Farrell, M., Finch, E., Gossop, M., Stewart, D. & Welch, S. (2000) Supervised injectable versus oral methadone maintenance treatment for opiate addiction: randomised trial and six-month outcome data. *Addiction*, 95: 1631–45.

Strang, J., Sheridan, J. & Barber, N. (1996) Prescribing injectable and oral methadone to opiate addicts: results from the 1995 National Postal Survey of Community Pharmacies in England and Wales. *British Medical Journal*, 313: 270–2.

Zador, D. (2001) Injectable opiate maintenance in the UK – is it good clinical practice? *Addiction,* 96: 547–53.

11

The supervised injecting clinic – a drug clinic's experience of supervising the intravenous self-administration of prescribed injectable methadone

Mike Cummins

Background

Providing injectable medication as a treatment for opiate addiction has long been a subject of heated debate (Strang 1990), with clinical opinion divided as to whether doing so is an effective harm reduction intervention or is alternatively contributing to injecting drug users' injecting-related damage. Some clients claim that they could stop using illicit heroin if they were prescribed 'injectables', an argument that would seem to have been taken on board by NHS prescribers in Britain. Currently 9% of methadone prescriptions are in injectable formulation (ampoules), but there is, as yet, no clear evidence to suggest improved outcomes where injectable methadone is prescribed (Strang *et al.* 1996). There is an acknowledgement that there may be a small section of the treatment population who may benefit from an injectable prescription (Department of Health 1999), although research is required to examine the role and efficacy of injectable opioid prescribing and to develop criteria to indicate for whom such prescribing might be appropriate (Department of Health 1998).

If providing injectable medication has been a divisive issue, the topic of providing a place for users to inject is even more so. Nevertheless, it is a consideration currently being explored by the European Monitoring Centre for Drugs and Drug Addiction. Users' rooms provide an environment in which drugs can be consumed under hygienic and supervised conditions, thus reducing the transmission of infectious diseases and the risk of fatal overdose (European Monitoring Centre For Drugs and Drug Addiction 2000), and are being actively considered in at least five European countries. The UK Department of Health guidelines on the clinical management of drug misuse and dependence recommend that the means should exist to supervise and monitor, in a clinical setting, the administration of the drug in the early stages of treatment, and at later stages where concern over clinical progress arises (Department of Health 1999), but few such facilities exist in the UK and there is no official guidance on how they should operate.

A supervised self-administration intravenous injection clinic was established at the Maudsley in South London in 1996 as a clinical response to a perceived need and also to facilitate a randomized trial of supervised injectable versus oral methadone maintenance; the aim of the trial was to assess the feasibility and effectiveness of supervised substitution treatment using injectable methadone for intravenous opiate addicts. The purpose of this chapter is to describe some of our experiences in running this clinic and outline some of the clinical anxieties we have encountered during the operation of the service. These will be discussed as 'organizational procedures' and 'treatment issues'. The formal results of the study have been published separately (Strang *et al*. 2000) and will only be included in support of the description.

Organizational procedures

A senior psychiatric nurse (the author) was recruited specifically to manage the clinic. In recruiting to this position, understanding of the nature and importance of the proposed study was paramount, as was the ability to facilitate the clinical research work. Overall responsibility for the clinic was held by a senior consultant psychiatrist to whom the senior nurse was accountable. To meet drug administration regulations, two nurses were required to be present during opening times. The pre-existing methadone maintenance clinic provided this additional nursing cover whenever required. Administrative and pharmacy support was drawn from existing resources.

It was necessary to secure appropriate long-term accommodation, suitably modified to meet local infection control policies, equipped with cupboards approved for the secure storage of controlled medicines and for the storage of injecting equipment. The pharmacy department had to expand its controlled drug storage facilities. There are cost implications for providing medication in ampoules rather than oral form, additional costs for the injecting equipment, the safe disposal of needles, syringes and clinical waste and the increased staff time compared with the oral methadone supervision facility. When taken together, the increased cost of a supervised methadone injecting service was more than 3.5 times more expensive than its oral counterpart.

There were additional staff training costs: in discussions leading up to the opening of the clinic, staff expressed a range of anxieties and concerns about participating. The need to ensure safer injecting practices, while not entirely condoning this method of use, was seen as a challenge, as was the possible contribution to injecting-related harms, which the staff might witness. Supervising clients whose only venous access was the neck or groin or private part of the body was a concern, as was the possibility that supervised clients may have difficulty finding a vein; how long should the client be able to try, and what sort of injecting techniques were going to be deemed unacceptable? Safety with regard to blood-borne viral infection risk, increased overdose potential and ensuring that the staff involved were equipped with the knowledge and skills to deal with these were major concerns because injecting drug use is by far the most hazardous way of introducing drugs into the body (Strang *et al.* 1998). The local infection control nurse gave advice on specific issues, and local infection control guidelines were developed. All staff routinely receive cardiopulmonary resuscitation (CPR) training and our overdose protocol was amended to include guidelines for the administration of naloxone by nursing staff in the absence of a medical practitioner.

External training in intravenous cannulation and close supervision by senior nursing staff enabled the staff to gain the skills and knowledge to participate in the clinic. As the staff have became more familiar with the clinic and their role within it, anxiety decreased. Additional literature, especially *The Safer Injecting Briefing* (a comprehensive manual specifically aimed at promoting safer injecting) (Derricott *et al.* 1999) became available and was perceived to have immense value as an information resource.

Thought was given to the environment of the clinic: what should it feel like? How should it look? 'Environmental cues acquire the ability to elicit conditioned responses through the pairing of the cues with the pharmacological effects of the drug. These conditioned responses serve to increase the motivation for use of the drug' (Siegel 1999). It was decided that a very clinical feel would reinforce the fact that this was a treatment intervention rather than a 'shooting gallery' and help to disrupt some of the conditioned responses that may be present for some clients who have developed regular patterns or rituals when injecting. We chose one of our examination rooms, which had a hospital atmosphere. The room contained a sink for hand washing and for raising veins by soaking the injecting site in warm water. A large radiator was available for the purpose of ensuring room temperatures that would also assist with venous access, and a hand exerciser was provided to promote circulation and help in the task of finding veins. A free-standing lamp was provided to make it easier to find injecting sites. The furniture was easily washable.

Recruitment and selection to the research trial

We had concerns that the injectable treatment option could become a victim of its own popularity and that clients may be attracted to treatment for injectables alone and could drop out, if randomized to the oral arm of the study. To reduce the opportunity for this to occur we chose to limit recruitment to those clients who were presenting for routine treatment.

Clients were recruited to the trial by selection from initial referral data in line with the criteria listed below. Clients who met the entry criteria were informed about the trial and, if interested in participating, were offered a further appointment designed to gather further information on injecting practices and impart information on the limits of the service (for example, a limit was imposed on the number of attempts to gain venous access and the time available to do so). Suitability for this treatment option was determined by injecting-related criteria. We wanted to ensure that we were not increasing or encouraging injecting behaviour, so only clients who reported injecting on most days and for longer than three years were considered. Though willing to advise on the safest way to inject in any site a client is using, we were only willing to supervise intravenous injecting in the arms. The practical constraints on the time available to supervise injecting mean that clients need to achieve their injection quite quickly. Clients considered for the study identified being able to inject within ten minutes, in five attempts or less, in their arms. Even in a clinically clean environment and with advice available to improve injecting technique, there exists the potential for injecting-related damage and health risks. Given also that methadone ampoules are not specifically licensed for intravenous use, we felt it was important to reiterate these dangers to ensure that we obtained true informed consent. Those clients who were eligible and who remained willing to be involved in the study underwent a routine physical and psychological assessment by the medical consultant. Methadone doses were assessed over 3 days with oral methadone to find their optimal dose, after which they were randomized to either the oral or intravenous treatment option.

Criteria for consideration for supervised injectable methadone clinic

(1) >21 years old
(2) three-year history of injecting
(3) currently injecting => 4 days per week
(4) able to access veins in arms (fingertip to shoulder)
(5) regularly able to self-inject in 10 minutes or five attempts, whichever comes first
(6) is not pregnant
(7) has no severe physical or mental health problems, including alcohol problems
(8) is able and willing to give consent

The recruitment period lasted 18 months, during which time 331 clients were assessed against the selection criteria. One hundred and ten clients met the minimum criteria and were offered a follow-up assessment; 48% did not attend. Twelve per cent were assessed as inappropriate and 4% declined to participate. Of the 40 clients accepted into the study, 23 were randomized to the supervised, self-administered injectable treatment option, with the remainder being offered the usual supervised, oral methadone maintenance treatment in another part of the same building.

A large number of clients originally thought to be eligible were unable to meet the selection criteria: 66% of the total clients seeking treatment (221 of 331) described having no venous access left in their arms, though many of these clients were still injecting in their legs or groin. The 48% non-attendance rate for follow-up assessments, though undesirable, is comparable to that of the usual methadone maintenance treatment pathway at that time.

Assessment

The assessment process includes determining the appropriate (most tolerable) concentration of methadone ampoules for each client. Methadone is known to be an irritant to veins in high concentrations and is not licensed for intravenous use. Methadone ampoules are available in a variety of concentrations, the weaker the concentration the less irritating to the veins but the greater the volume, thus making injecting difficult for those who find the larger syringes cumbersome. Determining the initial concentrations to use can seem arbitrary if the client has no prior experience to guide them and can require 'fine-tuning' following client feedback. We often use a combination of concentrations based on each client's individual tolerance and preference.

After the initial assessment, interventions include identifying the best veins available for injecting, by assessing the position, how it feels to the touch, general health of different sites and associated risk factors. Harm reduction issues are discussed in the client's individual appointments outside of the supervised injecting times; a variety of media including information posters and leaflets, photographic slides of injecting-related damage and the opportunity to practise using an intravenous training arm are available.

At its busiest, the clinic has supervised 23 clients during two 2 hour sessions each day although this capacity was probably greater than could be competently managed. As the number of clients receiving this treatment steadily declined, staffing the clinic was creating pressure on oral methadone treatment resources. Once staff had built up confidence in this treatment and clients began to manage take-home ampoules with no perceptible detriment, clinic times were reduced to one 1 hour session on three days. In order to disrupt the conditioned response that may be aroused, the responsibility for drawing up the prescribed dose rested with the staff who were also required to supervise the self injection of the methadone, while recording the number of attempts and the injection site.

Treatment and supervision

Many clients express anxiety about injecting in front of the nursing staff who are still strangers to them at this point; they are also worried about injecting in such a clinical environment. To alleviate this, the first week or two of supervised injecting treatment is used for unobtrusive observation, with minimal input from the nurses. This period helps the clients to relax in the clinic and provides an opportunity to observe the clients' existing injecting technique, knowledge and competence. The exception to this approach is when a client's injecting behaviour causes a 'blood risk' to themselves or others; in this case one of the staff will intervene immediately.

Once a client has settled in, the staff would begin actively addressing issues that arose from the initial observation period. Some of the more common initial health promotion and harm reduction interventions include basic hand washing and personal hygiene education. Using gauze and plasters to stem bleeding and making the area safe for the next client is often the first behaviour to be addressed. Encouraging the rotation of injecting sites and education about the health risks from bad habits (such as licking needles, or wiping them on clothing prior to injecting) are also early interventions. All clients are given their own individual tourniquet for use in the clinic and another to take home. Supplies of syringes and a range of needle sizes are given to the clients as well as sharps containers. In addition, alcohol wipes, gauze swabs and plasters are given to the clients on request and these have proved popular.

No matter how skilfully done, injecting is an invasive procedure that causes damage and increases health risks. Injecting-related damage is monitored in a variety of ways. A pictorial record is kept, showing where access is attempted and which sites are successfully used. This information is used to track the rotation of injecting sites. Despite consistent advice on the benefits of regularly rotating sites, many of our clients choose to use a vein until it stops working and then move on to another. We monitor specific injecting-related damage at two monthly intervals using a simple four-point severity rating scale. Relying on subjective observation of injecting damage, the assessments are completed by the same member of staff to provide a consistent rating of 'none', 'minor', 'moderate' or 'severe' damage.

Observable injecting-related damage (abscesses, bruising, swelling, infection) was reduced for all of the clients, but venous access has continued to deteriorate regardless of the prompting of many clients to choose alternative routes of administration. Indeed, of the 11 study clients still in treatment at the time of writing, five clients have oral methadone only, four clients have a combination of intravenous or intramuscular and oral methadone. The remaining two clients receive all of their medication in injectable form. The option to 'mix and match' formulations this way is available to clients from the beginning of treatment. Clients are actively encouraged to experiment with alternatives to intravenous administration but the decision to do so remains theirs where possible. On very rare occasions, a clinical decision to change to intramuscular or oral methadone has superseded client choice for injecting-related health reasons or due to chronically poor venous access.

Some clients requested to draw up their own medication or to have more time to enjoy the effect of their injection after it had been accomplished, complaining that the environment was uncomfortable and 'spoilt the effect'. Others created new rituals around the preparation of their gauze swabs and plasters. A few of the clients began drawing out their injection with repeated, slow, deliberate flushing (drawing up blood and reintroducing it to the vein), long after the methadone had been infused. The ritual of preparing the plasters is something that we may have contributed to, having actively encouraged clients to organize themselves and their equipment to promote hygiene and minimize 'blood risk' behaviours. 'Flushing' was actively discouraged on the grounds that, though a correct technique to ensure the needle is still correctly in situ during the injection, it was both unnecessary once the injection was complete and increased the risk of infection.

Supervised intravenous treatment offers the opportunity to observe the immediate effect of the medication and, consequently, the client's level of tolerance. Oral methadone can take several hours to reach a peak effect, by which time our clients have long since left the premises; in stark contrast, injectable methadone has an immediate effect. Supervised intravenous treatment gives us the opportunity to observe the immediate effect of the medication and the client's level of tolerance. Following the injection, the majority of our clients described experiencing a metallic taste at the back of their throat, but otherwise there were no readily identifiable changes from our visual observations. There were exceptions to this on three occasions when a client became drowsy, heavy lidded and confused. We did not need to administer naloxone and oxygen, or use other emergency services on these occasions, but a registered nurse and medical staff monitored these clients' vital signs closely until the effect had reduced to a degree considered safe. This time varied from 20 minutes to three hours. On each of these occasions, the clients attributed their intoxication to illicit use of sedative drugs prior to attending the clinic, rather than due to being given too large a dose of their prescribed medication. This seemed consistent with the fact that they had been tolerant to the same dose of intravenous methadone a number of times previously (and since) and was later additionally supported by urine drug screening which returned a positive result for the illicit drugs described by the client. These occasions provided an opportunity to remind the clients of the increased danger of overdose from the potentiating interactions that can occur between separate drugs and also raised questions about the clients who were on oral methadone. As most clients on oral methadone leave the clinic within minutes of having their methadone, what unobserved interactions may be occurring after they have left the premises?

Client feedback

A patient satisfaction survey of the two treatment groups found that the clients who received supervised injectable methadone had significantly higher satisfaction ratings with the operation of the clinic than those on oral methadone maintenance (Strang *et al.* 2000). This included their ratings of treatment decisions, their overall perception of treatment, counselling sessions, time in treatment and the drug clinic's rules and regulations. However, despite this observation, a less reassuring picture emerged from a focus group for the injecting group clients, held one year into treatment. This elicited a range of areas of dissatisfaction. Foremost of these was frustration at the short period of time allowed for injecting and many expressed the view that the limit of only five attempts was harsh and unrealistic.

Another major theme that emerged was about the emotional discomfort experienced at having their injecting supervised; the general feeling was that it was an anxiety-provoking experience. One client stated that his injecting was an intimate process and went so far as to say that injecting under supervision was 'like someone watching you having a shit'. In addition, the criteria of a time limit, a maximum number of attempts and the constant 'nagging' about technique caused some clients to feel under enormous pressure to perform well, with an acute blow to self-esteem if unable to find a vein. Many described injecting as being important enough that they would use illicit heroin on the days when they had been unable to inject prescribed methadone in the clinic. This was attributed to feeling 'cheated' in some way, or due to a lack of faith in the ability of oral methadone to keep them comfortable until the following day. The clients described being very sensitive to changes in the staff facilitating the clinic, being able to relax more when being supervised by a smaller range of more regular staff and experiencing difficulty in front of 'new faces'. Whilst acknowledging that the supervised injecting clinic had been of some benefit, most clients identified that they would still sooner be given their ampoules to take away and that attending a drug clinic, which other drug users frequented, on a daily basis was an additional obstacle to achieving their treatment goals. Some clients believed that the methadone ampoules had contributed to the collapse of their veins due to its alleged irritant nature and they felt that diamorphine would be a better option. Others felt that they were experiencing fewer injecting-related problems than they had been experiencing with illicit heroin.

Conclusion

Drug misusers need careful advice on the health hazards associated with injecting. For those already injecting, the advice about not sharing any injecting equipment or any of the paraphernalia associated with injecting needs to be reinforced (Department of Health 1997).

A supervised injecting clinic offers a unique opportunity to observe clients' injecting technique and to engage them in harm reduction and health promotion interventions. Prior to this clinic, it may have been presumed that these clients would be 'expert' injectors, especially as the criteria for being considered for this clinic required at least a three-year history of injecting. The discovery that this was not the case should serve as an important reminder that we cannot afford to make assumptions about a client's knowledge or skill about injecting risk behaviours, even if there have been many previous episodes of treatment. Another important point to be recognized is that harm reduction is not harm cessation and that even with intensive staff time being spent advising on and monitoring injecting technique, venous access has continued to deteriorate for all of our clients.

The overall conclusion from our recent experience with this new clinic has been one of increasing confidence in the legitimacy of this treatment option, and that for some at the severe end of the spectrum, it has been able to contribute to positive treatment outcomes in a way that might not have been achievable with oral methadone maintenance treatment. However, the greater operational costs will probably prevent it from being widely provided. Furthermore, if our experience of deteriorating access is predictive for others, then intravenous methadone maintenance may not be a sustainable long-term option, even for many of those clients for whom it initially seemed appropriate. Though many of our clients have subsequently moved from intravenous injecting to oral or intramuscular routes, this has been due to their deteriorating access as often as it has been due to the achievement of planned changes in their desire to continue injecting.

It may be difficult for some organizations with long waiting lists for treatment to justify the additional resource implications, even if a limited supervised injecting service is a valid option for those clients who have a known history of poor outcomes with oral methadone treatment. Identifying those who would do well remains an elusive art that requires further study. In the meantime it will be necessary to rely on shrewd initial clinical judgement and careful individual outcome monitoring to ensure that the injectable maintenance treatment is indeed significantly contributing to the desired changes in behaviours.

References

Department of Health (1999) *Drug Misuse and Dependence – Guidelines on Clinical Management.* London: The Stationery Office.

Department of Health (1998) *Drug Misuse Research Initiative.* London: Department of Health.

Department of Health (1997) *Purchasing Effective Treatment and Care for Drug Misusers, Guidance for Health Authorities and Social Services Departments.* London: Department of Health.

Derricott, J., Preston, A.. & Hunt, N. (1999) *The Safer Injecting Briefing.* Liverpool: HIT.

European Monitoring Centre for Drugs and Drug Addiction (2000) *Annual Report on the State of the Drugs Problem in the European Union.* Luxembourg Office for the Official Publications of the European Communities.

Siegel, S. (1999) Drug anticipation and drug addiction. *Addiction,* 94: 1113–24.

Strang, J. (1990) The roles of prescribing. In: Strang J, Stimson GV, eds. *AIDS and Drug Misuse: The Challenge for Policy and Practice in the 1990's.* London: Routledge; 142–52.

Strang, J., Marsden, J., Cummins, M., Farrell, M., Finch, E., Gossop, M.,

Stewart, D. & Welch, S. (2000) Randomised trial of supervised injectable versus oral methadone maintenance: report of feasibility and 6-month outcome. *Addiction,* 95: 1631–45.

Strang, J., Bearn, J., Farrell, M., Finch, E., Gossop, M., Griffiths, P., Marsden, J. & Wolff, K. (1998) Route of drug use and its implications for drug effect, risk of dependence and health consequences: a review. *Drug and Alcohol Review,* 17: 197–211.

Strang, J., Sheridan, J. & Barber, N. (1996) Prescribing injectable and oral methadone to opiate addicts: results from the 1995 national postal survey of community pharmacists in England & Wales. *British Medical Journal,* 313: 270–4.

Section D: The risks

12
Dependence on methadone: the danger lurking behind the prescription

Gillian Tober

Methadone reduces a number of the problems associated with opiate, primarily heroin use. The question of what happens to dependence, whether on heroin or on methadone, remains unanswered. The importance of this question may not always be obvious. The lack of unanimity in the definition and measurement of dependence across substances may be one of the reasons that the question is rarely debated. Instead, attention has been focused on the use of methadone in replacing heroin, and the resulting more visible benefits of crime reduction and those other advantages which accrue from its association with greater life style stability. Such benefits have been shown to occur virtually immediately on commencement of a methadone prescription, and more particularly where methadone substitution results in the immediate and complete cessation of heroin use (see Chapter 23); however, there is also some evidence that the benefits abate over the longer term and this might be due to an increase in levels of dependence. Dependence has been shown to endure during abstinence and only gradually to diminish with the continuation of abstinence (Tober 2000). The question of what happens to dependence in the course of methadone substitution treatment will have important implications for clinicians as well as policy makers in deciding realistic targets against which to measure long-term outcomes. In this chapter the nature of dependence and change in dependence are examined, and it is suggested that some of the benefits of methadone may not endure in the longer term, due to a gradual reinstatement of high levels of dependence.

The existence of methadone treatment undoubtedly brings very large numbers of heroin users into the health services orbit. This is in stark contrast to the small numbers of users of cannabis or psycho-stimulant drugs, for whom no such drug substitution treatment is thought to exist. It is not just the severity of the addiction-forming potential of heroin that may account for this marked difference in the extent of help seeking; the pleasurable effects and the dependence-forming potential of methadone are likely to play a significant role.

The nature of dependence

Dependence has variously been referred to as a physiological, a bio-psycho-social or simply a psychological phenomenon. Perhaps the most common usage with reference to opioids is the physiological state, as the symptoms resulting from regular use are well documented and reliably predictable; the term dependence is often used as a shorthand to refer to these symptoms. However, from the point of view of understanding drug use and the ubiquity of relapse after cessation of use, this approach has little explanatory power. More helpful in explaining the range of phenomena associated with the natural history of opioid drug use is the psychological view in which physiological phenomena are understood to constitute the conditions of learning, both as stimulus for use and as source of reinforcement, rather than constituting the condition itself. The physiological consequences of regular opioid use, referred to as neuroadaptive processes (Edwards *et al.* 1982) do not, in themselves, determine future drug use as attested by studies of hospital patients treated for pain with opioid drugs. It is rather the beliefs about the drug and the relationship the user has with the drug that are more likely to result in the continuation of use past the point of its original purpose or in relapse following attempts to quit use. Thus the nature of dependence is determined by the pursuit of relief or avoidance of those physiological effects, rather than by the occurrence of the withdrawal phenomena themselves (Topp and Darke 1997). This distinction between dependence and neuroadaptation forms the basis for the development of the concept of substance dependence as a psychological phenomenon (Tober 1992). Descriptions of dependent use of stimulants, such as cocaine and amphetamine with their withdrawal-like effects, more properly described as rebound effects, the primacy of the pursuit of the effect and avoidance of the absence of the drug effect, give support to a psychological understanding of dependence.

Tabakoff (1990) has described the preoccupation of researchers with withdrawal symptoms, perhaps because they are readily observable and measurable, to the detriment of acknowledging the continued importance of the drug effect through all stages of neuroadaptive change. He also described the phenomena of tolerance and withdrawal as the consequence of the regular and heavy use of a substance, albeit that they have powerful reinforcement potential, as do the psychoactive effects of the drugs, and are likely to cue the dependent behaviour. In other words, it is not the presence of tolerance and withdrawal that is a part of dependence, but rather it is the behaviour, thoughts and feelings that are conditioned by them. Miller (1980) has referred to this as the cognitive interpretation of physiological events; Leventhal and Cleary (1980) have proposed a learning mechanism where certain emotional states are conditioned to the pharmacological effects and physiological consequences of substance use and it is the regulation of these emotional states which drives the drug-seeking or drug-taking behaviour. Solomon (1980) described a theory of addiction based on his work with

Corbit (Solomon and Corbit 1974) in which they developed the opponent process theory of acquired motivation. In this theory, drug use recurs in an attempt to counteract the opponent process, the inevitable but delayed consequence of taking the drug, which has the opposite hedonic quality to the effects of the drug. These are some of a number of operant explanations of drug dependence that support the observation that the pursuit of the effect and the maintenance of the effect of the drug may be as important, if not more important in driving the drug-seeking and drug-using behaviour as is the avoidance of the negative consequences of not using or stopping using (the experience of withdrawal symptoms). Raistrick *et al.* (1994), in theorizing about the nature of dependence when developing a scale capable of measuring dependence on a variety of substances (the Leeds Dependence Questionnaire), included markers of dependence that reflected the pursuit of the effect, maximization of the effect and maintenance of the effect in their attempt more comprehensively to account for the whole spectrum of types (positive and negative) and sources (physiological, pharmacological, psychological and social) of reinforcement rather than exclusively the negative type with a physiological source. The relative severity of dependence on different substances can be compared using this scale (Heather *et al.* 2001), as can differences in the course of change between different substance dependencies (Tober *et al.* 2000).

The relevance of this to the present discussion is in the way that methadone should be understood as a drug with considerable dependence liability, which is based on far more than the neuroadaptive state that results from its continued use. How does this dependence liability compare with that of heroin?

Psychology and pharmacology: dependence liability of heroin versus methadone

The reinforcement potential, and therefore the addiction-forming potential of a drug, is determined by a number of factors: its potency, the immediacy of the onset of its effect (not exclusively the property of the drug but a factor that can be varied by the method of its use), the predictability of its effect and its elimination half-life. Potency of the effect is the positive reinforcement potential of the drug, whereas the speed of onset of the effect, or the question of how quickly that reinforcing consequence occurs, is known to be an important factor in whether a consequence is reinforcing at all. In operant conditioning terms, the consequence which most immediately follows the behaviour has the strongest reinforcement potential. The predictability factor works in a less straightforward manner. The most potent reinforcement schedule is the partial one where reinforcement does not occur on every occasion, but either does or does not occur. Thus, predictability refers to this dichotomous range of outcomes; when it is the case that the outcome is highly variable, as for example in the case of LSD, the expectation of a specific effect is minimized and the behaviour therefore less reinforcing. The relevance of the elimination half-life is two-fold: the loss of the drug effect and/or the onset of a rebound effect or withdrawal symptoms are important determinants of whether further drug use is sought. Either of these factors operates as a source of negative reinforcement, that is, where the behaviour is strengthened because of its ability to avoid or reduce a negative consequence.

Heroin is deemed to score highest in its reinforcement potential, with its most potent of opioid effects and its shorter elimination half-life; onset of the effect will vary with method of administration and its predictability rating, or patho-plasticity (Edwards 1974), is comparable to the other opioids. By comparison, methadone can be judged to have lower positive reinforcement potential, being less potent in its effect and having a slower onset of effect, particularly when taken by the oral route. In oral preparation, the onset of the effect of methadone is delayed compared with injectable methadone and the peak experience, the positive reinforcement potential, is reduced. In its injectable form, methadone, with the enhanced speed of onset and higher peak experience of the effect that results from injecting the drug, is likely to have dependence-forming properties much closer to those of heroin taken either intravenously or intra-nasally. Indeed, higher rates of dependence have been shown to be associated with injecting heroin use compared with oral and intra-nasal use (Gossop *et al.* 1992). Whether dependence escalates as a result of injecting use, or escalating dependence motivates a change to injecting use (an increase in perceived need being matched by an increase in the immediacy and potency of the effect) remains unclear, but the likelihood is that both can occur. The longer elimination half-life of methadone means that the perceived need for it occurs less frequently and the expectation of reinforcement is reduced. These are some of the reasons why oral methadone is the drug of choice for substitution prescribing. Not only does it have lower reinforcement potential and therefore less dependence liability, but also it directly reduces dependence on heroin, in one respect. Insofar as heroin use is negatively reinforced by the fear or experience of withdrawal, methadone removes such fear and therefore removes the perceived need for drug seeking that emanates from this source. The fact that methadone has a milder psychoactive effect than heroin means that it will be less effective in replacing heroin for those whose use is primarily reinforced by pursuit of the effect of the drug and maximization of that effect, for people seeking to 'get a hit'. The lesser dependence liability of methadone may mean that it stands a greater chance of diminishing over time.

However, there also exists in the common view a perception that methadone is in fact more highly addictive than heroin: it is seen to be more difficult 'to come off' methadone than heroin and Sievewright and Lagundoye have addressed this finding in Chapter 8. This view stems from a perception of the severity and duration of the withdrawal syndrome, the negative reinforcement potential of methadone compared with heroin. In the case of methadone, the withdrawal syndrome is experienced as causing greater discomfort over a greater duration of time. The shorter elimination half-life of heroin results in more frequent drug-seeking behaviour, but the more severe withdrawal syndrome with greater discomfort that is reported in the case of methadone suggests that, although drug-seeking behaviour is less frequent, it may be more powerfully (negatively) reinforcing when it does occur. Is this a question of the relative potency of positive and negative reinforcement, which has been investigated experimentally and in animal laboratories, or is it more difficult than that? Though there is likely to be individual variation in the importance of types and sources of reinforcement, learning theory teaches us that the frequency and schedule of reinforcement is important. Furthermore, there is considerably more positive reinforcement potential (a considerably more pleasurable effect) to be derived from heroin compared with methadone use. The overriding view then is that heroin is probably the more powerfully reinforcing, and has the greater dependence forming and dependence maintaining potential of the two.

Reducing dependence on heroin by substitution of methadone

The conclusion that methadone has lower dependence liability than heroin is more theoretically than empirically derived (though the means exist to investigate this question empirically). Anecdotal and reported experience reinforce this view. But is it the case that methadone is the drug of choice for prescribing in substitution for heroin because it is simply easier (and therefore cheaper) to manage than heroin? Does it really reduce dependence on heroin and result, in itself, in a lower level of dependence?

Methadone substitution for heroin is likely to have the effect of reducing dependence overall because methadone has the lower reinforcement potential: less potency and a longer duration of the effect or elimination half-life are the main reasons for this reduced dependence liability. This is the case for oral methadone compared with heroin taken intra-nasally or intravenously. Methadone use, to the extent that it is reinforcing, exercises this reinforcing effect only once a day, compared with once every four hours or so in the case of heroin. Methadone is further likely to reduce use and therefore dependence on heroin because of the way it occupies opioid receptors so that, even where heroin use continues, its pleasurable effects are reduced. Thus the reinforcement of pleasure seeking is eliminated. At the same time the aversive consequences of losing the drug effect cease to occur through two different routes. Firstly, the pleasurable effect, not having been there, cannot to the same extent be lost, and secondly, the onset of withdrawal is prevented by the action of methadone.

Physiological and pharmacological events though are not the only source of reinforcement, albeit that they may become paramount as dependence increases in severity; methadone itself may not therefore be adequate to eliminate or reduce dependence on heroin. Environmental and social sources of reinforcement are equally well documented, as is the complexity which results from the fact that the environment is capable of triggering physiological reactions and pseudo-pharmacological effects that in turn become drug-taking stimuli and reinforcers. Russell *et al.* (1974) described a sequence in the development of sources of reinforcement with reference to nicotine dependence, commencing with social sources, followed by pharmacological and psychological sources and culminating in physiological sources. Chick and Duffy (1979) investigated the sequence of the onset of symptoms of dependence on alcohol and showed that, if particular symptoms develop, then they will develop in a particular sequence. They showed that tolerance and withdrawal, understood here as negative sources of reinforcement, were late onset symptoms; behavioural and psychological symptoms were likely to occur earlier. Edwards (1984) described different levels of explanation by distinguishing the idea of natural history – the sequential development of symptoms resulting from individual reactivity to alcohol – from career, whose phases and transitions may equally be determined by social and psychological factors external to, but influencing, the evolving pattern of drinking. Such variations in patterns of development of dependence are similar to the accounts given by those with heroin dependence where initiation of use has occurred in a social context.

An understanding of all sources of reinforcement as well as methods of conditioning is necessary in order to make sense of dependent behaviour and make adequate plans for its extinction. For example, when people refer to having a 'needle fixation' the likelihood is that, owing to the pairing of the ritual of injecting with the pleasurable effects of the drug, the injecting itself is experienced as having these positive effects, in what is described as a classical conditioning paradigm (Siegel 1988). Sight and handling of the injecting equipment can elicit pleasurable feelings or withdrawal-like feelings. Similarly with the presence of tin foil and other paraphenalia of use, dependent users describe the way the presence of such paraphenalia in the absence of the drug can elicit the experience of craving or withdrawal-type effects, and these phenomena have been demonstrated experimentally (Siegel 1999). Equally the presence of particular people who have been drug-taking associates or drug dealers has been experienced as a stimulus that elicits craving. An interesting tale was related by a young man attempting to give up his heroin use: his mother used to comfort him during times of withdrawal in such a way that the smell of the shampoo she used would elicit withdrawal-like symptoms and thereafter a sense of drug craving during times of abstinence.

The sum total of the severity of dependence or the reinforcement history of the use of a particular drug will likely depend on the properties of the drug, the nature of the original learning of its use and the environment in which it is used. Reduction in the degree of such dependence will need to take account of these factors. Regular methadone use, when part of treatment, more often occurs in the clinical context, and is likely to have fewer sources of reinforcement other than the purely pharmacological and physiological, compared with illicit heroin use. If this is the case, further support is provided for its utility and effectiveness as a dependence-reducing measure.

Changing the course of dependence

Understanding the specific sources and types of reinforcement for any individual is a complex matter indeed and rather than trust the accuracy of such analysis, many treatment programmes are designed to eliminate or at best reduce all likely sources of reinforcement for heroin and other illicit drug use. To the extent that the drug-taking ritual is itself a source of reinforcement, either directly as a social source or indirectly in the way that it can constitute a stimulus for withdrawal and craving, changing both the substance, its method of use and the conditions of its use is likely to eliminate some and diminish other sources of reinforcement. Changing the environment to exclude the presence of people and objects that elicit drug craving and withdrawal may eliminate some of the sources of drug anticipation and reinforcement. The prescription, dispensation and use of methadone as treatment of heroin dependence occurs in a clinical setting where many environmental reinforcers of use are absent. Cummins gives an example of this in Chapter 11 when he describes how people who inject in a clinical setting experience less of the pleasurable effect of the drug.

A more robust method of dealing with drug-taking triggers may be to learn new responses to them so that the drug-using response is replaced by a different response. In the 12-step movement, as embodied for example in Narcotics Anonymous, substitute prescribing is generally felt to be an insecure route to recovery (that is abstinence), and groups of addicts learn new responses in an environment of mutual support and encouragement. The assumption is that the external environment is impossible to control completely, thus avoidance is not always possible, nor does it result in new learning.

In addition to reducing environmental, pharmacological and social sources of reinforcement, many of the thoughts and activities that constitute the dependent behaviour can be reduced by the simple fact of making a substance legally available; obviating the need to find illicit sources of a drug may reduce preoccupation of thoughts about it; planning of daily activities around procuring and using the drug is no longer necessary. Thoughts and activities can be freed up for alternative pursuits, which will diminish the perceived need for drug use as alternative rewards are experienced. The provision of methadone with its long-acting effects makes more possible the pursuit of these alternative activities.

Might methadone perpetuate dependence?

What happens in the longer term? Dependence on different substances has been shown to continue to decline with increasing duration of abstinence (Tober 2000), but what happens in the face of continuing methadone use? One of the objections to the long-term prescription of methadone is that such treatment prolongs and strengthens dependence. The suggestion that it prolongs dependence, apart from the face validity of the argument, derives from a number of sources. In theorizing about motivation to give up problem drinking, McMahon and Jones (1996) have argued that negative expectancy for continued use (bad things will happen if I continue drinking) is as influential as positive outcome expectancy for abstinence (good things will follow if I give up drinking) in the decision to change drinking behaviour. The replacement of heroin with methadone removes many of the negative consequences that result from heroin use, and may therefore reduce the incentive for further change in opiate use, particularly where a moderate level of dependent behaviour is not perceived in itself to be a problem. Even those programmes with built-in disincentives for the prolonged use of methadone tend to reward stable use by relaxing monitoring and pick-up conditions of prescriptions (see Chapter 18 by Watson *et al.* and Chapter 19 by Roberts). The relationship between dependence and motivation remains unclear but, to the extent that dependence reflects the perceived difficulty in giving up a substance or in doing without a substance (Russell 1976), the dependent patient is likely to require an incentive to change before embarking on attempts to give up the dependent behaviour.

And what about the course of dependence with the continuing use of the drug? Is it not the case with methadone, as it is with heroin, that the neuroadaptive state eventually manifests itself in a perceived need for more of the drug? Is it not the case that pursuit of an effect will result in the desire for increased doses? Is the neuroadaptive state more stable in the long term than it is with heroin use? Long-term studies with repeated measurement of dependence are needed to resolve this question. There is then the case to consider with 'using on top'. Best has described the increase in levels of dependence as one of the problems of such continued use in Chapter 13, and this eventuality may well explain the finding reported by Finch in Chapter 23 that there was an increase in amount of heroin consumed in those who recommenced heroin use following methadone treatment.

Weighing up the odds

When the idea of a natural history of heroin addiction was mooted (Stimson and Oppenheimer 1982), it was backed by epidemiological evidence that, on average, five years of experimental and recreational use was followed by five years of regular, dependent and problem use with attempts, often successful, to quit. In the Stimson and Oppenheimer (1982) study of the long-term outcomes of heroin addicts attending drug clinics in London during the late 1960s, half of the people who achieved stable abstinence from heroin did so with the assistance of a methadone prescription and were deemed to be leading otherwise normal lives. The studies of the 1980s and 1990s predated the widespread prescribing of methadone as a measure of harm reduction, an attempt to stem the spread of HIV infection. More recently, methadone treatment has come to be seen as a method of reducing the spread of other more prevalent infections and of offending behaviour. It seems that the risk of prolonging the course of dependence is thought to be a small price to pay compared with the risk of overdose, infectious disease transmission and continuing crime occasioned by continuing heroin use. One line of argument is that, since methadone itself is not very reinforcing, people will simply be bored out of using it and request withdrawal from their prescription. There are, however, other possible eventualities.

Data from a cohort of long-term methadone patients show dependence scores that are, on average, higher than those recorded at first contact for the help-seeking population in general. It may be argued that long-term dependence, even increasing dependence without adverse consequences, is far preferable to the adverse consequences of regular relapse into heroin use. The questions that remain to be answered in long-term follow-up studies are whether escalation of dependence on methadone eventually leads to a resumption of heroin use, in other words is the need for sensation, for the psychoactive effect, reinstated? Do long-term users of methadone remain relatively free of other drugs, or is the use of other drugs re-introduced over time? Do the negative consequences gradually re-appear, or is the worst that happens an incessantly growing population of methadone addicts, with the attendant growing health service bill for methadone treatment, who are not troubled by restrictions on their movements, or by the enduring stigma of addiction? Further evidence is required, to replace political argument and personal preference, for the purpose of making rational treatment-planning decisions.

References

Chick, J. & Duffy, J. (1979) Application to the alcohol dependence syndrome of a method of determining the sequential development of symptoms. *Psychological Medicine*, 9: 313–9.

Edwards, G. (1984) Drinking in longitudinal perspective: career and natural history. *British Journal of Addiction*, 79: 175–84.

Edwards, G. (1974) Drug dependence and plasticity. *Quarterly Journal of Studies on Alcohol*, 35: 176–95.

Edwards, G., Arif, A. & Hodgson, R. (1982) Nomenclature and classification of drug and alcohol-related problems: a shortened version of a WHO Memorandum. *British Journal of Addiction*, 77: 3–20.

Gossop, M., Griffiths, P., Powis, B. & Strang, J. (1992) Severity of dependence and route of administration of heroin, cocaine and amphetamines. *British Journal of Addiction*, 87: 157–1536.

Heather, N., Raistrick, D., Tober, G., Godfrey, C. & Parrott, S. (2001) Leeds Dependence Questionnaire: cross-validation in a large sample of clinic attenders. *Addiction Research*, 9: 253–69.

Leventhal, H. & Cleary, P. D. (1980) The smoking problem: a review of the research and theory in behavioural risk modification. *Psychological Bulletin*, 88: 370–405.

McMahon, J. & Jones, B. T. (1996) Post-treatment abstinence survivorship and motivation for recovery: the predictive validity of the Readiness to Change (RCQ) and Negative Alcohol Expectancy (NAEQ) Questionnaires. *Addiction Research*, 4: 161–76.

Miller, P. (1980) Theoretical and practical issues in substance abuse assessment and treatment. In: Miller W, ed. *The Addictive Behaviors: Treatment of Alcoholism, Drug Abuse, Smoking and Obesity.* New York: Pergamon.

Raistrick, D. S., Bradshaw, J., Tober, G., Weiner, J., Allison, J. & Healey, C. (1994) Development of the Leeds Dependence Questionnaire. *Addiction*, 89: 563–72.

Russell, M. A. H. (1976) What is dependence? In: Edwards G, Russell M, Hawks D, McCafferty M, eds. *Drugs and Drug Dependence.* Hampshire: Saxon House.

Russell, M. A. H., Peto, J. & Patel, U. A. (1974) The classification of smoking by factorial structure of motives. *Journal of the Royal Statistical Society*, 137: 313–33.

Siegel, S. (1999) Drug anticipation and drug addiction. *Addiction*, 94: 1113–24.

Siegel, S. (1988) Drug anticipation and drug tolerance. In: Lader M, ed. *The Psychopharmacology of Addiction.* Oxford: Oxford University Press; 73–96.

Solomon, R. (1980) The opponent process theory of acquired motivation. The costs of pleasure and the benefits of pain. *American Psychologist*, 35: 691–712.

Solomon, R. & Corbit, J. D. (1974) An opponent-process theory of acquired motivation: temporal dynamics of affect. *Psychological Review*, 81: 119–45.

Stimson, G. & Oppenheimer, E. (1982) *Heroin Addiction*. London: Tavistock.

Tabakoff, B. (1990) One man's craving is another man's dependence. *British Journal of Addiction*, 85: 1253–4.

Tober, G. W. (2000) *The Nature and Measurement of Substance Dependence.* University of Leeds: PhD Thesis.

Tober, G. (1992) What is dependence and why is it important? *Clinical Psychology Forum*, 41: 14–16.

Tober, G., Brearley, R., Kenyon, R., Raistrick, D. & Morley, S. (2000) Measuring Outcomes in a Health Service Addiction Clinic. *Addiction Research*, 8: 169–82.

Topp, L. & Darke, S. (1997) The applicability of the dependence syndrome to amphetamine. *Drug and Alcohol Dependence*, 48: 113–18.

13
'Using on top' and the problems it brings: additional drug use by methadone treatment patients

David Best and Gayle Ridge

Introduction

The effectiveness of methadone treatment has been widely documented in a variety of studies both in the UK and abroad (Hubbard *et al.* 1989). Domains of success in methadone treatment include reduced heroin use, improved health and social functioning, reduced criminal activity and HIV-risk behaviours. Despite the documented success of methadone treatment, a proportion of clients in treatment continue to use illicit opiates and a variety of other psychoactive substances. Pre-admission use of one or more illicit drugs in addition to opiates has been reported in up to 60% of methadone clients (Dunteman *et al.* 1992) and estimates of continued use during treatment range between 20% and 70% (Belding *et al.* 1998; Stitzer *et al.* 1981). Methadone patients who abuse more than one illicit substance are more likely to be discharged early from treatment (Joseph and Appel 1985), are more likely to be involved with risk behaviours (Klee *et al.* 1990) and have generally poorer outcomes than those who abuse only opiates (Weiss *et al.* 1988).

In this chapter, the extent of this additional substance use is outlined along with an examination of its significance for treatment retention and outcome and its implications for researchers and clinicians. The use of other drugs may be problematic not only as a breach of the treatment contract but also as a predictor of wider lifestyle and social issues, and as a correlate of treatment disruption and societal cost. The chapter is structured to examine each of the main forms of continued substance use and will include a consideration of heroin, alcohol, benzodiazepines, methadone, cocaine, cannabis and cigarette smoking. Some of the key specific and general issues they raise will be highlighted, followed by a synopsis of the personal, social and political implications of 'using on top'.

Heroin

One of the primary aims of methadone treatment is a reduction of illicit opiate use and the elimination of risky injecting practices, goals for which there is considerable evidence of success. The Treatment Outcome Prospective Study (TOPS) showed that subjects who remained in treatment for at least three months reduced their heroin use from a pre-treatment mean of 70% to 30% during treatment (Hubbard *et al.* 1989). The National Treatment Outcome Research Study (NTORS) found a reduction in heroin use to less than half pre-intake levels in a sample of over 700 clients enrolled in methadone programmes (Gossop *et al.* 2000), and similar findings have been reported in other large-scale studies.

For many clients, heroin use does not come to a complete end with the start of methadone treatment. A significant proportion of clients continue to use opiates regularly and fail to respond to interventions. Best *et al.* (1999a) found that 71% of a cohort of methadone maintenance patients who had been receiving methadone for a mean of over three years had been using heroin on at least one occasion in the three months before interview, with 31% using on a daily basis. Similarly, Ball and Ross (1991) found that 29% of methadone treatment clients had used intravenously in the month before interview and Iguchi *et al.* (1997) reported that, three months into treatment, 54% of clients failed to submit an opiate-free urine specimen.

The impact of methadone treatment on heroin use is generally thought to be mediated by key aspects of prescribing such as methadone dosing, with a reported inverse relationship between methadone dose and heroin use. Higher doses of methadone have been associated with improved client retention (McGlothlin and Anglin 1981) and with greater reductions in heroin use (Ball and Ross 1991). However, this benefit is clearly not consistent and universal, and Magura and Lipton (1988) revealed that, at every methadone dose level, one-half of all clients failed to achieve heroin abstinence up to three years into treatment. Saxon *et al.* (1996) also failed to find a clear association between methadone dose and reduced heroin use and one study has even found a reverse association (Caplehorn *et al.* 1993).

Best *et al.* (1999a) found that the most common reason given for continued heroin use during treatment in a sample of daily heroin users was to manage withdrawal symptoms. However, two-thirds of the sample also reported hedonistic heroin use at some time during treatment. These results suggest that providing more adequate methadone doses may only be beneficial for a sub-sample of treatment users. It should also be noted that other factors apart from methadone dose have been found to affect treatment outcome. Clients who receive ancillary services and greater levels of counselling and support during treatment also showed markedly greater improvements in retention and outcome than those who received methadone alone (McLennan *et al.* 1993). Both of these findings illustrate the limitation of assuming that methadone treatment is an exclusively biological substitute – its impact on heroin use is mediated significantly by psycho-social factors such as individual motivation, treatment affiliation, commitment and the social support, education and employment opportunities provided as part of the treatment package.

Groups at particular risk of poor treatment outcomes were identified by Magura and Lipton (1988) as poly-drug users and younger clients. For these individuals, extra interventions may be required. While reductions in heroin use frequently occur in methadone treatment populations, the elimination of use will usually be predicated on other factors relating to long-term goals of the individual, the style and structure of the treatment programme and the perceived benefits of abstinence or use across a wide domain of contexts.

Thus, despite its critics, methadone treatment continues to be the most frequently used form of treatment for opiate addicts with broad gains in a range of treatment outcomes, particularly quantity and frequency of heroin use. However, these benefits are not universal and are likely to be mediated by other aspects of treatment and the individual characteristics of the user.

Alcohol

Concurrent use of opiates and alcohol occurs in a significant proportion of methadone clients (Ball and Ross 1991; Hubbard et al. 1989), with alcohol abuse more prevalent among drug users than in the general population (Rounsaville et al. 1982). A significant number of heroin addicts enter treatment with a history of alcohol abuse and many continue to use alcohol excessively during treatment. Prevalence rates for the incidence of alcohol abuse in treatment populations have been reported to vary between 20% and 50% (Hunt et al. 1986; Chatham et al. 1995). Best et al. (1998) found that more than 50% of a cohort of methadone maintenance patients had consumed alcohol in the previous month. Precise estimates of the extent of alcohol abuse and associated problems in methadone clients are complicated as a result of disparate measures used across studies, inconsistencies of definition and a frequent failure to differentiate between 'alcoholism' and 'alcohol abuse' (Hunt et al. 1986).

While alcohol abuse among methadone clients is a recognized problem, there has been some debate about whether clients increase or decrease their alcohol consumption during treatment. While a number of clients are diagnosed as alcoholic at treatment admission, Gelb et al. (1977) found that, for 29% of their sample, alcohol abuse began after entry to methadone treatment. A third of a sub-sample of methadone clients described as 'abusive pattern drinkers' in a later study report consciously 'boosting' their methadone dose with alcohol (Hunt et al. 1986). This may occur as a result of direct pharmacological interaction (e.g. interference with metabolic pathways of breakdown and inactivation) or it may relate to use of alcohol as a means of coping with the lifestyle changes prompted by the transition to regulated behaviour, devoid of the drama and demand of street drug use. Thus, alcohol can be characterized as both a substitute and a coping mechanism in the hinterland of maintenance treatment.

Concurrent opiate and alcohol use in methadone clients presents a number of problems both to the individual and to treatment personnel. Heavy drinkers are at risk of a variety of medical problems including cirrhosis and pancreatitis. Dually addicted clients have a higher incidence of medical complications, including general hepatic dysfunction and liver disease (Force and Miller 1974) and also an increased risk of mortality. These clients also show more evidence of psychological problems, including anxiety and depression, and are more likely to continue to abuse a range of illicit drugs compared with heroin users without a drinking problem (Marcovici et al. 1980).

Concomitant alcohol abuse has been found to be a contributing factor to overdose (Ruttenber and Luke 1984). Alcohol problems have been associated with a greater frequency of lifetime overdose in methadone-maintained clients. Those who had experienced three or more overdoses reported significantly more alcohol dependence than those who had overdosed only once or twice (Best et al. 1999b). Co-administration of other central nervous system depressants such as alcohol can substantially increase the likelihood of fatal outcome following injection of heroin due to the potentiation of the respiratory depressant effects of heroin (Joseph and Appel 1985). Methadone maintenance treatment, however, has been shown substantially to reduce the risk of overdose. Thus there may be a pay-off that, while methadone maintenance treatment may reduce overdose mortality risk, it may also be generative of problem drinking, which may augment overdose and related risk following treatment discharge or completion.

Excessive alcohol use in methadone treatment clients has been associated with poorer treatment outcomes (Weiss et al. 1988) and has been described as a contributory cause of treatment failure and discharge (Joseph and Appel 1985). These authors report that approximately one-quarter of methadone maintenance discharges were as a result of alcohol abuse. However, other researchers have failed to find an association between alcohol use and treatment outcome, describing concurrent alcohol use as a 'complicating but not independent aspect of methadone treatment' (Marcovici et al. 1980). Chatham et al. (1995) found that clients classified as alcohol-dependent at admission remained in treatment significantly longer and benefited more at one-year follow-up in terms of reduced opiate use and alcohol-related symptoms than those clients classified as not alcohol-dependent.

While the evidence on the impact of alcohol use during methadone treatment is inconsistent, the health problems associated with excessive drinking certainly give cause for concern amongst a population already compromised by their opiate addiction. Opiate and alcohol dependencies are not mutually exclusive and may be indicative of wider lifestyle problems for a proportion of methadone patients, particularly those on long-term maintenance. The health problems of heavy drinking in this population may be compounded by lifestyle factors that disrupt treatment adherence and disrupt the therapeutic process.

This may suggest the need for targeted interventions and education to prevent alcohol-related health deterioration and decreases in treatment compliance. It also offers a challenge to service providers who may regard the benefits in reduced risk behaviours (such as reductions in sharing of injecting equipment) and in politically defined outcome indicators (crime reductions) as of overriding importance when there is then a danger of turning a blind eye to the concomitant impairments in functioning and self-efficacy that are often seen in the heavy drinking methadone treatment population.

Thus alcohol misuse is a common characteristic of methadone treatment populations, and one that appears to remain stable or even increase over the duration of treatment, potentially reducing treatment effectiveness and retention and increasing risks for overdose and other adverse outcomes. It constitutes a significant issue for clinicians to address as a core part of methadone treatment.

Benzodiazepines

Illicit benzodiazepine use is also widespread among opiate users in treatment (Ball and Ross 1991). Estimated prevalence rates of illicit benzodiazepine use among untreated opiate users range between 25% (Klee et al. 1990) and 50% (Perera et al. 1987). Similarly, persistent use of benzodiazepines has been reported in 30–40% of methadone clients (Darke et al. 1993; Sunjic and Howard 1996). Darke et al. (1993) found that 37% of methadone-maintained clients in an Australian sample had used non-prescribed benzodiazepines in the month preceding interview, while Stitzer et al. (1981) found that up to 70% of methadone patients showed evidence of illicit diazepam use. Woody et al. (1975) have highlighted the fact that diazepam may be being used by clients to medicate psychiatric symptoms and not necessarily for hedonic effects, although the amounts are often outside the therapeutic range.

In a community-wide sample of Edinburgh drug users, three-quarters of whom were being prescribed substitutes, the majority were prescribed high doses of benzodiazepines in addition to prescribed opioids. Thirty-one per cent indicated that they had sold all or part of their prescription on one or more occasions in the last six months. Diverted temazepam and diazepam were two of the most common street drugs used by the sample (Haw 1992). The issue of diversion relates not only to the street value and effect of the substance involved but also to the arrangements for the management of dispensing, which is crucial in the development of local drug cultures. In this Edinburgh sample, the ready availability of diverted methadone, dihydrocodeine and benzodiazepines were critical to the shape of the illicit drug culture, and to the presenting characteristics of new treatment admissions and the illicit use profile of those currently in treatment. This exemplifies the ways in which prescribing policy can influence not only the likelihood of illicit use by treatment populations but also the form that non-prescribed drug use will take and the characteristics of local drug markets.

Perera *et al.* (1987) reported that drug users in treatment may use benzo-diazepines to boost the euphoric effects of methadone, although other laboratory investigations found no evidence of such an effect. The poor cor-relation between methadone dose and methadone serum levels of benzodiazepine-using clients, along with client reports that their methadone dose was inadequate, may indicate that some benzodiazepines are capable of accelerating methadone metabolism leading to sub-optimal substitution levels (Bell *et al.* 1990). It must be noted that this relationship was only seen in a small number of clients and that such an interaction has not been sup-ported by other researchers (Preston *et al.* 1986).

An additional abuse potential involves the intravenous use of benzo-diazepines. Perera *et al.* (1987) revealed that approximately one-third of the UK non-treatment sample had previously injected benzodiazepines. A small proportion of methadone maintenance clients in Sydney had injected ben-zodiazepines in the preceding month (Darke *et al.* 1993) and this creates clinical problems as the injection of benzodiazepines is associated with vas-cular morbidity and mortality. Intravenous use of temazepam has been associated with striking behavioural effects including short-term memory loss and disinhibition, which may be partly responsible for the risk-taking behav-iour reported in this group of drug users (Klee *et al.* 1990).

Benzodiazepine use may have a detrimental effect on a sub-group of clients. Darke *et al.* (1993) reported that non-prescribed benzodiazepine users do not respond as well to treatment as other patients and may require extra clinical attention. This group of clients are more likely to have injected recently, to have used more classes of drugs in the previous month and shared needles, even though they were on higher methadone doses and had longer treatment tenures. Benzodiazepine use has been linked to higher levels of poly-drug use (Darke *et al.* 1993) and is associated with both fatal and non-fatal heroin overdose. This may be indicative of a more dysfunctional group of methadone clients and strengthens the argument that illicit use not only creates health effects but also may point the way to sub-culture membership and low levels of treatment adherence that are intrinsically problematic.

In light of the risk-taking behaviour of benzodiazepine users in treatment it is evident that caution should be exercised when prescribing these drugs, both in terms of diversion risk and through creating a second form of depen-dence that may interfere with opiate treatment. The combination of non-prescribed benzodiazepine use with methadone represents a high risk for opiate overdose, may be a disinhibitor for other forms of risky drug use and sexual behaviour, and may be predictive of low rates of treatment adherence or completion.

In summary, benzodiazepine misuse is highly prevalent among drug users in treatment and may be indicative of an at-risk population of clients who may be susceptible to overdose and to treatment drop-out. However, it may also suggest inadequacies in the management of medication which are likely to generate short-term public health risks and longer-term effects on the evolution of drug cultures based on diverted (or non-prescribed) opiates and benzodiazepines.

Methadone

In addition to prescribed use, many drug users 'top up' their prescriptions with additional methadone acquired through illicit markets. However, there are remarkably few studies concerning the use of illicit methadone by patients in treatment. This is surprising as the studies that have been conducted report extensive evidence of use of illicit methadone. Furthermore, in the UK, Fountain *et al.* (2000) found a substantial and thriving illicit market in methadone, which varies in price and appeal according to the different available forms. Sunjic and Howard (1996) found that 44% of an Australian sample had used methadone illicitly prior to treatment but this decreased to 6% during treatment. Similar reductions in non-prescribed methadone use were reported by the National Treatment Outcome Research Study (NTORS) sample at one-year with a reduction to less than half of pre-intake levels (Gossop *et al.* 2000).

Best *et al.* (2000) found that non-prescribed methadone was used by 7% of methadone patients at treatment intake, but six months later this had increased to 25%, and was not related to heroin use. Similarly, it was actually clients on higher doses of prescribed methadone who were more frequent users of illicit methadone. While illicit methadone use will partly be explained by inadequate dosing (or at least by the perception of this by patients), the above study suggests a more complex pattern, embedded within poly-drug use and shaped by the local sub-cultures for drug use among methadone patients. The use of non-prescribed methadone, which has received inadequate attention, may well provide an insight into the illicit use cultures that develop around substitute prescribing treatment centres.

The prevalence of injection of methadone syrup reported by Darke and Hall (1995) (lifetime prevalence of 52% of methadone maintenance clients in Sydney) has not been reported in other countries. The role of diverted methadone in overdose also merits further investigation with Neale (2000) reporting that, of recent non-fatal overdoses, illicit diversion of methadone was particularly common amongst those enrolled in treatment. It is likely that, if illicit methadone use is a marker for non-compliance individually and is indicative of participation in a non-adherent treatment culture, then participation in such behaviours may well represent a significant risk for treatment failure and the concomitant problems of health and outcome.

Given the relatively high prevalence of non-prescribed methadone use and the associated risks, it may be necessary for prescribers to review policies regarding methadone dispensing management to ensure that patients are neither tempted to sell their prescriptions nor to supplement their prescribed dose through a 'grey' market of diverted methadone. Inadequate doses of prescribed methadone may be one, but not the only, reason for use of diverted methadone, and broader research investigation is needed to understand the role of non-prescribed methadone use both as a component of poly-substance use by treatment patients and as a marker of disrupted treatment adherence.

Thus, although the research evidence base is weak, illicit methadone use is widespread, not only as a means of redressing perceptions of inadequate dosing of prescribed methadone but also as a component of drug use and trading. Greater research activity is required to understand more clearly how methadone diversion operates and what are its long-term implications.

Cocaine

High prevalence rates of cocaine use have been documented in methadone patients, both before admission and during treatment. Strug et al. (1985) found cocaine use in one-fifth of methadone clients at four clinic sites in New York, while Ball and Ross (1991) reported pre-treatment cocaine use in half of all methadone clinic admissions. Patients in Magura's study used cocaine extensively during a methadone treatment period of up to three years (Magura et al. 1998) while Chaisson et al. (1989) found that 24% of cocaine users in methadone treatment began or increased use after starting treatment. Also, Hartel et al. (1995) found cocaine users in treatment had a greater likelihood (43.9%) of heroin use compared with non-cocaine users.

Rowan-Szal et al. (2000) found that heavy cocaine-using clients typically spent less time in treatment compared with occasional users, and cocaine users have also been found to have a greater likelihood of discharge from treatment (Condelli et al. 1991; Magura et al. 1991). Clients who used cocaine during treatment have also been reported to have more anti-social personality disorders and a greater risk of HIV infection (Grella et al. 1995).

Cocaine-using methadone clients have reported higher rates of criminal involvement, with cocaine use more strongly associated with acquisitive crime than heroin use in treatment populations. Hall et al. (1993) reported that crack use was strongly associated with acquisitive crime, while Best et al. (2001) also found cocaine the better predictor of acquisitive crime than heroin in a treatment-seeking population in London. The cost of cocaine use during treatment often leads clients to return to criminal involvement to finance the habit (Strug et al. 1985) and may maintain an engagement with street drug cultures.

Strug et al. (1985) have suggested that cocaine attenuates the effect of prescribed methadone, resulting in the use of illicit methadone or heroin to compensate for this diminished effect and that cocaine use may also be associated with a high rate of hepatic metabolism of methadone (Hartel et al. 1995). Other reports have suggested that methadone mellows the effect of cocaine (Kosten *et al.* 1988), or that cocaine use may often require subsequent use of a depressant such as heroin to manage the 'wired' feeling that follows cocaine use. Increased sexual risk taking (Grella *et al.* 1995) and higher risk of HIV-risk behaviours have also been documented, and may imply that illicit cocaine use can disrupt the opiate treatment process through a number of disparate mechanisms.

However, there is also consistent evidence that methadone treatment reduces the frequency of cocaine use. Ball and Ross (1991) found that 24% of clients enrolled in methadone treatment for more than six months used cocaine in the preceding month compared with 47% who had been in treatment for less than this period. Among the NTORS sample, significant reductions in the frequency of crack cocaine and cocaine powder use were found between intake and one-year follow-up in both reduction and maintenance programmes, with use reduced to less than half the pre-intake levels (Gossop *et al.* 2000). The best predictors of reduced cocaine use following methadone treatment initiation are reduced heroin use and reduced injecting (Dunteman *et al.* 1992). Magura *et al.* (1991) found decreases in cocaine use were as frequent as decreases in heroin use, perhaps because of the practice of simultaneous injection or 'speedballing'.

Cocaine use, particularly the use of crack cocaine, is associated with unpredictable behaviour, including violence, increased risk of acquisitive crime and elevated probability of mental health problems. These cocaine problems may sometimes also be markers for inadequate treatment compliance and erratic attendance. Methadone patients who are also regular cocaine users may have significantly greater treatment needs, and treatment objectives may have to be amended to deal with this additional drug problem, especially given the pivotal role of (crack) cocaine in the poly-drug using profile of many opiate addicts in (and beyond) treatment services.

In summary, cocaine use is often indicative of patients with more intensive treatment needs and wider ranges of problems, including criminality and mental health needs that may interfere with treatment implementation. As a consequence, it is critical that initial gains in cocaine reduction as a result of treatment initiation are sustained so that the chances of treatment compliance and success are not diminished.

Cannabis

The use of cannabis is widespread, and it is therefore no surprise that it is also used by clients in methadone treatment. Cannabis is widely used by heroin users both before admission and during methadone treatment. Thirty-five per cent of TOPS patients were daily marijuana users before entering treatment (Hubbard *et al.* 1989). Sixty-four per cent of existing methadone clients in an Australian study reported marijuana use in the preceding month (Darke *et al.* 1993) and 40% of clients in an American study consistently tested positive for cannabis use during a six-month period during treatment (Saxon *et al.* 1993).

Best *et al.* (1999c) found that daily cannabis users (about 40% of the sample) in methadone treatment were more likely also to report poor diet and higher levels of anxiety and depression, but lower levels of heroin, crack and alcohol use than infrequent or non-users of cannabis. Cannabis users may also appear to be more socially withdrawn and isolated (Saxon and Calsyn 1992), which may interfere with the wider social rehabilitation goals of treatment. However, whether these characteristics precede or follow regular marijuana use, or treatment entry, remains a matter of dispute.

At present, it remains uncertain whether cannabis use among methadone clients impedes treatment. Wasserman *et al.* (1998) found cannabis-using methadone patients to be more likely to resume opiate use than non-cannabis users. These results conflict with those from an earlier study which failed to find differences in treatment retention (Saxon *et al.* 1993). As a consequence, cannabis cannot be regarded as a component of non-adherent poly-substance use but may well be associated with other problems of physical or psychological health, which may require individual consideration by clinicians and further investigation by researchers.

Cigarette smoking

Cigarette smoking is widespread among methadone treatment populations (Darke and Hall 1995). Ninety-three per cent of a methadone maintenance sample reported smoking cigarettes during treatment, with an average of 17.6 cigarettes smoked per day (Harris *et al.* 2000). Increased levels of mortality amongst methadone patients who smoke (Hurt *et al.* 1996) and worse treatment outcomes have been documented. There may also be behavioural and pharmacological interactions between cigarette smoking and methadone use. Interactions between methadone and cigarettes have been reported by Chait and Griffiths (1984) who found methadone administration resulted in substantial, dose-related increases in rates of cigarette smoking by methadone-maintained smokers. Kozlowski *et al.* (1993) also found that cigarette smoking may be a relapse factor for the use of alcohol and other drugs during treatment.

Many clinicians are opposed to smoking cessation efforts amongst this population, believing that cessation efforts would create additional stress and may interfere with treatment outcomes (Bobo and Gilchrist 1983). Yet, the limited evidence does not support this belief. Harris *et al.* (2000) found that one-third of opiate users undergoing inpatient detoxification would have welcomed the offer of simultaneous or consequent help to quit or reduce smoking, and Hurt *et al.* (1996) found that approximately 11% of clients who received smoking cessation programmes during drug and alcohol treatment achieved and maintained tobacco abstinence one year after treatment compared with none of those clients who had not received the cessation programme. Abstinence rates of other substance use did not differ between the two groups.

Smoking is recognized as an important health problem and has been targeted in the UK in the *Health of the Nation* document (Department of Health 1992). Tobacco poses a mortality risk at least as great as opiates and, in an ageing population of maintenance patients, is a significant contributor to morbidity and mortality. Irrespective of the elevated relapse risk associated with cigarette smoking, it is a major morbidity factor for most methadone patients and as a consequence should be addressed by treatment providers within the extensive treatment window afforded by substitution treatment, however hesitant clinicians and patients may be.

Thus, while cigarette smoking is the most common form of additional substance use by patients in drug treatment, and a major morbidity and mortality risk, it is inadequately assessed and addressed within treatment services on the grounds of the unsupported assertion: 'one drug at a time'.

Conclusion

'Using on top' is a major problem confronting treatment agencies. A substantial proportion of patients continue to use heroin, alcohol and a variety of other drugs in addition to their prescribed methadone. The pattern of their 'use on top' will be shaped in part by the structure of the service, particularly in terms of procedures for limiting leakage of prescribed drugs and for measuring and responding to continued illicit use (through the implementation of contingency contracting procedures). In this way, specialist and non-specialist prescribing services have a symbiotic relationship with local drug markets, particularly those which grow up around a prescribing service, from which there may be leakage of methadone and benzodiazepines.

The challenge is to work out what can be done, and what should be done to address this 'using on top' phenomenon at an organizational level as well as at an individual treatment level. Methadone treatment alone will often be insufficient to address the issues of those with multiple substance-dependence problems and an extended range of therapeutic options may be required for those clients for whom standard care will not be effective. Additional drug use may be seen as functional, a functionality that will be amplified by the range of motives behind additional use – it will not be explained solely in terms of inadequate dosing. The findings that multiple drug use has been related to heroin overdose (Darke *et al.* 1996) and HIV risk (Grella *et al.* 1995) is further indicative of the compounding effect that 'using on top' may have on treatment failure. Some of these problems will be best tackled by looking at the operational aspects of the service and at the purchaser's (and society's) choice of therapeutic objectives, whilst others will be better addressed by more careful attention to individuals. It is increasingly clear that the current widespread practice of ignoring the problem of 'using on top' serves neither the interests of the individual nor of society and is no longer defensible.

References

Ball, J.C. & Ross, A. (1991) *The Effectiveness of Methadone Maintenance Treatment.* New York: Springer-Verlag.

Belding, M.A., McClellan, A.T., Zanus, D.A. & Incmikoski, R. (1998) Characterizing 'non-responsive' methadone patients. *Journal of Substance Abuse Treatment,* 15: 1–8.

Bell, J., Fernando, D. & Batey, R. (1990) Heroin users seeking methadone treatment. *Medical Journal of Australia.* 152: 361–4.

Best, D., Sidwell, C., Gossop, M., Harris, J. & Strang, J. (2001) Crime and expenditure amongst multiple drug misusers seeking treatment: the connection between prescribed methadone and crack use, and criminal involvement. *Journal of Clinical Forensic Medicine,* 6: 224–7.

Best, D., Harris, J., Gossop, M., Farrell, M., Finch, E., Noble, A. & Strang, J. (2000) Use of non-prescribed methadone and other illicit drugs during methadone maintenance treatment. *Drug and Alcohol Review,* 19: 9–16.

Best, D., Gossop, M., Stewart, D., Marsden, J., Lehmann, P & Strang, J. (1999a) Continued heroin use during methadone treatment: Relationship between frequency and use of reasons reported for heroin use. *Drug and Alcohol Dependence,* 53: 191–5.

Best, D., Gossop, M., Lehmann, P., Harris, J. & Strang, J. (1999b) The relationship between overdose and alcohol consumption among methadone maintenance patients. *Journal of Substance Use,* 4: 41–4.

Best, D., Gossop, M., Greenwood, J., Marsden, J., Lehmann, P. & Strang, J. (1999c) Cannabis use in relation to illicit drug use and health problems among opiate misusers in treatment. *Drug and Alcohol Review,* 18: 31–8.

Best, D., Lehmann, P., Gossop, M., Harris, J., Noble, A. & Strang, J. (1998) Eating too little, smoking and drinking too much: Wider lifestyle problems among methadone maintenance patients. *Addiction Research,* 6: 489–98.

Bobo, J. & Gilchrist, L. (1983) Urging the alcoholic client to quit smoking cigarettes. *Addictive Behaviors,* 8: 297–305.

Caplehorn, J.R.M., Bell, J., Kleinbaum, D.G. & Gebski, V.J. (1993) Methadone dose and heroin use during maintenance treatment. *Addiction,* 88: 119–24.

Chaisson, R.E., Bacchetti, P., Osmond, D., Brodie, B., Sande, M.A. & Moss, A.R. (1989) Cocaine use and HIV infection in intravenous drug users in San Francisco. *Journal of the American Medical Association,* 261: 561–65.

Chait, L. & Griffiths, R. (1984) Effects of methadone on human cigarette smoking and subjective ratings. *The Journal of Pharmacology and Experimental Therapeutics,* 229: 636–40.

Chatham, I.R., Rowan-Szal, G., Joe, G.W., Brown, B.S. & Simpson, D.D. (1995) Heavy drinking in a population of methadone maintenance clients. *Journal of Studies on Alcohol,* 56: 417–22.

Condelli, W.S., Fairbank, J.A., Dennis, M.L. & Rachal, J.V. (1991) Cocaine use by clients in methadone programs: significance, scope and behavioural intentions. *Journal of Substance Abuse Treatment,* 8: 203–12.

Darke, S. & Hall, W. (1995) Levels and correlates of poly-drug use among heroin users and regular amphetamine users. *Drug and Alcohol Dependence,* 39: 231–5.

Darke, S., Ross, J. & Hall, W. (1996) Prevalence and correlates of the injection of methadone syrup in Sydney, Australia. *Drug and Alcohol Dependence,* 43: 191–8.

Darke, S., Swift, W., Hall, W. & Ross, J. (1993) Drug use, HIV risk-taking and psychosocial correlates of benzodiazepine use among methadone maintenance clients. *Drug and Alcohol Dependence,* 34: 67–70.

Department of Health (1992) *The Health of the Nation.* London: HMSO.

Dunteman, G., Condelli, W. & Fairbank, J. (1992) Predicting cocaine use among methadone patients. Analysis of findings from a National Study. *Hospital and Community Psychiatry*, 43: 608–11.

Force, E. & Miller, J. (1974) Liver disease in fatal narcotism: Role of chronic disease and alcohol consumption. *Archives of Pathology*, 97: 166–9.

Fountain, J., Strang, J., Gossop, M., Farrell, M. & Griffiths, P. (2000) Diversion of prescription drugs by drug users in treatment: analysis of UK market and new data from London. *Addiction*, 95: 393–406.

Gelb, A.M., Mildvan, D. & Stenger, R.J. (1977) The spectrum of causes of liver disease in narcotics addicts. *Journal of Gastroenterology*, 67: 314–18.

Gossop, M., Marsden, J., Stewart, D. & Rolfe, A. (2000) Patterns of improvement after methadone treatment: One year follow-up results from the National Treatment Outcome Research Study (NTORS). *Drug and Alcohol Dependence*, 60: 275–86.

Grella, C.E., Anglin, M.D. & Wugalter, S.E. (1995) Cocaine and crack use and HIV-risk behaviours among high-risk methadone maintenance clients. *Drug and Alcohol Dependence*, 37: 15–21.

Hall, W., Bell, J. Carless, J. (1993) Crime and drug use among applicants for methadone maintenance. *Drug and Alcohol Dependence*, 31: 123–9.

Harris, J., Best, D., Man, L., Welch, S., Gossop, M. & Strang, J. (2000) Changes in cigarette smoking among alcohol and drug misusers during inpatient detoxification. *Addiction Biology*, 5: 443–50.

Hartel, D.M., Schoenbaum, E.E., Selwyn, P.A., Kline, J., Davenny, K., Klein, R.S. & Friedland, G.H. (1995) Heroin use during methadone maintenance treatment. The importance of methadone dose and cocaine use. *American Journal of Public Health*, 85: 83–8.

Haw, S. (1992) *Pharmaceutical drugs and illicit drug use in Lothian region*. Edinburgh: Centre for HIV/AIDS and Drug Studies.

Hubbard, R.L., Marsden, M.E., Rachal, J.V., Harwood, H.J., Cavanaugh, E.R. & Ginsberg, H.M. (1989) *Drug abuse treatment: A national study of effectiveness*. Chapel Hill: University of South Carolina Press.

Hunt, D.E., Strug, D.L., Goldsmith, D.S., Lipton, D.S., Robertson, K. & Truitt, L. (1986) Alcohol use and abuse: Heavy drinking among methadone clients. *American Journal of Drug and Alcohol Abuse,* 12: 147–64.

Hurt, R., Offord, K., Croghan, I., Gomez-Dahl, L., Kittke, T., Morse, R. & Melton, J. (1996) Mortality following inpatient addictions treatment: role of tobacco use in a community-based cohort. *Journal of the American Medical Association*, 275: 1097–103.

Iguchi, M.Y., Belding, M.A., Morral, A.R., Lamb, R.J. & Husband, S.D. (1997) Reinforcing operants other than abstinence in drug abuse treatment; an effective alternative for reducing drug use. *Journal of Consulting and Clinical Psychology*, 65: 421–8.

Joseph, H. & Appel, P. (1985) Alcoholism and methadone treatment: consequences for the patient and the program. *American Journal of Drug and Alcohol Abuse*, 11: 37–53.

Klee, H., Faugier, J., Hayes, C., Boulton, T. & Morris, J. (1990) AIDS-related risk behaviour, polydrug use and temazepam. *British Journal of Addiction*, 85: 1125–32.

Kosten, T.R., Rounsaville, B.J. & Kleber, H.D. (1988) Antecedents and consequences of cocaine abuse among opiate addicts: a 2.5 year follow-up. *Journal of Nervous and Mental Disease*, 176: 176–81.

Kozlowski, L., Henningfield, J., Kennan, R., Lei, H., Leigh, G., Jelinek, L., Pope, M. & Haertzen, C. (1993) Patterns of alcohol, cigarette and caffeine and other drug use in two drug abusing populations. *Journal of Substance Abuse Treatment,* 10: 171–9.

Magura, S. & Lipton, D. (1988) The accuracy of drug use monitoring in methadone treatment. *Journal of Drug Issues*, 18: 317–26.

Magura, S., Kang, S-Y., Nwakeze, P. & Demsky, S.Y. (1998) Temporal patterns of heroin and cocaine use among methadone patients. *Substance Use and Misuse*, 33: 2441–67.

Magura, S., Siddiaqi, Q., Freeman, R.C. & Lipton, D.S. (1991) Cocaine use and help-seeking among methadone patients. *Journal of Drug Issues*, 21: 629–45.

Marcovici, M., McClellan, A.T., O'Brien, C.P. & Rosenzweig, J. (1980) Risk factors for alcoholism and methadone treatment: A longitudinal study. *Journal of Nervous and Mental Disease*, 168: 556–8.

McGlothlin, W. & Anglin, M. (1981) Long-term follow-up of clients of high- and low-dose methadone programmes. *Archives of General Psychiatry*, 38: 1055–63.

McLellan, A.T., Arndt, I., Metzger, D., Woody, G., O'Brien, C. (1993) The effects of psychosocial services in substance abuse treatment. *Journal of the American Medical Association*, 269: 1953–9.

Neale, J. (2000) Methadone, methadone treatment and non-fatal overdose. *Drug and Alcohol Dependence*, 58: 117–24.

Perera, K., Tuley, M. & Jenner, F.A. (1987) The use of benzodiazepines among drug addicts. *British Journal of Addiction*, 82: 511–15.

Preston, K.L., Griffiths, R.R., Cone, E.J., Darwin, W.D. & Gorodetzky, C.W. (1986) Diazepam and methadone blood levels following concurrent administration of diazepam and methadone. *Drug and Alcohol Dependence*, 18: 195–202.

Rounsaville, B.,Weissman, M., Kleber, H. (1982) The significance of alcoholism in treated opiate addicts. *Journal of Nervous and Mental Disease*, 170: 479–88.

Rowan-Szal, G.A., Chatham, L.R. & Simpson, D.D. (2000) Importance of identifying cocaine and alcohol dependent methadone clients. *The American Journal of Addictions*, 9: 38–50.

Ruttenber, A. & Luke, J. (1984) Heroin-related deaths: New epidemiologic insights. *Science,* 226: 14–21.

Saxon, A.J. & Calsyn, D.A. (1992) Alcohol use and high-risk behaviours by intravenous drug users in an AIDS education paradigm. *Journal of Studies on Alcohol*, 53: 611–18.

Saxon, A.J., Wells, E.A, Fleming, C., Jackson, R. & Calsyn, D.A. (1996) Pre-treatment characteristics, program philosophy and levels of ancillary services as predictors of methadone maintenance treatment outcome. *Addiction,* 91: 1197–209.

Saxon, A.J., Calsyn, D.A., Greenberg, D., Blaes, P., Haver, V.M. & Stanton, V. (1993) Urine screening for marijuana among methadone-maintained patients. *The American Journal of Addictions,* 2: 207–11.

Stitzer, M.L., Griffiths, R.R., McLellan, A.T., Grabowski, J. & Hawthorne, J.W. (1981) Diazepam use among methadone maintenance patients: patterns and dosages. *Drug and Alcohol Dependence,* 8: 189–99.

Strug, D.L., Hunt, D.E., Goldsmith, D.S., Lipton, D.S. & Spunt, B. (1985) Patterns of cocaine use among methadone clients. *International Journal of the Addictions,* 20: 1163–75.

Sunjic, S. & Howard, J. (1996) 'Non-injectables': methadone syrup and benzodiazepine injection by methadone-maintained clients. *Drug and Alcohol Review*, 15: 245–50.

Wasserman, D., Weinstein, M., Havassy, B., Hall, S. (1998) Factors associated with lapses to heroin use during methadone maintenance. *Drug and Alcohol Dependence*, 52: 183–92.

Weiss, R.D., Mirin, S.M., Griffin, M.L. & Michael, J.L. (1988) A comparison of alcoholic and non-alcoholic drug abusers. *Journal of Studies of Alcohol*, 49: 510–15.

Woody, G.E., O'Brien, C.P. & Greenstein, R. (1975) Misuse and abuse of diazepam: An increasingly common medical problem. *International Journal of the Addictions*, 10: 843–8.

14
Methadone and opioid-related deaths: changing prevalence over time

Michael Farrell and Wayne Hall

Concern about opioid-related deaths became a focus for policy makers after a long period of policy dormancy. In the UK, the development of clinical guidelines for the management of drug dependence (Department of Health 1999) and publication by the Advisory Council on the Misuse of Drugs (ACMD) on the subject of reducing drug-related deaths (Advisory Council on the Misuse of Drugs 2000) have drawn attention to the need for tighter monitoring and reduced levels of diversion of methadone from treatment programmes.

A range of complex issues is involved in the problem of opioid-related deaths. The first is the natural history of opioid dependence; there are high rates of morbidity and mortality among individuals who are opioid dependent, with a general estimate of mortality of 1–2% in untreated individuals. This rate is estimated to be approximately 14 times higher than age-matched population controls (Advisory Council on the Misuse of Drugs 2000; Christopherson et al. 1998). Many individuals report poly-drug dependence with alcohol, benzodiazepines and psycho-stimulant use, exacerbating both the problem itself and its identification. The physical complications of drug misuse are well recognized and described (Farrell et al. 2000).

Mechanisms of opioid-related fatalities are hard to confirm; it is generally assumed that central toxicity, with respiratory depression from a single or multiple respiratory depressant substances, is the main mechanism (White and Irvine 1999). In addition, suffocation from aspiration of stomach contents is a significant danger with a range of central depressants. Much of the work on mechanisms of fatality is based on post-mortem studies dating back to the 1960s and 1970s and is speculative in nature; little work has been published on mechanisms of deaths for some time.

As with all opioid agonists, there is a risk of overdose death from methadone. A fatal dose of methadone in opioid-naïve or non-tolerant individuals has been reported to be in the range of 25–40 mg per day. Doses considerably higher than this may be required for the purposes of averting withdrawal symptoms in opioid-dependent persons, and doses usually in excess of 60 mg per day are required for maintenance purposes (Ward et al. 1998).

There are two major overdose risks arising from the use of methadone for maintenance purposes. For opioid-dependent and opioid-tolerant individuals, the major risks arise during the process of induction onto methadone maintenance. In people with impaired liver function, normal doses of methadone may accumulate over the first week of treatment to pro- duce toxicity and death (Drummer *et al.* 1992; Caplehorn 1998). People who exaggerate the extent of their opioid use when being assessed for methadone maintenance treatment may be given doses of methadone that prove fatal (Caplehorn 1998). In Australia, the estimated risk of these deaths is 0.2% per annum of patients inducted into methadone maintenance treat- ment (Zador *et al.* 1998).

Overdose deaths

The risk of opioid overdose death is substantially reduced among individuals enrolled in methadone maintenance treatment (MMT) (Caplehorn *et al.* 1994; Caplehorn *et al.* 1996; Gearing and Schweitzer 1974). Gearing and Schweitzer (1974) found that the mortality among 17,000 patients receiving methadone maintenance (7.6 per 1000 per annum) was similar to that in the general population (5.6 per 1000 per annum), significantly lower than that among persons who left methadone maintenance (28.2 per 1000 per annum) and opioid users who were not in any treatment (82.5 per 1000 per annum). An Australian study of 307 heroin users enrolled in a methadone maintenance programme in the early 1970s revealed that they were nearly three times more likely to die when they were not in methadone maintenance (Caplehorn *et al.* 1994). This was largely due to the reduced likelihood of those in methadone maintenance committing suicide or dying from a heroin overdose (Caplehorn *et al.* 1996). Zador *et al.* (1998) have more recently corroborated these findings.

Comparison of trends in the UK with trends in Australia revealed that both countries observed an increase in opioid overdose deaths over the period 1985–1995. The mortality rate throughout the period was 4 to 10 times higher in Australia than the UK, whether measured by the proportion of all deaths due to opioid overdose or by the population prevalence of opioid overdose deaths. The rate of the increase may have been greater in the UK in the lat- ter half of the period since the difference in rate narrowed substantially over the whole period.

There are four possible explanations to be considered:

(1) differences in classification systems
(2) differences in the prevalence of opioid dependence
(3) differences in the prevalence of heroin smoking, and
(4) the overall penetration and the mode of delivery of methadone treatment or other forms of agonist pharmacotherapy.

Each could explain some of the observed difference in opioid overdose mortality between the UK and Australia. However, variation in classification and variation in prevalence of opioid dependence or differences in route of administration are unlikely to be large enough to account for the differences between the two countries. The more interesting but also very speculative possibility that needs to be considered is that the differences between the UK and Australia in opioid overdose mortality reflect differences in the way in which methadone maintenance is delivered in the two countries. It may be, for example, that allowing any registered medical practitioner to pre-scribe methadone leads to a greater proportion of heroin-dependent persons being involved in methadone treatment and thereby being at lower risk of opioid overdose. If the proportion of opioid-dependent people receiving methadone was a large enough proportion of all opioid-dependent persons, then the overall rate of opioid overdose deaths would be reduced. One cost of the increased availability of methadone may be that more overdose deaths occur as a result of diverted methadone. This hypothesis would explain the lower rate of opioid overdose death in the UK than Australia and the higher proportion of opioid overdose deaths that involve diverted methadone. Overall, critical data that would allow for confident interpretation of the differences in the different settings are not available and we can only conclude currently that there is no available simple explanation of these differences.

Time trends in opioid overdose deaths and other drug-related deaths

Neeleman and Farrell (1997) reported a consistent rise year on year of opioid-related deaths in England and Wales from 1975 to 1993 with a nearly ten-fold rise in deaths from opioid toxicity. There have been similar rises in the rate of fatal opioid overdose in the Nordic countries (Steentoft et al. 1996), Spain (De la Fuente et al. 1995; Sanchez et al. 1995), Italy (Davoli et al. 1997), Austria (Risser and Schneider 1994), and the United States (United States Department of Health and Human Services 1997). The Advisory Council on the Misuse of Drugs reports that from 1980 onwards, deaths related to drug misuse increased very significantly for men and significantly but less so for women and from a lower baseline. This increase occurred slowly at first and then rose more steeply. Those in the age group 20–29 were most at risk and also demonstrated the most dramatic acceleration in deaths. The Advisory Council for the Misuse of Drugs report of an Office for National Statistics analysis which calculates 'years of life lost' suggests that in 1995 drug misuse accounted for 5% of male years of life lost or 40,550 years of life lost in comparison to 58,000 from road traffic accidents. They report that the figures for years of life lost through drug misuse are converging with traffic accident figures as the former goes up and the latter comes down (Advisory Council on the Misuse of Drugs 2000).

The extent of illicit methadone use

Data from the UK show widespread use of illicit methadone: the National Treatment Outcome Research Study (NTORS) found that 49% of clients of treatment agencies reported having used illicit methadone in the 90 days preceding intake (Gossop *et al.* 1998). Fountain *et al.* (1998) have reported the tactics used by UK opioid users to obtain methadone and other pre-scribed drugs for sale to other users; Darke *et al.* (1996a; b) found substantial use of diverted methadone among heroin injectors in Sydney, Australia in 1995.

England

Clark *et al.* (1995) reported on 18 overdose deaths involving methadone that occurred in Sheffield between 1991 and 1994. In all of these deaths methadone was regarded as the principal cause of death although other drugs were present in a substantial minority of cases. Of these deaths, 17 occurred in adults (14 of whom were male); ten deaths occurred among persons who had been prescribed methadone for opioid dependence, and seven of these deaths occurred within the first four days of treatment. In the eight deaths that occurred among persons who had consumed diverted methadone, most had obtained the methadone from friends or bought it on the streets.

Cairns *et al.* (1996) reported on 90 deaths that they attributed in whole or part to methadone and that occurred in Manchester between January 1985 and December 1994. These represented 15% of all deaths attributed to alcohol and other drug toxicity during the study period. In 52 of the 90 deaths, methadone was regarded as the sole cause of death, with the remainder involving other drugs, alcohol or both. The mean age at death was 26 years and 88% of cases were male. In 36 cases the methadone had been prescribed, in 32 it was diverted and in the remainder the source was unclear (although probably diverted). They present time-series data which suggest that the rate of methadone overdose deaths in Manchester has risen with the rate of prescribing in the city.

Scotland: Lothian and Borders regions

Obafunwa and Busuttil (1994) reported an analysis of 352 deaths attributed to drug overdose in the Lothian and Borders regions of Scotland between 1983 and 1991. Approximately one-third of these deaths (32%, *n* = 114) were attributed to opioids, and equal numbers of these were attributed to methadone (18) and heroin (18). There was an increase in the number of deaths attributed to methadone over the period and a decrease in the num-bers of deaths attributed to heroin. Deaths attributed to heroin peaked in 1984 and fell significantly after 1986 while deaths attributed to methadone increased over the period.

A later study examined 179 accidental and suicidal overdose deaths in the region between 1989 and 1994 (Bentley and Busuttil 1996). Methadone was found to be responsible for 30% of all overdoses (38 cases) and contributed to another 26 cases.

Edinburgh

Hammersley *et al.* (1995) reported an analysis of 12 drug-related deaths in Edinburgh in 1991/2. Two of these deaths involved methadone, one involved heroin and five involved more than one drug. In 1986 the Lothian and Borders regions of Scotland (within which Edinburgh is located) implemented a policy of strict policing to reduce supplies of heroin while making methadone more readily available on prescription to addicts who requested it.

Glasgow

Cassidy *et al.* (1995) reviewed 62 drug-related deaths in Glasgow during 1992. In the majority of cases, more than one drug was found post-mortem. Heroin was found in 37 cases, benzodiazepines in 49 cases and methadone in two cases, in both of which heroin and benzodiazepines were also detected. Benzodiazepines were found post-mortem in 89% of the heroin deaths.

The introduction of supervised methadone to Glasgow in 1992 was demonstrated significantly to reduce methadone-related deaths when compared with the larger area of Strathclyde where supervision was not introduced until later. This study is the most impressive evidence for the impact of controlled administration on methadone-related deaths.

Risk factors for methadone deaths

Many of the risk factors associated with methadone deaths appear to be similar to those associated with heroin overdose deaths. Males are much more likely to die as a result of a methadone overdose. In Britain in 1995, 82% of those whose death was classified as accidental methadone poisoning were male. Similar figures have been recorded in the USA (Chabalko *et al.* 1973; Greene *et al.* 1974a; Barrett *et al.* 1996) and Australia (e.g. Zador *et al.* 1996). The sex difference in death rate reflects the greater numbers of males who become dependent on illicit opioid drugs (e.g. Ball and Ross 1991; Darke and Hall 1995).

Age may also be a risk factor for methadone overdose. In comparison with heroin deaths, methadone deaths in some studies have occurred among younger people (e.g. Greene *et al.* 1974a; b) although not all studies report a difference (Swensen 1988). Poly-drug use, particularly the use of alcohol and benzodiazepines, is a significant risk factor for methadone overdose

(Caplehorn 1998; Cassidy *et al.* 1995; Gilhooly 1997), as it is for heroin over-dose deaths (Darke and Zador 1996).

In studies that have examined the issue, the majority of methadone overdose deaths have occurred among persons who were not enrolled in methadone maintenance at the time of their death (e.g. Barrett *et al.* 1996; Cairns *et al.* 1996; Clark *et al.* 1995; Williamson *et al.* 1997). Some studies suggest that methadone deaths among those who are not prescribed methadone occur in younger persons (e.g. Clark *et al.* 1995; Williamson *et al.* 1997).

Making sense of the data

Research on methadone-related deaths has been sporadic and often oppor-tunistic. Studies are often prompted by media reports about methadone-related deaths among persons not enrolled in methadone main-tenance. They have been of limited utility because small numbers of deaths have been studied, the criteria used for attributing the deaths to methadone have not been made explicit or standardized, and rarely has any attempt been made to calculate mortality rates. Some studies have compared opioid overdose rates in settings in which methadone is available with settings where it has not, or within the same setting after efforts have been made to reduce methadone diversion.

A major problem with the literature is the lack of specification of the criteria used to classify the cause of these deaths. This makes it difficult to decide what contribution methadone makes to deaths in which other CNS depres-sants (such as alcohol, heroin and benzodiazepines) are involved. It is also difficult to estimate the risks of methadone versus heroin since it is likely that any estimate based on the numbers in methadone maintenance will under-estimate the size of the population who use methadone. This problem is one that is common to research on all illicit drug deaths, including those attributed to heroin. Without these figures, it is difficult to estimate the relative dangers of methadone and other opioids. Nevertheless, studies suggest a number of hypotheses that deserve more rigorous evaluation.

The first hypothesis is that increased availability of methadone mainte-nance and relaxation of controls on supervision of methadone dosing may be risk factors for methadone overdose deaths involving diverted methadone. In settings in which access to methadone maintenance increased (e.g. Denmark in the 1980s, Washington DC in the early 1970s and Manchester UK in the late 1980s) or restrictions on dosing have been relaxed (e.g. Western Australia in the late 1970s), studies have reported an accompanying increase in opioid overdose deaths involving methadone.

In relation to the second hypothesis, methadone overdose deaths that occurred among people in methadone maintenance were much less common than those among people who were not enrolled in methadone maintenance and who used diverted methadone. Deaths among people enrolled in methadone maintenance were most likely to occur when patients were being inducted into methadone maintenance. Some of these occurred because patients exaggerated their history of opioid use, or because undiagnosed liver disease allowed methadone doses that were below the fatal dose to accumulate over a number of days. Deaths during induction can be reduced by better assessment of dependence, use of lower starting doses of methadone and greater supervision during the first week of treatment (Drummer et al. 1992).

A third hypothesis, as evidence from some studies suggests, is that those who die as a result of ingesting diverted methadone may be younger users who have a low tolerance to opioids and are not experienced in using an opioid drug with a much longer half-life than heroin. Those who die of over-doses attributed to heroin tend to be older dependent opioid users and poly-drug users (Darke and Zador 1996).

A fourth hypothesis is, as several studies suggest (e.g. Greene et al. 1974a; 1975; Swenson 1988), that methadone-related overdose deaths can be reduced by increasing restrictions on take-away doses and increasing supervision of methadone dosing. These restrictions have on occasion been followed by a decline in overdose deaths involving methadone (Washington, DC in the early 1970s and Western Australia in the early 1980s, Glasgow and Strathclyde in the 1990s and possibly England in 1999). It is difficult however, given the small number of deaths in these studies, to exclude the possibility that the apparent decrease in methadone-related deaths after the implementation of the restrictions has been due to regression to the mean. The restrictions on methadone availability typically follow media concern about apparent clusters of methadone deaths and any apparent reduction in deaths that follows these restrictions is attributed to them; the possibility that the decrease represents chance fluctuations in a low base rate has not been tested. It would be preferable to have data over a longer period, or in a larger population, from a planned change in prescribing to assess this hypothesis properly. In England, by 2001, after a period of increasing concern about methadone-related deaths and the publication of new guidelines, the methadone death rate had fallen by 30% but the heroin and morphine-related death rate had increased by 127%, from 11 deaths per million population in 1995 to 25 deaths per million population in 1999 (Office for National Statistics 2001). A number of explanations could be given for this change, the most likely initial cause being a rise in the incidence and prevalence of heroin dependence. However, given the size of the increase, it is unlikely to be accounted for entirely by the dramatic rise in prevalence, but additionally by the lack of a corresponding growth in access to methadone treatment, even possibly a restriction in access to methadone treatment through public and professional concerns surrounding methadone-related deaths. This phe-nomenon requires further study if it is to be correctly interpreted.

The fifth hypothesis is that there may be an inverse relationship between the number of heroin and methadone-related deaths, with reductions in heroin overdose deaths being partially offset by an increased involvement of methadone in opioid overdose deaths. There is a suggestion, arising from comparisons of mortality in Denmark and Norway, that making methadone freely available reduced overdose deaths among those enrolled in methadone maintenance. If the proportion of opioid-dependent people who are in methadone maintenance is a large enough proportion of all opioid-dependent people in the population, then it may reduce the number of opioid-related deaths. If, however, this is achieved by liberal use of take-away doses, methadone diversion may increase the proportion of opioid overdose deaths that are attributed in whole or part to methadone.

Finally there has been very limited exploration of the contribution that imprisonment and release from imprisonment may play in the overall mortal-ity rate of individuals who are opioid dependent. The week of release from prison has been reported as a period of substantially increased risk (Seaman *et al.* 1998). To date the patterns of short-term imprisonment have not been adequately explored as a possible significant contributory factor to overall methadone and other opioid-related deaths. The foregoing hypotheses should be regarded as being in need of testing as the available data in them-selves are inadequate to provide strong evidence.

Conclusions

Opioid overdose deaths in general, and methadone overdose deaths in par-ticular, have increased and subsequently decreased in the UK over the past decade. The overall rate of opioid overdose deaths in the UK is substantially lower than Australia but the proportion of deaths to which methadone makes a contribution appears to be higher in the UK than Australia; in many cases these deaths occur among illicit opioid users who use diverted methadone. It is difficult to be sure on the basis of available data, but it seems likely that the way in which methadone maintenance, and possibly methadone reduc-tion, are delivered in the UK partly explains the high proportion of UK overdose deaths to which methadone makes a contribution. It is not always possible to distinguish between accidental deaths and suicide but it is likely that at least a small proportion are suicide deaths where methadone is the intentional overdose agent. Such issues need to be considered as part of an overall suicide prevention strategy.

The challenge facing the Health Service in the United Kingdom, as else-where, is to develop a system that maximizes access to methadone treatment for opioid-dependent people while reducing the risk of methadone overdose death from the illicit use of diverted methadone. It is desirable to reduce the diversion and recreational use of methadone, as this seems to be associated with a substantial proportion of opioid overdose mortality. The aim must be to do so in such a way that it does not adversely affect the access of heroin-dependent persons to methadone treatment.

Since the increased focus on methadone-related deaths, there have been a number of policy initiatives ranging from increasing levels of supervised methadone dispensing, increasing the level of supervision in the early phase of treatment, increasing education and training focused on general practitioners and increasing vigilance in the approach to initial methadone induction. There has also been increased attention to the need for education of users and families about the risks of overdose and methods for resuscitation, including methods of assisted respiration and the supply of naloxone to people inducted into methadone treatment. The other key new development is the introduction of buprenorphine for the management of opioid dependence. Mixed agonist–antagonist properties of the drug make it less likely to result in overdose toxicity. If buprenorphine becomes a key agent in the management of opioid dependence it may contribute to a falling opioid-related death rate.

Finally the challenge is to maximize access to good quality treatment, which includes good induction procedures and good monitoring and follow-up procedures that will help to minimize the risk of death.

References

Advisory Council on the Misuse of Drugs (2000) *Reducing Drug Related Deaths.* London: The Stationery Office.

Ball, J.C. & Ross, A. (1991) *The Effectiveness of Methadone maintenance Treatment: Patients, programs, services, and outcomes.* New York: Springer-Verlag.

Barrett, D., Luk, A., Parrish, R. & Jones, T. (1996) An investigation of medical examiner cases in which methadone was detected, Harris County, Texas, 1987–1992. *Journal of Forensic Sciences*, 41: 442–8.

Bentley, A. & Busuttil, A. (1996). Deaths among drug abusers in South-east Scotland (1989–1994). *Medical Science Law*, 36: 231–6.

Cairns, A., Roberts, I.S.D. & Benbow, E.W. (1996) Characteristics of fatal methadone overdose in Manchester, 1985–1994. *British Medical Journal*, 313: 264–5.

Caplehorn, J.R.M. (1998). Deaths in the first two weeks of methadone treatment in NSW in 1994: Identifying cases of iatrogenic methadone toxicity. *Drug and Alcohol Review*, 17: 9–17.

Caplehorn, J.R.M., Dalton, S.Y.N., Haldar, F., Petrenas, A.M. & Nisbet, J.G. (1996) Methadone maintenance and addicts' risk of fatal heroin overdose. *Substance Use and Misuse*, 31: 177–96.

Caplehorn, J.R.M., Dalton, S.Y.N., Cluff, M.C. & Petrenas, A.M. (1994) Retention in methadone maintenance and heroin addicts' risk of death. *Addiction*, 89: 203–7.

Cassidy, M., Curtis, M., Muir, G. & Oliver, J. (1995) Drug abuse deaths in Glasgow in 1992 – a retrospective study. *Medical Science Law*, 35: 207–12.

Chabalko, J., LaRosa, J. & DuPont, R. (1973) Death of methadone users in the District of Columbia. *The International Journal of the Addictions*, 8: 897–908.

Christopherson, O., Rooner, C. & Kelly, S. (1998) Drug-related mortality: methods and trends. *Population Trends*, Autumn: 1–9.

Clark, J.C., Milroy, C.M. & Forrest, A.R.W. (1995) Deaths from methadone use. *Annals of Clinical Forensic Medicine*, 2: 143–4.

Darke, S. & Zador, D. (1996) Fatal heroin overdose: A review. *Addiction*, 91: 1757–64.

Darke, S. & Hall, W. (1995) Levels and correlates of polydrug use among heroin users and regular amphetamine users. *Drug and Alcohol Dependence*, 39: 231–5.

Darke, S., Ross, J. & Hall, W. (1996a) Overdose among heroin users in Sydney, Australia: II. Responses to overdose. *Addiction*, 91: 413–17.

Darke, S., Ross, J. & Hall, W. (1996b) Overdose among heroin users in Sydney, Australia: I. Prevalence and correlates of non-fatal overdose. *Addiction*, 91: 405–11.

Davoli, M., Perucci, C.A., Rapiti, E., Bargagli, A.M., D'Ippoliti, D., Forastiere, F. & Abeni, D. (1997) Persistent rise of mortality of injecting drug users in Rome. *American Journal of Public Health*, 87: 851–3.

De la Fuente, L., Barrio, G., Vicente, J., Bravo, M.J. & Santacreu, J. (1995) The impact of drug related deaths on mortality among young adults in Madrid. *American Journal of Public Health*, 85: 102–5.

Department of Health (1999) *Drug Misuse and Dependence – Guidelines on Clinical Management*. London: The Stationery Office (http//www.doh.gov.uk).

Drummer, O.H., Opeskin, K., Syrjanen, M. & Cordner, S.M. (1992) Methadone toxicity causing death in ten subjects starting on a methadone maintenance program. *The American Journal of Forensic Medicine and Pathology*, 13: 346–50.

Farrell, M., Hawkins, D. & Brettle, R. (2000) Physical complications of drug abuse. In: *The Concise Oxford Textbook of Medicine.* Oxford: Oxford University Publications.

Fountain, J., Griffths, P., Farrell, M., Gossop, M. & Strang, J. (1998) Diversion tactics: how a sample of drug misusers in treatment obtained surplus drugs to sell on the illicit market. *International Journal of Drug Policy*, 9: 159–67.

Gearing, F. R. & Schweitzer, M. D. (1974) An epidemiologic evaluation of long-term methadone maintenance treatment for heroin addiction. *American Journal of Epidemiology,* 100: 101–12.

Gilhooly, T.C. (1997) Reduction in use of temazepam is a factor in deaths related to overdose. *British Medical Journal*, 315: 1463–4.

Gossop, M., Marsden, J. & Stewart, D. (1998) *NTORS at One Year: Changes in substance use, health and criminal behaviour one year after intake.* London: Department of Health.

Greene, M., Brown, B. & DuPont, R. (1975) Controlling the abuse of illicit methadone in Washington, DC. *Archives of General Psychiatry*, 32: 221–6.

Greene, M., Luke, J. & DuPont, R (1974a) Opiate overdose deaths in the District of Columbia. Part II: Methadone related fatalities. *Journal of Forensic Sciences*, 19: 575–84.

Greene, M., Luke, J. & DuPont, R. (1974b) 'Opiate overdose' deaths in the District of Columbia I. Heroin-related fatalities. *Medical Annals of the District of Columbia*, 43: 175–81.

Hammersley, R., Cassidy, M. & Oliver, J. (1995) Drugs associated with drug-related deaths in Edinburgh and Glasgow, November 1990 to October 1992. *Addiction*, 90: 959–65.

Neeleman, J. & Farrell, M., (1997) Fatal methadone and heroin overdoses: time trends in England and Wales. *Journal of Epidemiology and Community Health*, 51: 435–7.

Obafunwa, J. & Busuttil, A. (1994) Deaths from substance overdose in the Lothian and Borders Region of Scotland (1983–1991). *Human & Experimental Toxicology*, 13: 401–6.

Office for National Statistics (2001) Deaths related to drug poisoning: England and Wales, 1995–99. *Health Statistics Quarterly*, 9: 70–2.

Risser, D. & Schneider, B. (1994) Drug related deaths between 1985 and 1992 examined at the Institute of Forensic Medicine in Vienna, Austria. *Addiction*, 89: 851–8.

Sanchez, J., Rodriguez, B., De La Fuenta, L., Barrio, G., Vincente, J., Roca, J., Royuela, L. & the State Information System on Drug Abuse (SIT Working Group) (1995) Opiate and cocaine mortality from acute reactions in six major Spanish cities. *Journal of Epidemiology and Community Health,* 49: 54–60.

Seaman, S. R., Brettle, R. & Gore, S. (1998) Mortality from overdose among injecting drug users recently released from prison: database linkage study. *British Medical Journal*, 316: 426–8.

Steentoft, A., Teige, B., Holmgren, P., Vuori, E., Kristinsson, J., Kaa, E., Wethe, G., Ceder, G., Pikkarainen, J. & Simonsen, K.W. (1996) Fatal poisonings in young drug addicts in the Nordic countries: a comparison between 1984–1985 and 1991. *Forensic Science International*, 78: 29–37.

Swensen, G. (1988) Opioid drug deaths in Western Australia: 1974–1984. *Australian Drug & Alcohol Review*, 7: 181–5.

Ward, J., Mattick, R.P. & Hall, W. (1998) *Methadone Maintenance Treatment and other Opioid Replacement Therapies.* Amsterdam: Harwood Academic Publishers.

White, J. M. & Irvine, R. J. (1999) Mechanisms of fatal opioid overdose. *Addiction*, 94: 961–72.

Williamson, P.A., Foreman, K.J., White, J.M. & Anderson, G. (1997) Methadone-related overdose deaths in South Australia, 1984–1994: How safe is prescribing? *Medical Journal of Australia*, 166: 302–5.

United States Department of Health and Human Services (1997) *Drug Abuse Warning Network. Annual Medical Examiner Data 1995.* Rockville: MD, United States Department of Health and Human Services.

Zador, D., Sunjic, S. & Basili, H. (1998). Deaths in methadone maintenance treatment in New South Wales, 1990–1995. In: Hall W, ed. *Proceedings of an International Opioid Overdose Symposium.* National Drug and Alcohol Research Centre Monograph Number 35. Sydney: National Drug and Alcohol Research Centre.

Zador, D., Sunjic, S. & Darke, S. (1996) Heroin related deaths in New South Wales in 1992. Toxicological findings and circumstances. *Medical Journal of Australia*, 64: 204–7.

15
The play, the plot and the players: the illicit market in methadone

Jane Fountain and John Strang

Largely unseen and extensively unrecognized, there is a substantial illicit market in the UK of diverted supplies of the methadone prescribed to drug users to treat their drug dependence. Methadone ampoules and unconcentrated methadone mixture can both be found on the illicit market. Rarer are methadone tablets, which are infrequently prescribed, and the concentrated methadone mixture which is usually administered under supervision.

The play

Reports of the proportion of drug users in treatment who sell their prescribed drugs range from 5% to 34% (Whynes *et al.* 1989; Parker and Kirby 1996) and studies that ask for the sources of drugs used by misusers support the view that there is a substantial market in diverted prescription drugs (McDermott and McBride 1993).

The data in this chapter derive from a study by Fountain *et al.* (1996; 1998; 1999; 2000) on the use of diverted prescription drugs by chronic drug users and the operation of drugs marketplaces in London where these substances are traded. Qualitative methods were used to gather data from a small number of networks of chronic poly-drug users in several drugs marketplaces. In total, the study involved approximately 100 drug users.

The plot

The diversion of methadone may in principle occur at any point in its manufacture, transportation, delivery, storage, and dispensation. However, studies over many years reveal that drug users in treatment are the primary diverters (Vista Hill Psychiatric Foundation 1974; Burr 1983; Spunt *et al.* 1986; Fountain *et al.* 2000). Sales are conducted by a large number of individuals, each diverting some of their own prescribed drugs (Edmunds *et al.* 1996; Parker and Kirby 1996).

The majority of drug users in treatment who acquire methadone which is surplus to their own requirements use either or both of two methods

(Fountain *et al.* 1998): they obtain prescriptions from more than one drug treatment service ('multiple scripting', often inaccurately known as 'double scripting') and/or they obtain a larger dosage and/or a wider variety of drugs than they use ('overscripting'). Thus they may exaggerate the amount of drugs used in order to obtain a larger prescription for substitutes than needed, use false identities in order to obtain more than one prescription, claim to be a temporary resident to get a 'one off' prescription, or exploit prescribers judged to be 'easy' (Burroughs 1953; McKeganey 1988; Jones and Power 1990; Wheeldon 1992; Seivewright *et al.* 1993; Fountain *et al.* 1998).

There appears to be substantial geographical variation in the type and amount of diverted methadone. Major reasons for this are local prescribing policies, the availability of illicit drugs, and the patterns of drug use of buyers and sellers. Over- and under-supply can occur in the same marketplace on the same day, since trade relies on the surplus supplies of many individual sellers; several individuals collecting two-week supplies of methadone from a pharmacy on the same day can create a glut, but a shortage can quickly follow when it is sold (Burr 1983). As the supply of diverted methadone differs between markets, so does demand. In some markets, methadone is not a marketable commodity (Whynes *et al.* 1989), whilst others trade primarily in it (Edmunds *et al.* 1996).

'Marketplaces' are central to the distribution of diverted methadone, and typically evolve near drug treatment agencies, needle exchanges, and those pharmacies which dispense prescriptions to drug users in treatment. Drug trading hours often reflect those of these agencies (Burr 1983; Jones and Power 1990). In some areas, methadone and illicit drugs are bought and sold in the same marketplace, whilst in others, they are traded in separate locations (Edmunds *et al.* 1996). The legality of ownership of the methadone (i.e. by the named recipient) facilitates the operation of marketplaces where they are traded. Potential buyers and sellers can linger with impunity until the point of sale. It has been reported that the police rarely discover diverted prescription drugs because distribution is contained within networks of drug users trading in personal prescriptions (Parker and Kirby 1996). Marketplaces have shown themselves to be remarkably resilient, and their reaction to disruption has often been simply to relocate nearby (Burr 1983; Edmunds *et al.* 1996).

The price of methadone on the illicit market can fluctuate according to supply and demand, although that for unconcentrated methadone mixture appears to have been stable for many years at £10 per 100 mg. The cost of the larger-than-usual 50 mg methadone ampoules ranges from £8 to £15, and from £4 to £5 for the less widely available 10 mg ampoule. Concentrated methadone mixture and methadone tablets are not available on the illicit market often enough for there to be a standard price. Drawing on data from the London study, it is possible to postulate some general principles about the determinants of the price of methadone on the illicit market:

- Methadone is cheaper than its equivalent in illicitly manufactured heroin.
- Injectable methadone is more expensive than the oral formulations. The relative scarcity of injectables on the illicit market may further add to their cost. In the UK, for example, ten times more prescriptions are written for oral methadone mixture than for injectable methadone ampoules (Strang *et al.* 1996; Strang and Sheridan 1998).
- High dose units are cheaper per mg than low dose units: thus, a 10 mg methadone ampoule can cost as much as £5, whilst a 50 mg ampoule can cost as little as £8 in times of plentiful supply.

The players

The players in the diverted methadone market can be divided into two groups: sellers and buyers. Many switch roles at different times, or play these two roles simultaneously, most often selling their prescribed methadone mixture in order to buy methadone ampoules.

The sellers

Individuals are likely to change their motives for selling their prescribed methadone according to their current drug-using pattern, treatment status and financial situation. A crude typology of sellers consists of the substitutors, the fundraisers, and the retired criminals.

The substitutors
Substitutors are drug users who are receiving treatment with methadone but do not like it and sell it to buy heroin and/or other licit and illicit substances. Examples of this dissatisfaction can be seen in the quotes from the following clients:

> *Sarah: It's awful to not give people what they need. I mean I can't understand the system in a country, where it's supposed to work, and people are given this green liquid and told 'This is enough for you, this is as much as we are going to give'. And these people are having to say 'Yes, thank you, but actually I'm a heroin addict'. I mean it really does not make any sense, does it?*

> *Harriet: ...this green unpleasant-tasting liquid, that is not terribly good for you.*

> *Edward: ...I told them [at the clinic] I was using smack [heroin] and that I wasn't taking any methadone, but...I've ended up with a methadone script, so by rights they've actually given me a methadone habit. I mean, they could have left me on the smack, but [the doctor] said it was too expensive.*

The fundraisers

The fundraisers are drug users receiving private treatment who are raising funds to pay their prescription and dispensing fees. A prescription from a National Health Service practitioner had a standard fee of £5.90 per item (or was free to those on a low income) but the cost of private treatment not only was considerably more but also could vary. In London, where the majority of private treatment was located, the initial consultation and assessment from a private practitioner was typically around £50, plus £25 per week for the consultation that resulted in the prescription. The total cost, depending on the drug, dosage, formulation, and the pharmacy's prices, could reach £125 a week. Herbie and Sally describe how Herbie's private prescriptions could be financed:

> **Herbie:** If I sold the lot I could sell it for, say £550 a week...I pay £100–120 for it – £25 to the doctor, £70 odd...

> **Sally:** ...to the chemist. So it's costing about a hundred pounds a week to actually buy, but the amount [of prescribed drugs] he's getting, he could go and sell easily down the [marketplace] and make triple the amount easily.

> **Herbie:** It works out cheaper than heroin...

> **Sally:** ...he earns enough to, like, cover his script...

> **Herbie:** ...and I end up with a little bit of money in my pocket.

The retired criminals

Some sellers can best be described as retired criminals – drug users in treatment who sell their prescribed drugs rather than commit other crimes to fund their heroin use. Their appearance, physical capabilities, and reputations in local shops means that burglary, mugging and shoplifting are not viable income sources, as explained by these two methadone sellers:

> **Derek:** ...half the people that go to [marketplace] can't go into any of the shops round there...Soon as their faces are seen, the hooter [alarm] goes off – they are that well-known. That did happen to me when I went into Superdrug once...I was told never to go in there again. Another time, my mate went in there and I waited outside, but they recognised me from outside and knew that I was with him, so then they slung him out.

> **Mike:** ...with a list [criminal record] as long as my arm, my sentences are going up and up and up, so I'm trying not to do any thieving now...I'm not really a violent person – I don't want to be going out mugging and stuff like that...

The buyers

The unknown and variable impurity and the high cost of illicit heroin means that some (but probably not the majority of) drug users prefer methadone, although, as discussed shortly, buyers of diverted methadone usually use it in combination with other drugs to obtain the desired effect. An additional significant attraction of methadone to the purchaser is that it is manufactured in standard doses in recognizable packaging.

The buyers of diverted methadone do not generally use the drug (particularly the oral formulation) for its pleasurable effects. Rather, its main roles in poly-drug-using repertoires are as a cheap, safe and pure medication to reduce withdrawal symptoms and as a base for drug cocktails (Lauzon *et al.* 1994; Chatham *et al.* 1995; Rettig and Yarmolinsky 1995). Combinations, about which the user may be discerning or not, can include methadone and other prescribed opioids, illegally-manufactured drugs (such as heroin and cocaine), alcohol, cyclizine, benzodiazepines, and stimulants (cocaine, amphetamine sulphate, and dexamphetamine sulphate). Some respondents in the London study expressed a great deal of enthusiasm for experimenting with different combinations of substances.

In the UK, the most economical method for a drug user to obtain methadone is to get an NHS prescription. As described above, if the prescribed dosage is less than they are trying to obtain, then overscripting or multiple scripting is another 'cost-free' option. If yet more methadone is sought, two options exist: to buy it on the illicit market, or to obtain a private prescription, which is more likely to be for the preferred variety, dosage, and formulation (Strang *et al.* 2001; *Pharmaceutical Journal* 1997). The latter is the cheaper option if an individual can secure a sufficiently large dose to make re-sale realistic in order to raise the necessary fees: for example, in London, the cost of a private prescription for four 50 mg methadone ampoules per day (a frequently prescribed amount) is around £100 per week. On the illicit market, these would cost £224–£420. However, some drug misusers could not accumulate the initial £100 as the single sum every week. An alternative is to buy from the illicit market several times a week, according to the cash available, where they can obtain single ampoules at £8–£15 each.

Patterns of use of diverted methadone are varied. They range from regular and heavy use, to occasional use as a 'treat', an experiment, or in an emergency such as buying methadone to avoid withdrawal symptoms when no heroin is available. Thus buyers are not necessarily regular and the amounts of methadone purchased from the illicit market vary from a single dose of methadone occasionally to two weeks' supply regularly. In addition, an individual is likely to change his or her reasons for purchasing methadone according to their current drug-using pattern, treatment status, and financial situation. Bearing these differences in mind, methadone buyers can be categorized as the supplementers, the treatment avoiders and the substitutors.

The notion that those who buy methadone on the illicit market are engaged in self-treatment is then also considered.

The supplementers

An insufficient dose (real or perceived) of methadone can occur at the start of treatment, particularly if the addict has high expectations that it will address all of their drug needs and will stop cravings for other drugs (Dole *et al.* 1966; Preston 1996). It can also occur during treatment, if the dosage is reduced too quickly and if tolerance to the drugs prescribed – and/or those used in addition – increases. Two supplementers explain:

> **Paul:** ...they don't believe the amount of drugs you can take these days...like when I first got registered...I had to sit in a room with [drugs worker] whilst I did the crossword in The Mirror, The Star etc. I had to take these drugs all at once in case I went clunk. Obviously I didn't. It wasn't half the amount that I wanted or needed. I don't get stoned off my prescription – it just keeps the wolf from the door.

> **Edward:** ...it's a vicious circle in one way, because they don't give out enough for a start. A lot of people are driven onto the streets [to buy extra drugs] from these demands that the clinics make.

The treatment avoiders

There are several reasons why those who are drug dependent and buy diverted prescription drugs do not arrange their own prescriptions. These include an unwillingness – especially of women with children – to submit to official attention, and their experiences from previous treatment episodes which have left them disillusioned with services (McKeganey 1988; Sheehan *et al.* 1988; Stimson *et al.* 1995; Department of Health 1996; Powis *et al.* 1996). Harriet is one of these:

> I would never get registered because I didn't want my name down on any government list – that's another very common thing especially with organized junkies who have got a straight job, like a nurse or something like that, because of all the prejudices that go with it. The reason I don't want my name down on that list is partly because I do want a reasonably straight job – that's why I'm doing my degree – and also for my child. As soon as you say 'junkie' you become a bad, irresponsible parent in the eyes of everybody, even people that should know better like doctors etcetera. I didn't tell them when I was pregnant that I was using. I came off on my own rather than say that, because I knew the minute that I said I was using, my name would be put down on the lists, and my child's name would be put down.

The substitutors

NHS drug treatment services are reluctant to prescribe injectable formulations to drug users in treatment, and successive government documents have emphasized the caution that should be associated with the prescribing of such injectable drugs (Advisory Council on the Misuse of Drugs 1993; Department of Health 1991; 1999). However, this policy stimulates demand from the illicit market for injectable methadone, even though buyers may already be receiving a prescribed supply of the same drug in an oral form. The prescription of the client below had been changed from an injectable to an oral formulation of methadone:

Interviewer: So you haven't got any amps on a script now, then?

Maurice: No, but I can get them. But I don't get them legally...That's what I said to them up there [at the clinic] – 'You're just defeating the object. You stop my amps so I just go out and buy brown [heroin] or I go and buy amps off of someone else.'

The self-treaters?

It has been suggested that some of those buying diverted methadone are engaged in self-treatment (Langrod *et al.* 1974; Spunt *et al.* 1986; Gossop *et al.* 1991) and that the benefits of prescription drugs are therefore reaching an out-of-treatment population. However, 'self-treatment' suggests that users are embracing the same therapeutic objectives and are mimicking the therapeutically based decisions of treatment agencies. The supratherapeutic amounts and the combinations of prescription drugs used by some who buy them on the illicit market are not generally purchased with such therapeutic objectives, and would not be available to them in these forms and doses via legitimate treatment sources (Ruben and Morrison 1992; Seivewright and Dougal 1993; Strang *et al.* 1993). Nevertheless, some users of diverted prescription drugs have assimilated the harm reduction advice emanating from drug treatment services and disseminated by the drug users' grapevine. Ironically, the knowledge that illicit drugs and injecting are dangerous probably increases the demand for the 'safer' methadone from the illicit market (Edmunds *et al.* 1996).

The finale

It is generally accepted that some diversion of drugs prescribed to drug users in treatment is unavoidable (Department of Health 1996), and the literature on diversion control argues that the energy and ingenuity which some drug users devote to obtaining drugs to divert can thwart control attempts unless all avenues are closed simultaneously (National Institute on Drug Abuse 1993). When restrictions are placed on only one substance or one source of supply, buyers may find a substitute or experiment with new combinations of drugs or routes of administration to achieve the desired effect (Klee *et al.* 1990; Strang *et al.* 1992; 1993; Fountain *et al.* 1999).

Implicit in the UK *Guidelines on Clinical Management* (Department of Health 1999) is the notion that good prescribing practice minimizes diversion.

However, when substitute prescribing is included as an option for treating drug users, the level of concern and decisions made about the potential for diversion depend on whether the policy-making community is more concerned with treating addicts than preventing them selling drugs. However difficult, the objective should be the identification of the most health-conferring balance between caution against overprescribing (despite the possibility that the patient may sell the surplus on the illicit market) and caution against underprescribing (and maybe prompting the patient to 'top up' from the illicit market). The application of this balanced judgement is the challenge.

Acknowledgement

The study and literature review from which the data for this paper were taken were funded by the Department of Health, England. The views expressed, however, are those of the authors.

Some sections of this chapter were first published in Fountain, J., Strang, J., Gossop, M., Farrell, M. & Griffiths, P. (2000) Diversion of prescribed drugs by drug users in treatment: analysis of the UK market and new data from London. *Addiction*, 95: 393–406.

References

Advisory Council on the Misuse of Drugs (1993) *AIDS and Drug Misuse Report: Update.* London: HMSO.

Burr, A. (1983) Increased sale of opiates on the black market in the Piccadilly area. *British Medical Journal*, 287: 883–885.

Burroughs, W. (1953) *Junky.* London: Penguin.

Chatham, L.R., Rowan-Szal, G.A., Joe, G.W., Brown, B.S. & Simpson, D.D. (1995) Heavy drinking in a population of methadone-maintained clients. *Journal of Studies on Alcohol*, 56: 417–22.

Department of Health (1999) *Drug Misuse and Dependence – Guidelines on Clinical Management.* London: The Stationery Office.

Department of Health (1996) *The Task Force to Review Services for Drug Misusers, Report of an independent review of drug treatment services in England.* London: Department of Health.

Department of Health (1991) *Drug Misuse and Dependence, Guidelines on Clinical Management.* London: HMSO.

Dole, V.P., Nyswander, M.E. & Kreek, M.J. (1966) Narcotic blockade. *Archives of Internal Medicine*, 118: 304–9.

Edmunds, M., Hough, M. & Urquia, N. (1996) *Tackling Local Drug Markets*, Crime Detection and Prevention Series Paper 80. London: Home Office Police Research Group.

Fountain, J., Strang, J., Gossop, M., Farrell, M. & Griffiths, P. (2000) Diversion of prescribed drugs by drug users in treatment: analysis of the UK market and new data from London. *Addiction*, 95: 393–406.

Fountain, J., Griffiths, P., Farrell, M., Gossop, M. & Strang, J. (1999) Benzodiazepines in polydrug-using repertoires: the impact of the decreased availability of temazepam gel-filled capsules. *Drugs: Education, Prevention and Policy*, 6: 61–9.

Fountain, J., Griffiths, P., Farrell, M., Gossop, M. & Strang, J. (1998) Diversion tactics: how a sample of drug misusers in treatment obtained surplus drugs to sell on the illicit market. *International Journal of Drug Policy*, 9: 159–67.

Fountain, J., Griffiths, P., Farrell, M., Gossop, M. & Strang, J. (1996) *A Qualitative Study of Patterns of Prescription Drug Use amongst Chronic Drug Users.* Report prepared for the Department of Health. London: National Addiction Centre.

Gossop, M., Battersby, M. & Strang, J. (1991) Self-detoxification by opiate addicts: a preliminary investigation. *British Journal of Psychiatry,* 159: 208–12.

Jones, S. & Power, R. (1990) Observation to Intervention: drug trends in West London. *International Journal of Drug Policy*, 2: 13–15.

Klee, H., Faugier, J., Hayes, C., Boulton, T. & Morris, J. (1990) AIDS-related risk behaviour, polydrug use and temazepam. *British Journal of Addiction*, 85: 1125–32.

Langrod, J., Galanter, M. & Lowinson, J. (1974) Illicit methadone abuse. In: Senay E, Shorty V, Alksne H, eds. *Developments in the Field of Drug Abuse*; National Drug Abuse Conference, 1974. Cambridge Massachusetts, Schenkman; 461–6.

Lauzon, P., Vincelette, J., Bruneau, J., Lamothe, F., Lachance, N., Brabant, N. & Solo, J. (1994) Illicit use of methadone among IV drug users in Montreal. *Journal of Substance Abuse Treatment*, 11: 457–61.

McDermott, P. & McBride, W. (1993) Crew 2000: peer coalition in action. *Druglink*, 8: 13–14.

McKeganey, N. (1988) Shadowland: general practitioners and the treatment of opiate abusing patients. *British Journal of Addiction*, 83: 373–86.

National Institute on Drug Abuse (1993) *Impact of Prescription Drug Diversion Control Systems on Medical Practice and Patient Care, NIDA Research Monograph 131*. Rockville Maryland: National Institute on Drug Abuse.

Parker, H. & Kirby, P. (1996) *Methadone Maintenance and Crime Reduction on Merseyside*. Crime Detection and Prevention Series Paper 72. London: Home Office Police Research Group.

Pharmaceutical Journal (1997) News item. Volume 259, July 26.

Powis, B., Griffiths, P., Gossop, M. & Strang, J. (1996) The differences between male and female drug users: community samples of heroin and cocaine users compared. *Substance Use and Misuse*, 31: 529–43.

Preston, A. (1996) *The Methadone Briefing.* London: ISDD.

Rettig, R.A. & Yarmolinsky, A. (eds) (1995) *Federal Regulation of Methadone Treatment*. Washington DC: National Academy Press.

Ruben, S.M. & Morrison, C.L. (1992) Temazepam misuse in a group of injecting drug misusers. *British Journal of Addiction*, 87: 1387–92.

Seivewright, N. & Dougal, W. (1993) Withdrawal symptoms from high dose benzodiazepines in poly drug users. *Drug and Alcohol Dependence*, 32: 13–23.

Seivewright, N., Donmall, D. & Daly, C. (1993) Benzodiazepines in the illicit drugs scene: the UK picture and some treatment dilemmas. *International Journal of Drug Policy*, 4: 42–8.

Sheehan, M., Oppenheimer, E. & Taylor, C. (1988) Who comes for treatment?: drug misusers at 3 London agencies. *British Journal of Addiction*, 83: 311–20.

Spunt, B., Hunt, D.E., Lipton, D.S., Goldsmith, D.S. (1986) Methadone diversion: a new look. *Journal of Drug Issues*, 16: 569–83.

Stimson, G.V., Hayden, D., Hunter, G., Metrebian, N., Rhodes, T., Turnbull, P. & Ward, J. (1995) *Drug Users' Help-Seeking and Views of Services*, A report prepared for The Task Force to Review Services for Drug Misusers. London: Department of Health.

Strang, J. & Sheridan, J. (2001) Private prescribing of methadone to addicts:

comparison with NHS practice in the south east of England. *Addiction*, 96: 567–77.

Strang, J. & Sheridan, J. (1998) National and regional characteristics of methadone prescribing in England and Wales: local analyses of data from the 1995 survey of community pharmacies. *Journal of Substance Misuse*, 3: 240–6.

Strang, J., Sheridan, J. & Barber, N. (1996) Prescribing injectable and oral methadone to opiate addicts: results from the 1995 national postal survey of community pharmacies in England and Wales. *British Medical Journal*, 313: 270–2.

Strang, J., Seivewright, N. & Farrell, M. (1993) Oral and intravenous abuse of benzodiazepines. In: Hallstrom C, ed. *Benzodiazepine Dependence*. Oxford: Oxford University Press; 129–42.

Strang, J., Seivewright, N. & Farrell, M. (1992) Intravenous and other abuses of benzodiazepines: The opening of Pandora's box? *British Journal of Addiction*, 87: 1373–5.

Vista Hill Psychiatric Foundation (VHPF) (1974) Methadone diversion. *Drug Abuse and Alcoholism Newsletter*, 3: 4.

Wheeldon, N.M. (1992) Wolff-Parkinson-White syndrome mimicking myocardial infarction on ECG-exploitation by a heroin addict. *British Journal of Clinical Psychology*, 46: 269–70.

Whynes, D.K., Bean, P.T., Giggs, J.A. & Wilkinson, C. (1989) Managing drug use. *British Journal of Addiction*, 84: 533–40.

Section E: Service delivery

16
A primary care based specialist service

Susanna Lawrence

St Martins Practice is an inner city group practice in Chapeltown, Leeds. The Addiction Service is a stand-alone service operating within the general practice setting, delivering care to 100–150 problem drug users per annum. The vast majority of clients attend for management of opiate addiction, and substitute prescribing of methadone is widely employed. All clients are registered with the practice for general medical services, as are family members in many cases.

The addiction team combines full-time specialist staff with members of the primary care team who commit a proportion of their working week to the Addiction Service. The two services are closely integrated. The model effectively combines the accessibility and holism of primary care with some of the treatment benefits of specialized care. The service model is an appropriate choice for areas of high drug using activity, such as exist in any city and many rural areas. In 2000, the practice was awarded Beacon status for its Addiction Service.

Background to the service

In the mid-1980s, one of our patients was diagnosed HIV positive. He was (and still is) an intravenous drug user, and chose to confide in his family doctor. In consultation with the local specialist service, he commenced prescribed methadone, dietary supplements, and clean needle exchange. Word got around, other drug users booked appointments to come and discuss their drug use, and the foundations of the St Martins Practice Addiction Service were laid.

Chapeltown has a long-standing reputation as the centre of the illegal drug trade for the city and has all the familiar hallmarks of inner city deprivation. The Index of Social Conditions held by the Department of the Environment places Chapel Allerton Ward (which includes Chapeltown) amongst the 10% most deprived wards in the country. Jarman indicators scoring high are single parent status, unskilled and unemployed, overcrowding and ethnicity. 1991 Census information defines the Chapeltown population as 50% white, 20% African Caribbean, 25% Asian; at least 11 different ethnic communities co-exist alongside one another. The age distribution of residents is skewed to the left, with 56% of the population under 30 years of age, compared with 41% for the whole of Leeds.

The health profile of the locality is predictable: there is a high incidence of mental illness, teenage pregnancy, and smoking-related diseases, as well as drug and alcohol misuse. Premature death from coronary heart disease is amongst the highest in the city. Primary care is thus under considerable pressure to deliver services to a mobile, heterogeneous population with high levels of morbidity, and significant language and cultural differences. The primary health care workforce within Chapeltown is unusual for a deprived locality, in that there are adequate numbers of general practitioners (GPs) (a large proportion single handed), although recruitment of nursing and administrative staff can be difficult. There has been little enthusiasm for managing drug misuse in primary care, with lack of capacity for managing both clinical and behavioural problems cited as the main objections.

St Martins Practice has much in common with other local practices, providing health care to a representative practice population in a challenging environment exacerbated by historic under-resourcing. There are also some differences. Owing to various circumstances (including two arson attacks) the partnership was forced to undergo rapid change in the early 1990s. Over a period of just a few years, the practice population doubled in size, and the partnership grew from two to six doctors. This rapid expansion allowed us to create a partnership that was unusually ideologically aligned. The practice has a history of innovation and attracts health professionals who actively choose to work in the inner city. There is a commitment to flexible working and creating a healthy working environment, as a consequence the practice enjoys a higher retention rate than can generally be expected in a deprived area.

St Martins has a practice philosophy created and owned by all members of the practice team, whether clinical or administrative. Of relevance to our work with substance misusers is the open door policy of accepting all patients within our practice area irrespective of need, health or social circumstance. Before the Addiction Service was formally created, a significant number of patients with problem drug use were registered with the practice, receiving general medical services. This situation reflected the view of the practice team that drug misusers had equal rights of access to appropriate primary health care, regardless of whether or where they were receiving treatment for their addiction. With commitment from all members of the practice team, the management of problem drug use gradually became incorporated into the provision of general health care. Protocols of care have been developed for harm minimization interventions, substitute prescribing, detoxification regimens, and relapse prevention. The service has become increasingly standardized and broadened out to include related areas of health care: management of pregnant drug users, child protection, hepatitis B and C and sexual health.

In 1996, the service was formally recognized by the Health Authority as a secondary care addiction service delivered in a primary care setting, according to government guidelines (Department of Health 1999). The guidelines support the provision of secondary care within general practice where it is more convenient for the patient, cost effective, safe, and of a recognized standard. The GPs are required to have relevant experience, to co-operate with approval and audit processes, and to deliver a service that is complementary to General Medical Services. The contract is locally determined; the St Martins Addiction Service is contracted to deliver care solely to patients currently registered with St Martins Practice. The Addiction Service workforce is made up of members of the practice team, both administrative and clinical, in addition to a full-time addiction therapist. Essentially the Addiction Service and the practice are two different agencies but deliver care to the same population, by the same workforce, in the same building. The workload of the addiction service is relatively stable, with around 100 clients in active treatment at any one time: about 2% of the practice population. A balance exists between the two services, which suggests that this is the optimum proportion: the volume of addiction clients is both big enough to benefit from a specialist workforce and small enough to co-exist alongside the general population without compromising either service.

Description of the service

The St Martins model aims to combine the attributes of a specialist service and primary care to deliver a safe, manageable and clinically effective service. The health care interventions are tailored to address the hierarchy of treatment goals as defined by the Advisory Council on the Misuse of Drugs (Advisory Council on the Misuse of Drugs 1984; 1993). Thus, while the absolute goal of abstinence is held for all patients, interventions are chosen to reflect the patient's clinical condition.

All patients who disclose drug use receive harm reduction and health promotion interventions. As far as possible these interventions are offered at the first consultation, in the knowledge that this may be the patient's only contact with the service. Further goals regarding stabilisation and reduction of drug use, and subsequently detoxification, abstinence and relapse prevention, are agreed following a comprehensive assessment of the patient's clinical and social needs, knowledge, expectations, and motivators for changing their drug using behaviour.

In the course of the assessment, which is regarded as a process rather than an event, formal recognition is given to the need to establish a therapeutic relationship as a key intervention in maximizing outcomes. Safety and authenticity are addressed through urine toxicology analysis and confirmation of involvement from other agencies. Prochaska and DiClemente's transtheoretical model of change (Prochaska and DiClemente 1984) is employed to assess the client's current status, inform the treatment plan and identify appropriate interventions. The client and addiction therapist establish a treatment agreement, which includes operational details such as appropriate use of emergency appointments, as well as substitute prescribing. Health promotion and harm reduction interventions include immunization against hepatitis B, screening for hepatitis B and C, general health promotion (nutrition, dentition), advice regarding safer sex and safer injecting, and free condoms. Close liaison with the local hepatology unit ensures continuity and access for investigation and treatment of patients diagnosed hepatitis C positive.

The co-existence of the Addiction Service alongside general practice offers maximum opportunity for immediate intervention following disclosure, and minimizes duplication of effort. All members of the clinical team are involved in recruiting patients into the Addiction Service, and indeed initiate the work with the client. A single set of records is kept, incorporating the easily identifiable addiction assessment and treatment record alongside the general clinical notes. Tasks identified are allocated as shown in Table 16.1.

Table 16.1 Allocation of assessment and treatment tasks.*

Appointment	Task	Team member
First contact (opportunistic or patient request)	Establish help seeking request Outline drug history Harm reduction – safer injecting, safer sex, hepatitis screening and immunization Obtain urine sample Request proof of address Obtain permission to contact previous clinician	Practice nurse (new patient health check or other contact) GP Midwife/health visitor/district nurse/addiction therapist
Assessment interview	Detailed drug history Current health problems Social history Client's treatment goals Motivators for change Formulation of management plan Treatment agreement Follow-up health promotion	Addiction therapist
Subsequent appointments	Update Review treatment goals Appropriate therapeutic intervention	Initially weekly with addiction therapist Weekly or fortnightly with prescribing doctor As needed with doctor for general medical services

* Reproduced from Lawrence 2000, *Drugs: Education, Prevention and Policy*.

Pharmacological and psychological interventions are integrated to provide a package of care, delivered by GP and addiction therapist, designed to maximize treatment outcomes (Carroll 1997). The majority of clients receive a treatment package equivalent to the 'standard methadone service' described by McClellan *et al.* (1993): methadone plus counselling. A few clients (less than 5% of opiate users) receive long-term methadone maintenance with minimal psycho-social support, if the more intensive approach has failed to secure a reduction in opiate use.

In order to meet the needs of a population that is geographically, rather than clinically, selected, it is important that the service is able to accommodate a wide range of health care needs. The client group includes chaotic drug users, experimenters, pregnant and young users, patients with co-morbidity. Non-drug users also benefit: family members, carers, and abstinent former drug users are invited to use the service.

The success of the service relies on a fairly strict adherence to protocols. The protocols not only address aspects of prescribing, but also require that each step of the management plan is negotiated and agreed with the client. Substitute prescribing is commenced only once the client has been fully assessed, and urine toxicology tests confirm opiate use. Methadone mixture is the only substitute opioid prescribed for stabilization and maintenance, and daily supervised consumption is the norm. The maximum starting dose is 40 mg methadone/day. Lost or stolen prescriptions are not replaced under any circumstances. Clients who are prescribed methadone are stabilized on the minimum dose necessary to prevent withdrawal symptoms; most clients achieve stability on methadone doses of 30–60 mg/day, and the average daily dose of methadone is 40 mg. Higher 'blocking' doses are occasionally prescribed for clients with a history of heavy street opioid use or those with high-risk behaviours associated with drug use.

Once stabilization of drug use is achieved, social needs such as housing, employment, finances and child care are focused on, as well as general health care, such as nutrition, contraception and dental treatment. Detoxification is delayed until there is agreement by therapist, client and carers that the client has adequately prepared. Three different detoxification regimens are employed: methadone reduction, dihydrocodeine crossover and reduction, and symptomatic management. The choice is governed largely by patient preference, and is always negotiated. An agreed, small formulary of drugs is used for symptomatic treatment (including lofexidine); all benzodiazepines except chlordiazepoxide are avoided.

The clinical effectiveness of treatment is measured using a range of treatment outcomes, which include both hard and soft data (see Chapter 6 for further discussion of outcome measures). A great emphasis is placed on client-defined treatment goals, and outcomes are measured against the goal of interventions employed (see Table 16.2).

A total of 133 clients (generating 153 treatment episodes) attended the programme in the year 1997–1998. The mean duration of engagement with

Table 16.2 Treatment goals and outcome measures.*

Treatment goals	Treatment outcome measures
Harm reduction	Cessation of intravenous drug use Modification of injecting behaviour Death
Health promotion	Hepatitis B immunization Hepatitis C status Safer sex Increased understanding re drug use
Stabilization of drug use	Controlled drug use Improved social relationships New employment
Maintenance on prescribed medication	Reported cessation of problem drug use Negative urine toxicology Reduction of prescribed dose
Detoxification	Cessation of substitute prescribing Cessation of drug misuse
Abstinence	Drug-free after one, three and six months

* Reproduced from Lawrence 2000, *Drugs: Education, Prevention and Policy*.

the service was 11 months. The male:female ratio was 3:1; less than 20% of the cohort were from minority ethnic groups. A total of 117 (88% of the cohort) identified opiates as a problem drug; just over half of these injected drugs. All these clients received harm minimization interventions, including information and counselling regarding safer injecting and hepatitis/HIV screening. Seventy-nine per cent agreed to hepatitis C screening; of these 61% were hepatitis C positive. Sixty-eight clients (51.1%) achieved initial treatment goals; 49 (36.8%) underwent successful detoxification and achieved abstinence. Follow-up through the abstinence phase is predictably inconsistent, but approximately half those undergoing detoxification attended for relapse prevention, and continued to be drug free. Fourteen (10.5%) did not achieve any defined goal.

Twenty-one (15.7%) patients were removed from treatment: 17 went into custody, 4 were asked to leave following criminal behaviour (forging prescriptions, selling methadone). All remained on the practice list for general medical care. Two patients died whilst on the programme: one from natural causes, one from a drugs overdose.

The bigger picture – an integrated approach to service delivery

It is the volume of demand for Addiction Services that has driven the political agenda to advocate the development of addiction services within primary care (Department of Health 1996). The clinical needs of the client group, however, also support this model. First, methadone treatment in general practice can be as safe and effective as for patients in a specialist setting (Gossop *et al.* 1999; Weinrich and Stuart 2000). In addition, the style of primary care services is well suited to the delivery of addiction services in general and methadone treatment in particular. The care of drug misusers echoes that of other relapsing and remitting conditions, such as asthma, where effective primary care management is executed by a multidisciplinary team offering health promotion, harm reduction, and the medical management of the chronic condition and the acute exacerbation. The longitudinal continuity and ready access offered by primary care suits the needs of the drug using client group (Cabinet Office 1998) and the skills employed in the management of drug misuse, such as motivational interviewing, are equally applicable to any other area of health promotion.

The social inclusion agenda, central to the government's white paper *The New NHS* (Wilson *et al.* 1995) and NHS National Plan (Department of Health 1998), is advanced by the integration or co-existence of addiction services within primary care. Service user feedback at St Martins specifically cites the anonymity, convenience and safety of using a primary care based service. However, it is not just the addiction clients who derive benefit: the quality of general practice is improved. Routine questioning at each new patient health check informs every new client that addiction and violence are recognized as valid health issues. One of the unrecognized strengths of primary care based addiction services is the added value reaped by family members, particularly children. Child health and child protection issues can be raised informally and problems identified early.

In the main, the limitations of the model are those experienced by any specialist service delivered in the locality setting: restriction of patient choice and professional isolation. The St Martins model offers a more restricted range of treatment options than that available in a specialist setting, and issues such as preferred gender of therapist cannot be addressed. Particularly difficult behaviour, usually violence, results in the exclusion of the occasional client from the scheme due to the relative vulnerability of staff working in a primary care setting. Professional isolation is significant: the primary care team relies on professional support to be delivered across disciplines, and it is vital that addiction therapists working in primary care create external links with their own professional group.

Wider changes across the city

No addiction service can operate effectively in isolation from other agencies. At St Martins Practice this was recognized early on, and good relationships were established with other specialist organizations. During the formative years of the service, most of the team attended training courses at the specialist NHS addiction agency, the Leeds Addiction Unit, establishing many common core principles of clinical practice. This has proved to be an excellent basis on which to shape future collaborative working between the two organizations. The success of the working relationship relies on common beliefs – namely that primary care based services are safe, effective and necessary, that a consistent approach is required throughout the city of Leeds, and that adequate training of primary care clinicians is the route to establishing such services.

Representatives from the two organizations have worked together on two major service development initiatives led by the Health Authority: the Leeds GP shared care training scheme and the Leeds Addiction Treatment Strategy. Indeed, there is opportunity for further collaboration, for instance in developing a consistent approach to treatment outcomes, developing a city-wide research and development agenda, disseminating and evaluating new treatment options.

Initially, the impact of the St Martins model on primary care across the city was slow, and arguably counterproductive. St Martins was viewed locally as a maverick practice, possibly allowing other practices to dismiss the care of drug users as anomalous, rather than a necessary component of inner city primary health care. Although the St Martins Addiction Service has been adequately funded now for several years, the willingness of the St Martins team to do the work as part of core general practice disenfranchized some local practices who saw it as breaking ranks with grass roots political opinion. In addition, the commitment to take all comers within the practice area allowed other local GPs to opt out by directing addicted patients to the Practice. St Martins was also slow to engage with the few other practices across the city who were managing addiction patients. The change came about in the mid-1990s, when the Health Authority initiated the development of a shared care training scheme for GPs across the city. The three-day training module was designed with major input from St Martins and the Leeds Addiction Unit, and equips GPs to deliver a standardized methadone programme with the support of an addiction therapist employed and supervised by the Leeds Addiction Unit. There is a strong emphasis during the training of recognizing the realities of general practice, and an expanding network of participating practices across the city. Nominated pharmacists within the city supervise methadone consumption, minimizing street diversion and maximizing compliance and benefits (Hutchison *et al.* 2000).

In more recent years, a second primary care service has been contracted by the Health Authority to deliver a secondary care addiction service. A range of service models in primary care has thus developed across Leeds, allowing for different levels of interest, expertise and capacity to be accommodated, whilst delivering an increasingly standardized package of care across the city. This approach underpins the Leeds Addiction Treatment Strategy, which aims to offer a consistent quality of care to drug users regardless of the point of contact. The city-wide strategy identifies the St Martins model as appropriate for areas of high drug usage within the city. It is envisaged that a third 'hotspot' service will be developed, that areas of intermediate usage are covered by the shared care scheme, and areas of low usage serviced by outreach locality clinics from the Leeds Addiction Unit. This is a fine example of collaborative working that also goes outside the NHS.

And for the future...

The advent of primary care groups and trusts creates new structures for developing consistency of care. There are possibilities for primary care trusts to commission specialist services, such as addiction services, from primary care providers within the locality. The St Martins model could also be adapted to deliver addiction services to patients registered with other local GPs in the locality. Whilst this application addresses the variation in commitment within primary care, it is important to recognize that the considerable benefits of integrating the individual client's addiction services with their general health care would be lost if the model were applied in this way. Sexual health and hepatitis screening are obvious examples, but less tangible issues such as social inclusion, family health, opportunistic follow-up are arguably of equal or greater importance. Nonetheless, it is vital for the development of effective networked services that primary care groups and trusts design mechanisms for delivering the national agenda. Addiction is a health inequalities issue, and has been identified as such in the national plan. The St Martins model could be best utilized as one of a range of service configurations that take into account the geographic distribution of drug using populations. A stand-alone service within primary care is appropriate for areas of high activity, and effectively addresses the service need whilst protecting the health care needs of the general population. The risk of overwhelming general practice by a group of high demand patients is minimized by offering a dedicated addiction service, and the benefits of integrated care are preserved.[1]

References

Advisory Council on the Misuse of Drugs (1993) *AIDS and Drug Misuse Update Report.* London: HMSO.

Advisory Council on the Misuse of Drugs (1984) *Prevention.* London: HMSO.

Cabinet Office (1998) *Tackling Drugs to Build a Better Britain: The Government's Ten-Year Strategy for Tackling Drugs Misuse.* London: The Stationery Office.

Carroll, K.M. (1997) Integrating psychotherapy and pharmacotherapy to improve drug abuse outcomes. *Addictive Behaviors,* 22: 233–45.

Department of Health (1999) *Drug Misuse and Dependence – Guidelines on Clinical Management.* London: The Stationery Office.

Department of Health (1998) *The New NHS: Modern, Dependable.* London: The Stationery Office.

[1]Data included in this chapter were originally presented in Lawrence (2000).

Department of Health (1996) Health Service Guidelines 96/31: *A National Framework for the Provision of Secondary Care within General Practice.* London: The Stationery Office.

Gossop, M., Marsden, J., Stewart, D., Lehmann, P. & Strang, J. (1999) Methadone treatment practices and outcome for opiate addicts treated in drug clinics and in general practice: results from the National Treatment Outcome Research Study. *British Journal of General Practice,* 49: 31–4.

Hutchinson, S.J., Taylor, A., Gruer, L., Barr, C., Elliot, L., Goldberg, D.J., Scott, R. & Gilchrist, G. (2000) One-year follow-up of opiate injectors treated with oral methadone in a GP-centred programme. *Addiction,* 95: 1055–68.

Lawrence, S. (2000) Models of Primary Care for Substance Misusers: St Martins Practice, Chapeltown, Leeds – secondary provision in a primary care setting. *Drugs: Education, Prevention and Policy,* 7: 279–91.

McClellan, A.T., Arndt, I.O., Metzger, D.S., Woody, G.E. & O'Brien, C.P. (1993) The effects of psychosocial services in substance abuse treatment. *Journal of the American Medical Association,* 269: 1953–9.

Prochaska, J. & DiClemente, C. (1984) *The Transtheoretical Approach: Crossing the Traditional Boundaries of Therapy.* Homewood, Illinois: Dow Jones-Irwin.

Weinrich, M. & Stuart, M. (2000) Provision of methadone treatment in primary care Medical Practices. *Journal of the American Medical Association,* 283: 1343–8.

Wilson, P., Watson, R. & Ralston, G.E. (1995) Supporting problem drug users: improving methadone maintenance in general practice. *British Journal of General Practice,* 45: 454–5.

17

A central assessment service with widely disseminated delivery in primary care

Fiona Watson, Linda Mays and Judy Bury

Introduction

Since the mid-1980s, government policy has been to encourage primary care physicians' (general practitioners' (GPs')) involvement in the care of drug users. In 1993 a report from the Advisory Council on the Misuse of Drugs (Advisory Council on the Misuse of Drugs 1993) emphasized the central role of GPs again but noted that there was little evidence of any significant increase in the number becoming involved in this work. Studies that have found GPs to be reluctant to work with drug users (e.g. Glanz 1986; McKeganey and Boddy 1988; Clarke 1993), also suggest they may be more willing if support were available (Glanz 1986). McKeganey and Boddy stress the need to explore other approaches to client management such as the use of practice policies (McKeganey and Boddy 1988), whereas Clarke emphasized the importance of training for GPs (Clarke 1993), as did the 1993 Advisory Council on the Misuse of Drugs report.

The recently published *Guidelines on Clinical Management* (Department of Health 1999) state that shared care is a rational model to improve service delivery, utilizing different skills in the most effective manner. This document also states that medical practitioners should not prescribe in isolation but should seek to liaise with other professionals who will be able to help with factors contributing to an individual's drug misuse and that a multidisciplinary approach is essential.

An outline is given of the methods used in Lothian to harness the enthusiasm of GPs to care for drug users by sharing care between themselves and a statutory drug service. The usefulness of facilitation by a specialist team in ensuring that GPs remain committed to this work will also be described.

Background: the Lothian experience

Edinburgh and the Lothians comprise the city of Edinburgh, East Lothian, Midlothian and West Lothian. These cover a large and varied geographical area and a variety of populations, ranging from isolated, small, rural communities through mixed, urban/rural areas to multiply deprived inner city estates. Local government is devolved to these four areas and each has its own Drug Action Team (DAT). Three of the DATs include alcohol and of these, one also includes nicotine. All four areas have their own unique characteristics and identity.

The population is approximately 750,000, divided roughly 60:20:10:10 between Edinburgh city, West Lothian, Midlothian and East Lothian respectively. This ratio was used historically by Lothian Health in the allocation of resources and currently tends to dictate the allocation of resources, to the DATs.

During the mid-1980s it became apparent that two epidemics were occurring simultaneously in Lothian – an epidemic of intravenous drug use and an epidemic of HIV infection, which was spreading rapidly among intravenous drug users (Robertson *et al*. 1986). This situation led to a variety of responses including the establishment of the Community Drug Problems Service (CDPS) and the Primary Care Facilitator Team (PCFT) for HIV/AIDS.

The Community Drug Problems Service (CDPS)

The Community Drug Problem Service was established in 1988. The high prevalence of HIV infection in Edinburgh dictated its main aims: to promote harm reduction to drug users by the provision of substitute prescribing but with an ultimate goal of abstinence (Greenwood 1992). From the outset a shared-care model working with GPs was encouraged. The CDPS offered assessment, drug titration and keywork while the GP provided the ongoing substitute prescribing. Latterly, some direct provision of substitute prescribing was undertaken in the CDPS for clients who were difficult to contain in general practice in the primary care setting, e.g. patients with severe and enduring mental health problems.

The Primary Care Facilitator Team

In 1989 Lothian Health Board appointed a doctor with general practice experience to the post of Primary Care Facilitator (HIV/AIDS) for three sessions a week. By 1992 the team had expanded with the addition of a full-time administrator, a practising GP and a former health visitor, to concentrate on the non-medical members of the primary care team.

The facilitators encouraged primary care teams to become more involved in preventing HIV infection and caring for those already infected by using various means including: running courses for GPs; organizing practice visits to provide information, training and support; and distributing regular information sheets.

Between 1989 and 1994, as more practices became involved in caring for drug users, the work of the team expanded to include drug facilitation, not just as one aspect of HIV prevention, but in its own right. By 1995, one of the stated aims of the PCFT was 'Working alongside the CDPS, to support primary care teams to work more effectively with drug users' (Bury 1995a).

In October 1995, a pilot scheme, 'Supporting Practices Caring for Drug Users in Lothian' was established and subsequently monitored by the PCFT. The scheme offered, and still offers financial support and training to practices providing care to drug users over and above general medical services. Practices are required to submit information on a quarterly basis about the drug users for whom they are claiming. Practices are also visited on a regular basis to support and encourage doctors to bring their care of drug users in line with the guidelines set out in the handbook *Managing Drug Users in General Practice*, issued in December 1995 (Bury 1995b).

Service developments

Initially, the CDPS was a centralized service within the city. However, over time, a decision was made to establish sector teams in line with the Mental Health sectors, creating seven sectors throughout Lothian. Small, multidisciplinary teams provided assessment and care to drug users, liaison with GPs and service development. This method for delivery of service was considered appropriate for a number of years.

Surveys of GPs in Lothian were carried out in 1988, shortly after the CDPS was established, and again in 1993, to ascertain GP involvement and confidence in managing drug users. Between 1988 and 1993 the proportion of GPs prescribing for drug users more than doubled from 36% to 73% (Ross *et al.* 1994). The proportion of GPs with above-average confidence in managing drug users also increased from 16% to 34%, while the proportion lacking confidence fell from 49% to 30%. It is likely that the existence of the CDPS, in the context of the epidemic of HIV infection, contributed to encouraging GPs to become involved, and the PCFT helped to maintain that enthusiasm. There was evidence, however, of an inequality of distribution in prescribing practices. By 1993, 17 out of 76 practices in Edinburgh were each prescribing for more than 20 drug users, and two practices in particular were each prescribing for more than 100 drug users. In contrast, a small number of practices established 'No Prescribing' policies. They either continued to offer general medical services only, (although the drug user was usually unlikely to consult under these conditions) or they seemed reluctant to have drug users on the list at all.

Signs of strain

Gradually over time, the progressive increase in the cumulative number of clients presenting to the service placed considerable strain on the organization and the individuals who worked in the CDPS. Between 1993 and 1998 the financial resources available for the CDPS remained relatively static and during this period medical staffing was reduced to address an over-spend in the staffing budget. The CDPS annual referral rate rose from 138 in 1988 to 1806 in 1999. Drug misuse continued and continues still to be a substantial and growing problem, with a significant and profound impact on the health and social functioning of many individuals (Department of Health 1999).

To cope with the increasing demand, all clinicians undertook the role of keyworker, and the size of individual caseloads increased. In 1998 the average individual caseload size in the CDPS was 61 clients. The accepted national average at that time was 35. Waiting lists were also developing in some sectors and it was apparent that, without change in a short period of time, these lists would be lengthy.

A further GP survey was undertaken in 1997 to gain some measure of GP opinion regarding working with drug users, substitute prescribing and views on the CDPS (Watson 2000). This survey showed that some GPs would not prescribe for drug users and that others had reached their capacity. In terms of CDPS service delivery, the top priority for GPs was good quality assessment of referrals within a short time frame. Up until that time, although providing good quality assessment, the CDPS's main focus had been to provide long-term key-work in the belief that this was the best method of supporting GPs. Following the survey, two service developments were piloted: a dedicated assessment team to service the city of Edinburgh and a locality clinic providing substitute prescribing support to GPs who would not prescribe or who had reached capacity.

At the time of writing, the clinical staff complement in the CDPS consisted of two consultant psychiatrists, two part-time hospital doctors, one nurse/operational manager, ten senior grade community psychiatric nurses, six nurses at more basic levels, one pharmacist, a part-time psychologist and a part-time social worker. The clearly defined medical role involved prescribing, advice on prescribing and a significant input in mental and physical health care issues. The nursing role overlapped to some extent with other professions; however, in the main, the nurses provided most of the therapeutic interventions. The specialist nurse had an important role to play in developing a consultative model of work which provided support and peer supervision for the non-specialists, in particular the general practitioners (Kennedy and Faugier 1989).

In November 1999, a study was undertaken to investigate and evaluate the redesigned staff resources within the city sectors. The results of this showed that in 1999 the staff complement had increased, whereas medical time had decreased due to a lack of interest in advertised posts. Referral rates had increased, caseload size had declined, waiting lists had reduced significantly and total key-work activity as measured by number of contacts was reduced by 20%. Although there had been an increase in staff, it did not amount to an increase of 20%. Outside the assessment team, staff activity and caseload size varied markedly and there were differences in delivery of service and policy between sectors. The sector teams were small and when staff were on extensive leave or when vacancies arose, major problems of cover occurred within the sector. Clients increasingly had to wait lengthy periods of time to be seen in these areas. The remaining staff in the sector were expected to manage these clients when they already had full case-loads. Waiting lists for allocation to keyworker increased and the clients waited even longer to be seen. The study indicated that the introduction of a sessional dedicated assessment clinic had contributed greatly to the reduction in caseloads and activity and there was enough evidence to support its continuation and development.

Introduction of a new way of working

The change in delivery of service proved to be a major task which was almost a year in preparation. Negotiating with the Trust, external agencies and individual staff proved to be time consuming but very necessary to assist all parties in investing in the change. The GPs were kept informed of proposed changes and progress thereof by regular correspondence and the service annual report. Requests for forbearance on their part during the transition period were by and large received sympathetically.

The assessment clinic

An assessment clinic was established to undertake comprehensive assessment of clients who live within the boundaries of the City of Edinburgh. Good assessment is essential to the continuing care of the client. It can engage clients in treatment and begin a process of change even before full assessment is complete (Department of Health 1999).

Five whole-time clinicians offered an assessment service with a routine appointment within 2–3 weeks of receipt of referral and the facility to offer more urgent appointments when necessary. The clinic operated mainly in the city centre but other locality sites were used on a sessional basis. This improved access for the clients and facilitated communication with GPs and other agencies. Occasionally (but in very exceptional circumstances), a client may have needed to be assessed at home; this could be accommodated if, for safety reasons, two staff members were able to undertake the visit.

During the transition period between models, the waiting time was considerably longer than that mentioned above and a significant backlog of referrals developed. While this was stressful for some of the staff and undoubtedly unsatisfactory for both clients and GPs, it was unavoidable in the circumstances. The end result, however, was a consistent and equitable service where postcode had no bearing on the service received.

The assessment process

The Maudsley Addiction Profile (Marsden *et al.* 1998) was used to facilitate consistency of approach. It was also useful when inducting staff new to the field. Ideally, this instrument was on a database and accessed live during the assessment process, facilitating audit, evaluation of service provision and outcome measurement. Initial assessment covered a brief drug use history, current drug use, injecting behaviour, criminal history and social circumstances. A specimen for urinalysis was collected and a drug use diary given to the client to complete and return at their next appointment. Risk behaviour was identified and advice given about safer sex and safer injecting if appropriate. A summary of the assessment was then sent to the GP within seven days.

At initial assessment, the client could be given the appointment for full assessment. This saved considerably on administration time and acknowledged the often temporary nature of a client's address. All full assessments were then discussed by the assessment team and a decision made as to whether the client could proceed to a substitute prescription or required a management meeting with a doctor. This would be arranged for any client whose management needed to address a particularly high risk or high priority, in the case of pregnant clients, where there was concurrent physical illnesses not being managed elsewhere and in the case of high dose users. Psychiatric assessment could be undertaken by one of the consultant psychiatrists in the team.

The planning appointment

This appointment was designed to plan treatment and may include discussion of the methadone programme, tolerance testing or home detoxification. Staff would ensure that the client fully understood the plan of action and was in agreement with it. For those clients commencing methadone treatment, the initial dose of methadone was decided by the prescribing doctor; the client was then booked onto the methadone programme, usually within two to three weeks. A contract was then signed, a copy of which was given to the client. A letter was sent to the GP outlining the plan of action.

The methadone programme

At the time of writing, five new clients started on the methadone programme each week. An audit of the 10-month period from June 1999 to March 2000 indicated that a total of 154 clients started the programme, of whom 128 (83%) successfully completed. One did not attend, 2 died, 3 went to prison and 19 were asked to leave, either for unacceptable behaviour in the clinic or for consistent use of opiates in addition to pre-scribed methadone. A client may have stayed on the programme for a period of one to five weeks depending on what was required for stabilization. For example, heroin injectors often required more than three weeks and someone whose starting dose did not need any change often required only one week.

Clients were seen for daily, supervised consumption of methadone during the week and were given prescriptions to have their methadone supervised on Saturday and dispensed on Saturday for Sunday at a local pharmacist. As there were only three pharmacists in Edinburgh who dispensed and supervised methadone on a Sunday, it was usual to arrange for supervision on those days only if the dose exceeded 100 mg of methadone or if there were other particular concerns about the client. Clients were assessed jointly by the prescribing doctor and the pharmacist on five occasions during a three-week programme to allow accurate titration of dose. On the other days, the pharmacist alone supervised administration of the medication and no changes were made. This service was delivered exclusively at the city-centre clinic.

Modified versions of this service were delivered at rural sites, including a district general hospital in West Lothian; considerable use was made of com-munity pharmacists to supervise administration of methadone, particularly in rural areas but also in Edinburgh city. While this had benefits in terms of safety and preventing diversion of medication, it had particular disadvantages in rural areas with small communities. Problems of confidentiality and identifi-cation of clients constituted a continual challenge.

The Methadone Education Group

Every client who attended the methadone programme or for tolerance test-ing was expected to attend the Methadone Education Group, which took the form of a nurse-led discussion. Again, this service was delivered centrally although the information could also be delivered in booklet form to suburban and outlying areas.

Tolerance testing

Following assessment, the client may have been deemed suitable for a single tolerance test, rather than daily attendance at the methadone programme. Clients who attended for tolerance testing needed only to attend for a single morning, followed by a period of supervised administration in a local pharmacy. To prevent clients having to travel long distances from rural areas, tolerance testing could be carried out by the general practitioner in the primary care setting.

Completion and follow-up plans

Following a final review by the initial prescribing doctor, a letter was written to the GP advising her or him of:

- the final dose of methadone
- any significant incidents and the client's progress through the programme
- the results of urine toxicology
- current prescribing plans including current local dispensing pharmacy.

The GP should be asked to take over the prescribing unless it is clear that he or she was not prepared to, or if the client's circumstances suggested that central prescribing was appropriate.

The appropriate care pathway was then identified in collaboration with the client. Those requiring keyworker support were allocated to a keyworker for a specific, time-limited intervention. This service could be provided in the city-centre clinic, a GP surgery, a local social work office or the client's home.

Discussion

The redesigned CDPS has moved from a sector model for all services to one providing a combination of central and local services. A dedicated, mainly centralized assessment team provides services to the city of Edinburgh, with some use of locality sites and a dedicated keyworker team offering specific, time-limited interventions centrally, locally and on a domiciliary basis. In the rural sectors the original model still prevails, mostly for reasons of geography and maintaining accessible services. Working in conjunction with the PCFT, the emphasis has been to support the primary care team, in particular the primary care physicians, in caring for drug users and to provide equitable, accessible services to drug users themselves. To date, unlike the experience in other areas (Tantam et al. 1993), this shared care model has been successful in involving large numbers of primary care doctors in the shared care of this group.

The changes made in response to the 1997 GP questionnaire, in particular the development of the dedicated assessment team, have resulted in reduced waiting times, streamlined and standardized assessment, and reduced caseload size, and have provided a flexibility of response that was hitherto lacking in the city. However, in the perceptions of both the primary care doctor and the client, it has become a less personal service. The primary care doctor does not have a familiar community psychiatric nurse to whom the client can relate and a client may see at least two different workers in the course of the assessment process. In spite of this, the attendance rate appears to have been unaffected by the change. A more crucial factor affecting attendance was undoubtedly the waiting time, and hence reducing this may have offset other factors.

Liaison with the general practice doctor is a vital component for shared care working and this is maintained as far as possible by regular correspondence and telephone contact. A duty worker, available during office hours, can answer GP telephone enquiries. The PCFT undertakes regular visits to GP surgeries for continuing advice and support. Primary care facilitators have experienced difficulties in liaison with the CDPS about individual practice when there has not been an identified worker in the assessment team.

Conclusion

Supportive liaison between the specialist addiction service and primary care is crucial to the effective operation of the overall service. The existence of a specialist, statutory service which initiates care is then able to encourage GPs to take over the care of drug using patients, in the context of the advice, support and training offered by the PCFT. The result has been active, continuing liaison with GPs, which in turn improves the quality of care provided to drug users. The model has proved productive in terms of streamlining and standardizing assessment, facilitating referral of clients to the appropriate care pathway. The skills of workers were clearly defined and utilized in a manner that produced benefit for the clients and enhanced job satisfaction. These changes require continuing audit and evaluation in the light of changing trends in drug use, client profile and demands on primary care medicine. The model described is designed to allow for greater flexibility to respond to further changes.

References

Advisory Council on the Misuse of Drugs (1993) *AIDS and Drug Misuse Update.* Department of Health, London: HMSO.

Bury, J. (1995a) Supporting GPs in Lothian to care for drug users. *International Journal of Drug Policy,* 6: 267–73.

Bury, J. (1995b) Handbook: *Managing Drug Users in General Practice.* Lothian: Lothian Health.

Clarke, A.E. (1993) Barriers to GPs caring for patients with HIV/AIDS. *Family Practitioner,* 10: 8–13.

Department of Health (1999) *Drug Misuse and Dependence – Guidelines on Clinical Management.* Norwich: HMSO.

Glanz, A. (1986) Findings of a national survey of the role of GPs in the treatment of opiate misuse: views on treatment. *British Medical Journal,* 293: 543–5.

Greenwood, J. (1992) Services for problem drug users in Scotland. In: Plant M, Ritson B, Robertson R, eds. *Alcohol and Drugs.* Edinburgh: University Press Edinburgh.

Kennedy, J. & Faugier, J. (1989) *Drug and Alcohol Dependency Nursing.* Oxford: Heinemann.

Marsden, J., Gossop, M., Stewart, D., Best, D., Farrell, M., Lehman, P., Edwards, C. & Strang, J. (1998) The Maudsley Addiction Profile (MAP): a brief instrument for assessing treatment outcome. *Addiction,* 93: 1857–68.

McKeganey, N.P. & Boddy, F.A. (1988) GPs and opiate-abusing patients.

Journal of the Royal College of General Practitioners, 38: 73–5.

Robertson, J.R., Bucknall, A.B., Welsby, P.D., Roberts, J.J.K., Inglis, J.M., Peutherer, J.F. & Brettle, R.P. (1986) Epidemic of AIDS-related virus (HTLV-III/LAV) infection among intravenous drug abusers. *British Medical Journal,* 292: 527–9.

Ross, A., Von Teilingen, E., Bury, J., Porter, M. & Huby, G. (1994) *Experience of Lothian GPs with Drug Users and People with HIV Infection: 1988–1993.*

University of Edinburgh: Department of General Practice.

Tantam, D., Donmall, M., Webster, A., Strang, J. (1993) Do GPs and general psychiatrists want to look after drug misusers? Evaluation of a non-specialist treatment policy. *British Journal of General Practice,* 43: 470–4.

Watson, F. (2000) Models of primary care for substance misusers: the Lothian experience. *Drugs: Education, Prevention and Policy,* 7: 223–34.

18
A centrally co-ordinated city strategic approach

Richard Watson, Jane Jay and Laurence Gruer

Introduction

During the 1980s, Glasgow experienced a marked increase in the prevalence of injecting drug use, involving the injection of pharmaceutical drugs such as buprenorphine and temazepam (Sakol *et al.* 1989) as well as heroin (Hammersley *et al.* 1990). Prior to, and through the early stages of what came to be called an epidemic, the treatment response was small-scale and largely excluded treatments involving the prescription of methadone (Paxton *et al.* 1978). By 1991 there were about 8500 injecting drug users in the Greater Glasgow area, which has a population of about 900,000 (Frischer *et al.* 1993). Most lived in areas of marked socio-economic deprivation, injected heroin and often used other drugs, especially benzodiazepines. At least 70% had hepatitis C, though only 1% had HIV infection (Gruer 1993). There were also many other serious health, social and legal consequences.

Health service response

A 1992 survey showed that three-quarters of the 221 general practices in the Greater Glasgow Health Board had patients known to be injecting drugs. There was very little methadone prescribing, but much prescribing of diazepam, dihydrocodeine, temazepam and buprenorphine (in the 400 mcg Temgesic preparation). The latter two drugs were often injected. Several psychiatrists treated patients with addiction problems but mainly dealt with alcohol and, because of some negative experiences in the 1970s, none prescribed methadone on a maintenance basis (Paxton *et al.* 1978).

Some general practitioners in the city were prescribing methadone on their own initiative. A few saw patients in special clinics, often with support from local drugs workers and obtained payments for this under the national health promotion arrangements in force at that time. A group of prescribers, known as MUGs (Methadone Users Group), began meeting informally. In conjunction with a public health consultant and others they drew up a scheme to encourage responsible prescribing and pay practices for the additional work involved, which they successfully argued was beyond the general medical services normally required of a general practitioner.

This scheme built on a model of proven efficacy and feasibility as described in Wilson *et al.* (1994). Wilson and his colleagues described the development and success of methadone maintenance treatment clinics run entirely in two general practices in Glasgow. Based on the success of this model, combined with other published evidence of methadone prescribing in nearby Edinburgh and elsewhere (Greenwood 1990), the Health Board was convinced that methadone maintenance treatment was the way forward.

The Greater Glasgow Health Board General Practitioner Drug Misuse Clinic Scheme

The scheme was established in May 1994 and a review body was formed to supervise it. This had a membership of three general practitioners, the director of the Glasgow Drug Problem Service, the health board medical prescribing adviser, and a consultant in public health medicine. Clear criteria were established, and continue to operate, for participation in the scheme (Gruer *et al.* 1997) (see box).

Criteria for participation in the Drug Misuse Clinic Scheme

- Participating general practitioners are allowed 5–20 patients each.
- Oral methadone 1 mg/1 ml is the only permitted opiate substitute.
- GPs may prescribe a reducing course of diazepam. They may not prescribe temazepam.
- Supervised consumption of daily dispensed methadone in a local pharmacy should be arranged whenever possible. This should normally continue for at least a year.
- All patients should receive regular additional counselling and support from a drug worker or appropriately trained nurse. Ideally this takes place in a dedicated clinic in the GP surgery.
- GPs must attend at least two approved post-graduate training seminars per year.
- Audit data should be recorded at each patient attendance.

General practitioners wishing to join the scheme are asked to complete a form on which they indicate the number of patients they wish to treat, their proposed arrangements for consulting and counselling, whether they can arrange for supervised consumption of methadone and whether participation in the scheme has the agreement of the other members of the practice. Applications are considered at quarterly meetings of the review body who may seek further information by telephone, correspondence or a visit to the practice. If the application is successful, and the large majority are, then the general practitioner signs a formal agreement and is issued with a guidance pack. An educational visit by a doctor experienced in running clinics in the scheme is offered to new members.

General practitioners are paid for a notional clinic of 10 patient attendances at a rate based on the hospital practitioner scale. At the outset, a maximum of three attendances per month per patient can be claimed. Thus a general practitioner with 20 patients can claim for up to 60 attendances per month, worth £370. Doctors who have been in the scheme for more than a year can claim for up to 40 patients each, but with the same ceiling of 60 attendances per month. This is based on the assumption that patients at established practices are generally more stable and therefore need to be seen less often.

Specialist support

The Glasgow Drug Problem Service (GDPS) was established in January 1994 as a primary care based service to provide help with initial assessment, stabilization of drug users and assistance with problem cases. It was modelled on a similar service in Edinburgh (Greenwood 1990). Patients were referred by a general practitioner who must agree to continue a methadone prescription once the patient has been started on this by the GDPS. The service is run by doctors who are mainly general practitioners with a special interest in drug addiction and a team of specialist nurses. At the time of writing, patients are seen at clinics held in 12 health centres sited around the city.

Supervised consumption of methadone

The widespread supervision of methadone consumption in community pharmacies was pioneered in Glasgow (Scott *et al*. 1994) (see Chapter 19 for further detail). It was widely supported by general practitioners and pharmacists as well as the Health Board. All parties were concerned that in areas with large amounts of unsupervised methadone dispensing there was significant leakage of prescribed methadone onto the illicit market and large numbers of methadone-related deaths. The high level of supervision achieved in Glasgow has successfully minimized the number of methadone-related deaths and has been praised in both the UK and abroad (Weinrich and Stuart 2000).

At first, supervision was provided voluntarily by pharmacists. As it became more widespread, pharmacists in areas with high prescribing found that their workload was increasing considerably. In April 1995 the Health Board began paying pharmacists for this service and supervision was strongly encouraged from 1996 onwards; over 80% of Glasgow's pharmacies now take part. All participating pharmacists complete a distance-learning package for which they are remunerated.

The topic of methadone-related deaths was explored in detail by Scott *et al.* (1999). Their confidential enquiry into methadone-related deaths uncovered substandard care in 18 cases of the 32 deaths in Glasgow in 1996. Consumption of illicitly obtained methadone was the largest single cause and was implicated in 13 of the deaths. This is a continuing area of national concern with 674 methadone-related deaths reported in England and Wales in 1997 (Advisory Council on the Misuse of Drugs 2000).

Between 1992 and 1998 the number of patients prescribed methadone increased from about 140 to 2800. Methadone-related deaths rose from 3 in 1992 to 23 in 1996, falling to 8 in 1997 and 7 in 1998 (Advisory Council on the Misuse of Drugs 2000). By correlating the number of methadone-related deaths with the amount of methadone prescribed, it can be seen that the methadone-related death rate has declined since 1992 and particularly since 1996 when about 90% of prescriptions were supervised. Figure 18.1 compares the methadone-related death rate in Glasgow with that in the surrounding area of Strathclyde, where supervision was introduced in 1996, but remains patchy and incomplete.

However, such a high level of supervision does have its problems. Dispensing and supervision fees are by far the largest cost in the provision of methadone in Glasgow (see Table 18.1). Pharmacies in areas of high demand

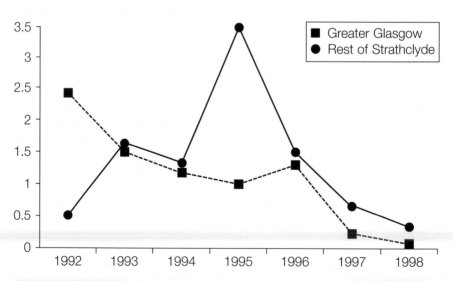

Figure 18.1 Methadone-related death rates per 100 patient years of treatment in Greater Glasgow and the rest of Strathclyde region, 1992–98.
Source: Advisory Council on the Misuse of Drugs 2000

Table 18.1 The cost of methadone prescribing in thousands of pounds sterling.

	1997–98	1998–99	1999–2000	2000–01 estimate
	(£,000)	(£,000)	(£,000)	(£,000)
Methadone	730	791	863	900
Dispensing fees	1295	1623	1740	2070
Supervising fees	284	393	530	540
GP fees	186	256	298	343
GDPS	730	730	720	740
Total	3225	3793	4151	4593

have large numbers of patients attending daily for methadone (sometimes over 100) and many pharmacists feel unable to accept any further patients. Many general practitioners report difficulty in arranging supervision for new patients. In several areas, some local people, shopkeepers and property developers have objected to the large numbers of people attending daily. Many patients resent having to attend daily to take their methadone in public. Indefinite daily supervision might hinder rehabilitation and discourage patients from taking up treatment. Details of the dispensing and supervision of prescriptions issued under the scheme are found in Table 18.3.

Counselling and social support

Many practices have drug workers visiting once or twice a week. This has the advantage of facilitating communication between doctor and drug worker. The drug worker usually sees the patients every one to four weeks. The doctor will see them regularly at initiation of treatment, when there is a problem, for blood sampling or for review at intervals of no greater than three months. When patients have to attend to collect their prescription, attendance is better than at appointments for counselling only. A few practices use the practice nurse or health visitor to run clinics. An alternative approach has been taken by a few practices in which the general practitioner sees patients at a local drug project. Some doctors prefer this as it means fewer drug users attend the surgery, but it does take the doctor away from other duties at the surgery.

Although the joint clinic arrangements outlined above are the preferred models, they are not a compulsory part of the scheme. Doctors must ensure that some counselling is made available to patients, but this may take place at drug projects away from the surgery. Payment to general practitioners is made, however, only for attendances at the surgery or at clinics elsewhere at which the general practitioner is present. A survey in 2000 revealed that only about 30% of patients were receiving social support and counselling.

Table 18.2 Approximate number of patients receiving methadone in Greater Glasgow in September 2000.

Service	Patients
GP Drug Misuse Clinic Scheme	2900
GPs not in the scheme	400
Glasgow Drug Problem Service	300
Glasgow Drug Crisis Centre	40
Department of Infection	40
Women's reproductive health service	30
Barlinnie Prison	30
Alcohol and Drugs Directorate	30
Total	3770

Results of the scheme – review of seven years

Thirty-nine GPs in 22 practices joined at the scheme's inception in May 1994, and by March 2001 there were 166 GPs from 92 practices. Numbers of patients treated by individual practices varied from 5 to over 100. Thus, although many practices had two or more doctors in the scheme, some saw far more patients than the maximum 40 per GP for which they can claim payment.

Doctors in the scheme are not the only ones to prescribe methadone in Glasgow. A snapshot survey in September 2000 estimated that there were 3770 patients then being treated with methadone in Glasgow, of whom 77% were treated by doctors in the scheme (see Table 18.2).

Methadone dose

Table 18.3 shows that the average daily dose of methadone prescribed by doctors in the scheme has fallen over the years to its current level of 49 mg. This is well below the often quoted level of 60 mg and above which is associated with greater treatment retention and lower levels of illicit drug use (Ball and Ross 1991; Caplehorn and Bell 1991; Payte 1997) and there are concerns that many general practitioners in Glasgow are not using sufficiently high doses.

Benzodiazepines

Many drug injectors in Glasgow also misuse benzodiazepines and some may begin doing so only after they are started on methadone. This has been reported elsewhere (Darke *et al.* 1994). To some extent this may represent self-medication to aid the insomnia and anxiety that many complain of, but there is a suggestion that benzodiazepines enhance the subjective effects of methadone (Preston *et al.* 1984). The use of benzodiazepines has been

Table 18.3 Comparison of seven years of the Greater Glasgow GP Drug Misuse Clinic Scheme.

	1994/5	1995/6	1996/7	1997/8	1998/9	1999/ 2000	2000/1
GPs in scheme	54	75	99	103	124	158	166
(% of all GPs in GGHB)	(11.5)	(12)	(16)	(15)	(20)	(25)	(26)
Practices in Scheme	–	41	50	58	78	90	92
(% of all practices in GGHB)		(21)	(23)	(26)	(36)	(41)	(42)
Total number of patients	1244	1613	1873	2606	3586	3456	4031
Total number of visits	18,143	24,756	31,561	37,120	45,776	50,170	60,125
Average daily dose of methadone (mg)	54	54	54	53	50	48	49
% of methadone prescriptions that are dispensed daily	92	97	91	91	89	88	90
% of methadone prescriptions where consumption is supervised	65	91	88	90	88	87	90

linked to higher levels of needle sharing, higher levels of poly-drug use, an increased chance of injecting illicit drugs during methadone maintenance and higher levels of criminal activity, as well as poorer health and social functioning (Darke *et al.* 1992).

Whether benzodiazepines should be prescribed remains an unanswered question. There are large variations between practices in the scheme. In 2000–2001, 11% of practices never prescribed them while some did so at over 70% of attendances. Diazepam was prescribed at 13% of attendances and nitrazepam at 4%. As reasons for not prescribing, doctors state that they fear diversion on to the illicit market or replacing intermittent misuse with daily use. Prescribing of benzodiazepines to a few individuals can lead to requests from others who may not have a genuine clinical indication. These issues are thoughtfully discussed by Seivewright (2000).

Outcome

The use of methadone in Glasgow has been the subject of a major research study (Hutchinson *et al.* 2000). Over 200 drug injectors were followed up for a year from the time they began treatment with methadone. Patients who stayed in treatment and received methadone continuously for one year showed major beneficial reductions in risky behaviours:

- daily heroin injecting declined from 78% to 2%
- overdose in the previous six months declined from 24% to 2%

- average daily drug spend declined from £50 to £4
- average monthly number of property crimes declined from 13 to 3.

However, only 29% (58) of the cohort remained continuously on methadone for 12 months, and only 50 of those were interviewed at 12 months. Discontinuation of treatment was most often due to imprisonment (39% of those discontinuing) or sanctions by the prescriber (33% of those discontinuing). The remainder left voluntarily or the reason was not given.

During the first two years of the scheme, participating GPs were obliged to complete the Opiate Treatment Index questionnaire every six months for each patient. This 19-page document is used to audit outcomes. Many participants found it too time consuming to complete, and there was insufficient clerical support to enter the data at the Health Board, so this requirement was dropped. Currently data on each attendance are recorded in clinic logs that are then submitted quarterly as evidence for payment. These data are then computerized and used to produce an annual report on the scheme as a whole and reports for individual practices. The reports do not give outcome measures other than continuation in the scheme and reasons for discontinuation. A new audit tool is being developed.

Costs

Table 18.1 shows the costs of methadone prescribing. These are the costs directly borne by the Health Board and include prescribing outwith the scheme. They clearly do not fully represent the cost of GP time and do not take account of social work costs. Glasgow City Council Social Work Department estimates that they spent £1.4m in 1999–2000 supporting clients on methadone. This represents 45% of expenditure by the City Council on non-residential addiction services.

The Health Service costings give an average cost of about £1200 per patient per year. The additional cost of social care has been estimated at £1800 per client per year, although only 30% of patients are in contact with social work services at any point in time.

Strengths of the scheme

The GP scheme allows a large number of people to be treated within the primary care system close to where they live. The scheme is much more flexible and cost effective than conventional specialist clinic services. Arranging supervision of methadone consumption in community pharmacies increases patient compliance and reduces illegal diversion and overdoses. At their best, joint clinics between GPs and drug workers can combine health and social care effectively.

Problems

A large number of individuals are unable to access the programme; in the year 2000, it was estimated that at least 1250 more people in Glasgow would benefit from treatment. There is inconsistent provision via general practice, with variable standards, as development around Glasgow has been patchy and unco-ordinated. There are excessive numbers of patients in some practices, while others refuse to treat any, and there is insufficient community pharmacy capacity in some areas. Local residents, traders and developers have been known to object to the use of pharmacies by large numbers of drug users.

Many patients dislike prolonged supervision and there is sometimes insufficient social care available. There are few opportunities for people on methadone maintenance to undergo adequately supported detoxification, with rehabilitation and relapse prevention.

Proposals for further development: expansion of the scheme

At the time of writing there are plans to expand and strengthen the GP scheme. In 2001, the Primary Care Trust took over responsibility for the scheme and the Glasgow Drug Problem Service was given responsibility for its management. The payment scheme for GPs may be adjusted to encourage experienced GPs to take on more patients and to encourage new GPs to join the scheme. This could be linked to increased training and support from a team of experienced doctors and nurses employed to visit practices and deliver training courses.

However, there are also cautionary voices pointing out that about 20% of GPs in Glasgow refuse to prescribe any methadone and many others appear reluctant to take on new opiate-dependent patients. They suggest that an increase in centralized prescribing, through the GDPS or through new, locally based, structures may be the only way forward.

Increase in methadone dispensing and supervising capacity

There is concern that the capacity for local pharmacists to dispense and supervise the consumption of methadone is limited and that this may limit any further increase in methadone prescribing. The possibility of supervising consumption at new sites, such as drug projects, is being explored. This would offer a greater degree of privacy than is possible at community pharmacies and would encourage attendance at the projects where social support is available. Methadone could continue to be dispensed by the community pharmacies with individually labelled doses being brought to drug projects. However, this would have major implications for staffing, space and security at the drug projects.

Phased reduction in supervision for stable patients will also be explored. Patients who have been free of illicit drug use and criminal activity for a specified period of time, and who have a stable social situation, might initially be permitted supervision on three days per week with take-home doses for the other days. This could progress to weekly dispensing if progress continues. A working group will develop guidelines and the situation will be carefully monitored to avoid any increase in methadone diversion and deaths.

Special groups

Special schemes to treat the homeless and prostitutes are underway. The Drug Treatment and Testing Orders, an alternative to imprisonment for drug-related offenders, have been piloted in Glasgow with the GDPS being one of the care providers. Treatment with methadone or abstinence-orientated treatments are the two main options.

Increase in social care support and training and employment opportunities

For many patients, the key to genuine rehabilitation lies in housing, training and employment, all beyond the control of the prescribing doctor. City of Glasgow Social Work Services recently announced a substantial increase in the number of drug workers supporting the scheme. The aim is to provide all clients receiving methadone with an average of 15 minutes' contact with a drug worker every fortnight. Substantial additional investment is also being made available to provide more people on methadone with realistic opportunities for education, training and legitimate work.

Conclusion

Our experience shows that it is possible for primary care practices to prescribe methadone to a large number of opiate-addicted patients and to do this effectively without a large number of methadone-related deaths. To achieve this end, a high degree of supervised consumption is required. Such a service requires encouragement, training, support and funding from the health authority. A major investment in social care is also needed if the potential for rehabilitation is to be realized. Although the costs are substantial, the health gains and reduced costs to society resulting from the treatment of drug misuse are much greater.

References

Advisory Council on the Misuse of Drugs. (2000) *Reducing Drug Related Deaths*. London: Stationery Office.

Ball, J.C. & Ross, A. (1991) *The Effectiveness of Methadone Maintenance Treatment: Patients, programs, services, and outcome.* New York: Springer-Verlag.

Caplehorn, J.R.M. & Bell, J. (1991) Methadone dosage and retention of patients in maintenance treatment. *Medical Journal of Australia,* 154: 195–9.

Darke, S., Swift, W., Hall W. & Ross, M. (1994) Drug use, HIV risk-taking and psychosocial correlates of benzodiazepine use among methadone maintenance clients. *Drug and Alcohol Dependence,* 31: 31–6.

Darke, S., Baker, A., Dixon, J., Wodak, A. & Heather, N. (1992) Drug use and HIV risk taking behaviour among clients in methadone maintenance treatment. *Drug and Alcohol Dependence,* 29: 263–8.

Frischer, M., Leyland, A., Cormack, R., Goldberg, D., Bloor, M. & Green, S. (1993) Estimating the population prevalence of injecting drug use and infection with human immunodeficiency virus among injecting drug users in Glasgow, Scotland. *American Journal of Epidemiology,* 138: 170–81.

Greenwood, J. (1990) Creating a new drug service in Edinburgh. *British Medical Journal,* 300: 587–9.

Gruer L. (1993) *Drug Misuse and Health in Glasgow.* Glasgow: Greater Glasgow Health Board.

Gruer, L., Wilson, P., Scott, R., Elliott, L., Macleod, J., Hawden, K., Forrester, E., Hinshelwood, S., McNulty, H. & Silk, P. (1997) General Practitioner centred scheme for treatment of opiate dependent drug injectors in Glasgow. *British Medical Journal,* 314: 1730–5.

Hammersley, R., Forsyth, A. & Lavelle, T. (1990) The criminality of new drug users in Glasgow. *British Journal of Addiction,* 85: 1583–94.

Hutchinson, S.J., Taylor, A., Gruer, L., Barr, C., Hills, C., Elliott, L., Goldberg, D.,

Scott, R. & Gilchrist, G. (2000) One-year follow up of opiate injectors treated with oral methadone in a GP-centred programme. *Addiction,* 95: 1055–68.

Paxton, R., Mullin P. & Beattie J. (1978) The effects of methadone maintenance with opioid takers. A review and findings from one British city. *British Journal of Addiction,* 132: 473–81.

Payte, J.Y. (1997) Methadone dosage and outcome. In: *Effective Medical Treatment of Heroin Addiction.* National Institute of Health (NIH) Consensus Conference, November 17–19: 1997, Bethesda MD. Available at: *http://odp.od.nih.gov/consensus/cons/ 108/108_abstract.pdf:123–126*

Preston, K.L., Griffiths, R.R., Stitzer, M.L., Bigelow, G.E. & Liebson, I.A. (1984) Diazepam and methadone interactions in methadone maintenance. *Clinical Pharmacology and Therapy,* 36: 534–41.

Sakol, M.S., Stark C. & Sykes, R. (1989) Buprenorphine and temazepam abuse by drug takers in Glasgow – an increase, (letter). *British Journal of Addiction,* 84: 439–41.

Scott, R.T.A., Jay, M.J.H., Keith, R., Oliver, J.S. & Cassidy, M.T. (1999) A confidential enquiry into methadone-related deaths. *Addiction,* 94: 1789–94.

Scott, R., Burnett, S. & McNulty, H. (1994) Supervised administration of methadone by pharmacies. *British Medical Journal,* 308: 1438.

Seivewright, N. (2000) *Community Treatment of Drug Misuse: More Than Methadone.* Cambridge: Cambridge University Press.

Weinrich, M. & Stuart, S. (2000) Provision of methadone treatment in primary care medical practices; review of the Scottish experience and implications for US policy. *Journal of the American Medical Association,* 283: 1343–8.

Wilson, P., Watson, R. & Ralston, G. (1994) Methadone maintenance in general practice: patients, workload, and outcomes. *British Medical Journal,* 309: 641–4.

19
Supervised consumption of methadone in a community pharmacy

Kay Roberts

Introduction

Ten years ago it was unusual in the UK for patients treated for opiate dependence to receive their methadone supplies in instalments. It was even more unusual for the doses to be taken under supervision, either in a pharmacy or elsewhere. In the intervening years it has become almost commonplace for methadone to be dispensed in daily instalments and for patients to consume their daily dose under the supervision of the dispensing pharmacist. Supervised consumption of methadone is now recommended for the first three to six months of treatment (United Kingdom Anti-Drugs Co-ordination Unit (UKADCU) 1998; Department of Health 1999; Advisory Council on the Misuse of Drugs 2000).

This chapter aims to describe why these changes have taken place and what benefits have accrued through this practice. In addition, consideration will be given to the lessons that have been learnt and to some recommendations for future development of services to drug misusers within a community setting.

Background

There is currently no requirement under UK Misuse of Drugs legislation for methadone, or any other controlled drug, to be supplied in instalments or to be consumed under supervision. This is not the same elsewhere. In the USA, for instance, community pharmacists are not permitted to dispense or supply methadone for the treatment of addiction. Methadone is supplied, with a few exceptions, on a daily basis under supervised consumption at a 'methadone programme', although it is possible to 'earn' the right to take home doses, provided certain criteria are fulfilled. The right usually depends on evidence of good behaviour over a period of time and can include an annual 'holiday' allowance. By contrast, perhaps as a result of the vast distances between townships, treatment services in Australia depend to a great extent on supervised consumption of methadone in community pharmacies. Indeed in two Australian states, Queensland and Victoria, dispensing of methadone through pharmacies is virtually the only means of access for a very large number of dependent patients. Indeed, in some Australian cities, such as Adelaide or Melbourne, the pharmacy may have a separate entrance so that both methadone consumption and needle exchange services can be accessed as discretely as possible.

One of the main driving forces that led to a change in practice in the United Kingdom was the growing concern that prescribed methadone was 'leaking' into the illicit market and possibly contributing to a marked increase in methadone deaths (Frischer and Gruer 1992; Frischer et al. 1997; Stone et al. 1989). Of particular concern were a number of reports of inadvertent ingestion of methadone by small children (Beattie 1999; Benbow et al. 1997; Cairns et al. 1996).

The need for a new system

In Glasgow during the late 1970s and early 1980s methadone had been prescribed extensively without adequate levels of support or monitoring facilities. Paxton et al. (1978) concluded that there was little evidence to support the claims that methadone maintenance would prevent illicit drug use, enhance treatment contact, reduce mortality, morbidity and crime and improve social adjustment, and asserted that the projected benefits of such treatment had been exaggerated. The practice was deemed to be ineffectual and even counterproductive and was abandoned. In the absence of specialist services during the late 1980s many primary care physicians (general practitioners (GPs)) in the city developed their own treatments, using a wide range of drugs in an inconsistent and unco-ordinated way. By the early 1990s it was recognized that there was need for a more co-ordinated approach, and a major review was undertaken to develop a future strategy for services to drug misusers (Greater Glasgow Health Board 1993). The final report proposed new service developments, including the setting up of a specialist service. Important objectives of the proposed strategy were to reduce the prevalence of injecting and the misuse of drugs. Methadone was recognized as the main therapeutic intervention as it possessed the best chance of success in terms of reducing morbidity and mortality, and primary care medicine (general practice) was identified as the most appropriate setting for treatment to be carried out.

The Greater Glasgow Health Board (GGHB), the Glasgow Drug Problem Service (GDPS) and the Area Pharmaceutical Committee (APC) all recognized that supervised consumption of methadone in pharmacies would be crucial to the success of the proposed scheme (Roberts et al. 1998). It was important not to recreate the earlier experience of the late 1970s when previous experiments with methadone fell into disrepute in the light of reports that methadone was being sold by patients and causing fatalities. It was thought that the local press and anti-methadone lobbyists would be monitoring progress carefully and the slightest indication that methadone was again leaking onto the streets and causing further deaths would result in negative reporting of the scheme.

By 2001, 78% (167 out of 213) of Glasgow's community pharmacies had a supplementary contract to supervise the consumption of methadone on their premises. Results from a Glasgow-wide survey undertaken in July 2000 indicate that over 3600 patients are visiting these pharmacies five, six or, in some instances, seven times each week (Greater Glasgow Drug Action Team et al. 2001). The number of patients seen at a pharmacy each day varies from 1 to 120. The results also indicate that 30% of the responding pharmacies felt unable to take on additional patients. Some of the reasons given were that: they had too many patients already; the pharmacy was too small; there would be a negative impact on other customers at the pharmacy, there would be an increase in shoplifting; the security of staff and stock would be compromised, and there would be negative feedback from local residents.

It is now recognized that the Glasgow scheme has been instrumental in promoting better compliance with methadone regimens and in reducing leakage of methadone onto the street market. Data from the Scottish Drugs Misuse Database demonstrate a stark difference between the number of reports of illicit methadone use in Glasgow compared with that in Edinburgh, which is a distance of 45 miles away. For 1999/2000, the database recorded 23% of individuals from Glasgow reporting prescribed methadone as their main drug compared with 2% reporting use of 'other methadone', i.e. illicit methadone. These figures compare with 17% of individuals in Lothian/ Edinburgh reporting prescribed methadone as their main drug and 11% of individuals reporting 'other methadone' (Information and Statistics Division 2000a). This is in spite of the fact that 86,777 prescriptions for methadone were dispensed by community pharmacies in Glasgow during the period compared with 22,920 prescriptions in Lothian/Edinburgh (Information and Statistics Division 2000b). The level of supervised consumption in Glasgow is considerably higher than that in Lothian/Edinburgh, though the level of supervision in Edinburgh has shown a steady increase in recent years.

Research undertaken in England and Wales by Sheridan et al. (1996) and in Scotland by Matheson et al. (1999) demonstrated that in 1995 a higher proportion of pharmacies were involved in the supply of controlled drugs than had been the case in 1985. Sheridan and colleagues further concluded that the network of community pharmacies represented an underused point of contact for the prevention of drug misuse (Sheridan et al. 1996); a positive attitude to the extension of their role in the prevention of HIV and in the treatment of drug misuse to include the supervision of methadone consumption on their premises was identified (Sheridan et al. 1997). Throughout the UK there was an upsurge of interest in the concept of supervised consumption of methadone. A survey, designed to assess the supervision of methadone by the community pharmacy and undertaken in 1997, was reported by Cairns and Hender (1999). The objectives of the survey were to describe the mechanics of schemes, the level of training provided and the degree of satisfaction on the part of commissioners, and to establish a benchmark for remuneration of pharmacists. The schemes surveyed were those set up by health authorities and health boards where pharmacists were being paid to supervise the consumption of methadone in their pharmacies. At the time their survey was undertaken, 22% of responding health authorities had schemes in operation and a further 37% were planning to introduce such a scheme in the immediate future (Cairns and Hender 1999).

The manner in which the various methadone services have been set up and administered varies considerably between health authorities (Luger *et al.* 2000; United Kingdom Anti-Drugs Co-ordination Unit 2000). However, some of the issues that have been raised are common to all and need to be taken into account when future services are being considered or when existing services are being reviewed.

Why is supervision necessary?

The most often quoted reasons for introducing daily supply and supervised consumption of methadone are to enhance compliance, to prevent leakage onto the street and accidental poisoning of small children. However, it must also be recognized that for some patients the opportunity to take their dose of methadone in a safe environment may mean that they will not be subjected to pressure from others to share or sell it.

Overall benefits of supervised consumption

- Introduction of a routine as a result of the requirement for daily, personal attendance at the pharmacy
- Assistance in compliance and avoidance of exceeding a daily dose
- Daily contact between the patient/client and a health care professional
- The opportunity to increase dosage safely
- Reduction of the potential for sharing of medication
- Reduction in selling (voluntary or involuntary)
- Reduction in the supply of methadone to the street market
- An opportunity to monitor progress of the patient/client
- Increased professional dialogue between the prescriber and the dispensing pharmacist
- Accessibility and the absence of waiting time
- The opportunity to accommodate a large number of patients/clients

---

For many patients in methadone programmes, the convenience of being able to obtain supplies of prescribed medication at the local pharmacy is an attractive option. It is normally possible to have a prescription dispensed in a pharmacy on six days of the week. Community pharmacies are often open longer hours than specialist drug centres, thus affording greater flexibility in collection times. The patient can generally go to a pharmacy of his or her choice. Being able to obtain prescribed methadone from a pharmacy rather than having to attend a specialized centre gives an enhanced feeling of normality and can reduce stigmatization. Pharmacists themselves are, in the main, keen to develop this extension of their role and recognize the importance of being potentially the only health care professional in a position to monitor the day-to-day progress of this group of patients.

Problems and solutions

Although a few health centre pharmacies are open on only five days per week, there is also an increasing number of large multiple pharmacies that are open seven days a week. However, most pharmacies do not open until 9.00 a.m. and may be closed by 5.30 or 6.00 p.m. These opening hours can produce difficulties for some patients on methadone programmes, especially if they are employed or have similar responsibilities. Problems can arise for the patient who does not wish the employer to know that they are receiving methadone for fear of losing their position, similarly for those attending training courses or employment programmes. The longer opening hours at supermarket pharmacies can go some way to resolving these issues. However, it is time that health authorities and the pharmaceutical profession began to consider further extending opening hours. Initiatives such as 'methadone buses' in rural areas, and in urban areas for the roofless and homeless or those without pharmacies might be considered; seven-day opening and extended hours for health centre pharmacies and increasing involvement of supermarket pharmacies could be to the benefit of a wide range of users of community pharmacies as well as to methadone patients. Such initiatives could be to the benefit of a wide range of users of community pharmacies as well as to methadone patients.

Privacy, or the lack of it, can be a major issue for those who are required to consume their doses of methadone in a pharmacy. Recent research undertaken by the Scottish Drugs Forum found that some respondents said that they 'felt safer' getting their prescription supervised, though a large majority said that they found the experience: embarrassing, degrading, terrible or unacceptable (Scottish Drugs Forum 2000). Improving levels of privacy in the pharmacy can be of benefit to all those seeking information and advice from the pharmacist. However, a balance needs to be struck between increasing the level of privacy and compromising the safety of the pharmacist and pharmacy staff.

It has been suggested that strict supervision programmes can discourage people from staying in treatment and that doctors should be allowed to use their clinical judgement so that patients are not treated like long-term prisoners just because they need methadone treatment (Nelles 2000). There is obviously a need to strike a balance between ensuring methadone is used safely and securely without making life so difficult for the patient that they leave the programme.

Confidentiality can be a major issue for the prescriber, the client and the pharmacist. Particular problems arise when the pharmacy offers a needle and syringe exchange service in addition to the supply of methadone. The Royal Pharmaceutical Society's Code of Ethics states that 'pharmacists must respect the confidentiality of information acquired in the course of professional practice relating to a patient and the patient's family. Such information must not be disclosed to anyone without consent of the patient or appropriate guardian unless the interest of the patient or the public requires such disclosure' (Royal Pharmaceutical Society of Great Britain 2001).

Stigmatization is another area of concern to patients. Research undertaken in Scotland during 1996 showed that many interviewees had experienced negative treatment, and that some pharmacists had demonstrated negative behaviour (Matheson 1998). Drug users preferred pharmacies in which they had experienced positive treatment. Stigma was a key issue for respondents, and a poor self-image combined with apparent negative treatment may provoke negative behaviour. Education of pharmacists to promote positive attitudes and education of methadone patients on what to expect from pharmacies would encourage co-operation and a more harmonious relationship, resulting in enhanced patient care.

Other issues that can have a negative impact on the pharmacy are:

- The number of methadone patients per pharmacy: is there a safe number of clients per pharmacy?
- Fears of other people in the community: methadone patients are one of the visible faces of substance misuse in the community.
- Perceptions of other users of the pharmacy: fear of methadone patients may result in further negative reactions and attempts to prevent the local pharmacy involvement in this work.
- Isolation of pharmacists from other members of the care team, the prescribing doctors and drug workers.
- The security of pharmacy staff and pharmacy stock.
- A negative impact on the rest of the pharmacy business.

Finally, it is often argued that paying pharmacists to dispense and supervise the consumption of methadone is not the most cost-effective way of providing this service. However, when comparisons are made between supply through a community pharmacy and supply from a hospital pharmacy or methadone clinic, it is essential to compare all the costs involved and not just the cost of the methadone alone. Such comparisons should take account of additional costs such as the cost of staff, heating and lighting, recording and dispensing time per item, increased security (controlled drugs cabinets, closed circuit television, panic buttons), containers, labels and other packaging requirements.

It is thought that not all these factors are taken into account when the pharmacists' fees are determined, either at the national or at the local level. In addition, the costs to the patient in terms of finance and time need to be recognized, as do the transport costs to a central dispensing point, whichever agency picks up the bill for these, and need to be balanced against the probably lower costs incurred when visiting the local pharmacy.

Good practice – examples from Glasgow and Berkshire

It is essential to the smooth and efficient running of a supervised methadone programme that there is a high level of communication and co-operation between the patient/client and the various elements of the care pathway. Two examples of good practice are the Glasgow Supervised Methadone Consumption Programme (United Kingdom Anti-Drugs Co-ordination Unit 1998) and the Berkshire Four Way Agreement (United Kingdom Anti-Drugs Co-ordination Unit 2000). The Glasgow methadone programme was set up in 1994 following a major review of services for drug misusers, undertaken jointly by the Health Board and Social Services (Greater Glasgow Health Board 1993). The review produced a strategic framework for services to drug misusers: as well as the development of specialist services, primary care physicians (general practitioners) and community pharmacists would play a key role in future provision. As a result of previous experience of methadone becoming available on the streets, the supervised consumption of methadone was an essential component of the new methadone programme. Remuneration of pharmacists for supervising consumption was introduced in 1995. At the time of writing, nearly 80% of Glasgow pharmacists had a specific contract with the Primary Care Trust to provide this service and 87.5% of methadone was taken under the direct supervision of a community pharmacist.

The Berkshire Four Way Agreement is a system for organizing the shared care and treatment of substance misusers for whom methadone mixture is prescribed, bringing together the general practitioner, the pharmacist, the drug counsellor and the patient. The scheme was developed in response to the Department of Health recommendations to improve access to primary care treatment for drug misusers and has been rolled out across the county (Berkshire Health Authority 2000; 2001).

Aims of the Berkshire programme

(1) To ensure that opiate users have access to substitute treatment through a structured reduction and maintenance programme using shared care arrangements.
(2) To ensure there is a support network for the primary health care teams ensuring a multi-disciplinary approach to treatment.
(3) To ensure there is shared care of the patient and shared exchange of information between all professionals.

The Berkshire scheme initially covered four Primary Care Groups (PCGs) and was then rolled out to cover the area's remaining four PCGs. It is crucial to the success of shared care schemes, such as those currently in place in Glasgow and Berkshire, that the patient/client is aware of and has agreed to the exchange of necessary information between members of the care team. There may, indeed, be occasions when it is necessary for the pharmacist to refer the patient/client back to the prescribing doctor, drugs worker or social services. It is also important that prescribers, drugs and social workers make contact with the dispensing pharmacist before the patient presents in the pharmacy for the first time. Early dialogue can prevent or reduce problems occurring in the future.

Within the pharmacy it is essential to provide as much privacy as possible for consumption of methadone to take place, without compromising safety. The whole process should be designed to protect dignity where possible. Care must be taken to ensure that the whole dose is swallowed. Talking to the patient can assist this process. In addition, the provision of a drink of water can ensure that the methadone mixture is swallowed and can also be used to rinse the mouth. Allowing the patient to use drink from a can of soft drink should be discouraged as rather than swallowing the contents of the can, the patient may instead eject the dose of methadone into the can for subsequent sale as 'spit methadone'.

Training

As this work is new to many pharmacists, it is essential that all involved receive the appropriate level of education, training and professional support. In the case of pharmacists continuing professional development, education and training is under the auspices of four centres of continuing or post-qualification education. A variety of distance learning materials is available and local centres provided ongoing direct learning. Relevant distance learning materials are currently available from both the Scottish and English Centres for continuing pharmaceutical education; locally published guidance is also available (Scottish Centre for Post Qualification Pharmaceutical Education 1999; 1996 and see Appendix).

Specialist support

Some shared care schemes, such as those in Glasgow and Berkshire, require participating pharmacists to complete a training programme before they can have a contract to supervise methadone consumption. Three health boards in Scotland have created specialist pharmacy posts to offer a high level of pharmaceutical expertise and support not only to participating pharmacists but also to all those involved in the local shared care programme. The Berkshire scheme has also been dependent on a high level of specialist pharmacy input.

Conclusions

Supervised consumption of methadone in pharmacies or elsewhere is an essential element of methadone maintenance provision. The advantages to the patient/client and to society include the increased benefit from improved compliance as well as the reduced potential for diversion to the illicit drug market and a reduction in methadone-related deaths. An increase in public confidence and support are further benefits of supervised consumption and in Glasgow following the initial negative reaction in the press, reintroduction of the practice of prescribing methadone was made possible by the implementation of supervision as well as other methods of monitoring. The success of supervised consumption schemes is dependent on the level of communication and collaboration between all the professionals involved and the patient. Supervised consumption programmes should not be so rigid that they result in a high level of attrition; efforts to retain patients on the methadone programme may ultimately result in preparation for detoxification. Communities and patients need to understand the rationale for supervised consumption of methadone. Lack of understanding within the community can lead to a public backlash against the programme which may not be in the best interests of the community, patients, prescribers, pharmacists or drug workers involved. Where understanding and community acceptance do prevail, then supervised consumption of methadone in community pharmacies allows the maximum number of patients to begin the long process of rehabilitation and reintegration without stigmatization and within the confines of their own community.

Appendix

Relevant distance learning materials available from the Scottish Centre for Post Qualification Pharmaceutical Education at Todd Wing, SIBS Building, University of Strathclyde, 47 Taylor Street, Glasgow.

- Scottish Centre for Post Qualification Pharmaceutical Education (1996) Pharmaceutical aspects of methadone prescribing.

- Scottish Centre for Post Qualification Pharmaceutical Education (1999) Pharmaceutical care of the drug misuser.

Locally published guidance:
- Guidelines for Supervision of Methadone Consumption in Pharmacies. Third Edition (2000) published jointly by Greater Glasgow Health Board, Primary Care Trust and Area Pharmaceutical Committee.
- Tayside Pharmacists Guide to the Management of Drug Problems: Supervised Self-Administration of Methadone (SSAM) (Tayside Health Board 1998).
- Guidelines for the Supervised Self Administration of Methadone in Community Pharmacists (Lothian Health 1997).
- Drug Misuse: The GP Guide (Wirral Community Healthcare 1997).
- Berkshire Substance Misuse Services: Guidelines to the 4 Way Agreement (2000) Berkshire Health Authority.

References

Advisory Council on the Misuse of Drugs (2000) *Reducing Drug Related Deaths*. London: The Stationery Office.

Beattie, J. (1999) Children poisoned with illegal drugs in Glasgow. *British Medical Journal*, 318: 1137.

Benbow, E. W., Roberts, I. S. D. & Cairns, A. (1997) Fatal methadone overdose (letter). *British Medical Journal*, 314: 975.

Berkshire Health Authority (2001) *Combined Annual Reports of the Berkshire Needle and Syringe Exchange Scheme and the Berkshire Four Way Agreement*, April 2000-March 2001.

Berkshire Health Authority (2000) *Berkshire Four Way Agreement: Annual report 1999/2000. Shared Care for Opiate Users in Berkshire*.

Cairns, C. & Hender, J. (1999) *Community Pharmacy Supervised Methadone Administration Schemes in the UK*. London: St George's Hospital, Pharmacy Academic Practice Unit.

Cairns, A., Roberts, I.S.D. & Benbow, E. W. (1996) Characteristics of fatal methadone overdose in Manchester, 1985–94. *British Medical Journal*, 313: 264–5.

Department of Health (1999) *Drug Misuse and Dependence – Guidelines on Clinical Management*. London: The Stationery Office.

Frischer, M., Goldberg, D., Mohammed, R. & Berney, L. (1997) Mortality and survival among a cohort of drug injectors in Glasgow, 1982–1994. *Addiction*, 92: 419–27.

Frischer, M. & Gruer, L. (1992) Mortality among injecting drug users in Glasgow: causes of death, the role of HIV infection and the possible impact of methadone maintenance. *AIDS News Supplement*, CDS Weekly Report (A.N.S.W.E.R) (Glasgow, CDS 92/13).

Greater Glasgow Drug Action Team, Glasgow City Council, Greater Glasgow Health Board (2001) *An integrated approach to restoring drug users to a positive place in their community. Annex A Review of the Methadone Programme in Greater Glasgow*.

Greater Glasgow Health Board (1993) *Drug Misuse and Health in Glasgow*. Glasgow: Greater Glasgow Health Board.

Information and Statistics Division (2000a) *Drug Misuse Statistics Scotland: 2000, Table 48-Main Drug*. pp. 68–9. Edinburgh: Information and Statistics Division, Common Services Agency.

Information and Statistics Division (2000b) *Drug Misuse Statistics Scotland: 2000, Table 85-Methadone mixture prescriptions: 1996/97–1999/00*. p. 121. Edinburgh, Information and Statistics Division, Common Services Agency.

Luger, L., Bathia, N., Alcorn, R. & Power, R. (2000) Involvement of community pharmacies in the care of drug misusers: pharmacy based supervision of methadone consumption. *International Journal of Drug Policy,* 11: 227–34.

Matheson, C. (1998) Views of illicit drug users on their treatment and behaviour in Scottish community pharmacies: implications for the harm-reduction strategy. *Health Education Journal,* 57: 31–41.

Matheson, C., Bond, M. & Morrison, J. (1999) Attitudinal factors associated with community pharmacists' involvement in services for drug misusers. *Addiction,* 94: 1349–59.

Nelles, B. (2000) Supervised consumption. *Newsletter Euro-Methwork*, 19: 9–10.

Paxton, R., Mullin, P. & Beattie, J. (1978) The effects of methadone maintenance with opioid takers. A review and some findings from one British city. *British Journal of Psychiatry*, 132: 473–81.

Roberts, K., Gruer, L., McNulty, H., Scott, R. & Bryson, S. (1998) The role of Glasgow pharmacists in the management of drug misuse. *International Journal of Drug Policy,* 9: 187–94.

Royal Pharmaceutical Society of Great Britain (2001) *Medicines, Ethics and Practice: A guide for pharmacists. Section 2 Code of Ethics and Standards. Part 2 Confidentiality. 25; 85.* London: Royal Pharmaceutical Society of Great Britain.

Scottish Centre for Post Qualification Pharmaceutical Education (1999) *Pharmaceutical Care of the Drug Misuser.* Glasgow: Scottish Centre for Post Qualification Pharmaceutical Education.

Scottish Centre for Post Qualification Pharmaceutical Education (1996) *Pharmaceutical Aspects of Methadone Prescribing.* Glasgow: Scottish Centre for Post Qualification Pharmaceutical Education.

Scottish Drugs Forum (2000) Users have their say on methadone programme. *Scottish Drugs Forum Bulletin*, 140: 2.

Sheridan, J., Strang, J., Taylor, C. & Barber, N. (1997) HIV prevention and drug treatment services for drug misusers: a national study of community pharmacists' attitudes and their involvement in service specific training. *Addiction*, 92: 1737–48.

Sheridan, J., Strang, J., Barber, N. & Glanz, A. (1996) Role of community pharmacies in relation to HIV prevention and drug misuse: findings from the 1995 national survey in England and Wales. *British Medical Journal,* 313: 272–4.

Stone, M., Stone, D. & McGregor, H. (1989) Intravenous drug misusers presenting to the accident and emergency department of a large teaching hospital: A failure of clinical management. *Scottish Medical Journal*, 34: 428–30.

United Kingdom Anti-Drugs Co-ordination Unit (2000) *Case Study: Berkshire Shared Care – Four Way Agreement, in Annual Report 1999/2000*. London: UKADCU.

United Kingdom Anti-Drugs Co-ordination Unit (1998) Enabling people with drug problems to overcome them and live healthy and crime-free lives: supervised consumption of methadone. In: *Tackling Drugs to Build a Better Britain: The Government's 10-year Strategy for Tackling Drug Misuse*; Guidance Notes, 27. London: UKADCU.

Section F: Special cases

20
A methadone programme for substance-misusing pregnant women

Ann Walker and James Walker

Introduction

As with all antenatal care, services for the substance-misusing pregnant woman should benefit both mother and baby (Hepburn 1993). They need to be all encompassing, accepting, non-judgemental and supportive. There should be fewer rules and restrictions than in other areas of addiction support, as the women will require antenatal care regardless of whether they agree to addiction management (Benson 2000). Many women who attend a clinic are new to addiction treatment and it is the pregnancy that brings them to the service. Pregnancy produces specific problems but also provides a unique opportunity to engage with them at a time of their lives when they are more susceptible to change (Daley *et al.* 1998). Stabilization of drug use and lifestyle using methadone is the mainstay of care as insistence on abstinence may deter women from engaging (Ottenjann 2000). Abstinence, however, must remain the longer-term, usually post-partum, goal. Such a treatment programme can allow development of coping and parenting skills. Babies that stay with the mother in the long term generally do better than those who are taken into care (MacMahon 1997). Mothers who keep their babies also tend to be more successful in improving their long-term outcome as they have a greater feeling of responsibility and consequence. As their lifestyle is often complicated by associated social, legal and environmental factors, it is important to organize the service to take advantage of this opportunity to involve all the relevant agencies in an integrated service (Hepburn 1998).

Specific problems of heroin addiction in pregnancy

The main clinical problems of heroin addiction in pregnancy are the direct drug effect on the baby and the reduced ability of the mother to look after her infant (Soepatmi 1994). There is no known teratogenic effect from opiates (Schneider *et al.* 1996). However, their use is associated with intrauterine growth restriction (IUGR) and premature delivery (Boer *et al.* 1994; Nair *et al.* 1994; Soepatmi 1994), a higher incidence of fetal distress and a greater need of neonatal care (Nair *et al.* 1994). Longitudinal studies have found an increased incidence of deficits in cognitive development and behavioural problems but no differences in motor development. However, it is difficult to separate the effects of the in-utero exposure to heroin from the problems of lack of neonatal nurturing (Ornoy et al. 1996). Children who are adopted from an early age into nurturing families do not develop differently from normal controls. This implies that if a mother is stabilized and succeeds in changing her lifestyle, the long-term outcome for the baby can be completely normal. However, an increased risk of sudden infant death syndrome (SIDS) has been observed (Kandall et al. 1993). This demonstrates that pregnancy care is only the starting point and there is a need for ongoing support after delivery (Vanbaar et al. 1994).

Methadone maintenance treatment is more successful within a strong supportive environment and is largely independent of the methadone dose or plasma concentration (Wolff et al. 1996). Therefore, the quality of the service may be the most important factor (Lejeune et al. 1997).

Methadone in pregnancy

Methadone use in pregnancy varies (Grella et al. 2000). In the USA, higher doses are used to block opiate receptors and reduce cravings whereas in the UK, the approach is often to find the lowest dose to prevent withdrawal symptoms. Risk and severity of neonatal abstinence syndrome (NAS) appear to be increased by methadone compared with heroin, but, despite this, methadone stabilization has considerable benefits for both the mother and her baby. Studies have shown improved weight and prolonged birth gestation with its use (McCarthy et al. 1999). It is difficult to tell whether these benefits result from the use of methadone, the reduction of other drug use, an improved lifestyle or a combination of all three.

Since methadone at therapeutic doses does not create euphoria, sedation or analgesia and has no adverse effects on motor skills, mental capability or employability, it is compatible with a reasonably normal lifestyle. Therefore, it is suitable for stabilization during pregnancy and short- to medium-term use after delivery to maintain stability. Although many will reduce their opiate use, only a few (between 10% and 25%) become drug free (Boer et al. 1994; Schneider et al. 1996). Those who are withdrawn from opiates often return to heroin use after delivery.

The amount of methadone required can be assessed in the usual way. There should be a clear history of daily use, withdrawal symptoms and positive urine toxicology. Dosage is then titrated against withdrawal scores until stabilization is achieved. The aim is to find the lowest dose of methadone that is compatible with an absence of withdrawal symptoms or cravings. The maximum dose used in the Leeds service is 80 mg per day, as is the case with the non-pregnant user. Because the metabolism of methadone in pregnancy is increased, leading to a shorter half-life, the dose can be split into a twice daily dose in later pregnancy to maintain a satisfactory steady state (Jarvis *et al.* 1999). This can increase the compliance without a need to increase the total dose (DePetrillo and Rice 1995).

Once stabilization is achieved and life style issues addressed, gradual reduction can begin. Because of the danger of miscarriage, this is more safely carried out between 12 and 30 weeks' gestation. After this, it is better simply to stabilize in preparation for labour and delivery. Reduction should be done slowly, by reducing daily dosage by 5 mg, no faster than every two weeks, in order to achieve the lowest sustainable dose without the mother resorting to heroin or suffering withdrawal symptoms (McCarthy *et al.* 1999). It is important to aim for the lowest maternal dose to reduce the possibility of NAS in the baby. Although not strictly dose-related, a dose of less than 20 mg is not usually associated with significant NAS, unless there is concurrent street drug use. Regular urine toxicology will allow accurate assessment of the success of the treatment programme and assist in the planning of dose adjustments (Wolff *et al.* 1996).

Alternatives to methadone

Because of the well-recognized limitations of methadone treatment, alternatives have been investigated. Recent trials in Baltimore and Vienna have studied the use of buprenorphine instead of methadone in the third trimester of pregnancy (Mello *et al.* 1993; Fischer *et al.* 1999). Patients already stable on a methadone treatment programme have been converted to an equivalent dose of buprenorphine. This conversion has been done as an inpatient, to allow close monitoring of the mother and fetus.

Early results have been encouraging, with no significant adverse effects found. The great advantage may be a reduction in the rate of NAS. At present the children are being closely followed up with regular monitoring of both physical and psychological development. So far, no clear detrimental effects have been found. If these results are confirmed by current randomized trials, drug-abusing mothers would be greatly encouraged to engage in treatment.

Integrated management

It is important to have a multidisciplinary approach. Programmes of antenatal care that provide social and behavioural support, along with medical care, have been shown to improve the health of the mother and the outcome of her pregnancy (Scholl *et al.* 1994), with comparable birth outcomes to match non-drug using mothers (Hepburn 1993; Siney 1994). The specifics of the care provided are probably less important than the quality of the care given.

As the aim is to encourage women into the service, clinic attendance should be as easy and non-threatening as possible. Good communication with the general practitioner, community midwife and health visitor is imperative as they can help in the engagement of the client and encourage her to take the first steps. A system centred on a reward structure is better than one that is based on punishment. The ultimate reward is being able to keep and care for her baby after delivery.

Individual risk assessment needs to account for the patterns of drug use, the environment, the social circle in which the woman lives, the degree of her awareness of the effects of her risk-taking behaviour, and the past involvement of social services with existing children. The support of partners and family members, and whether they themselves are drug abusers, can be decisive. Treatment for the partner, where appropriate, can significantly improve outcome. Once engaged into the service, there needs to be provision of a network of professionals both to assess any potential risk for the expected baby and also to provide support for the necessary lifestyle changes. At all times it is important to be realistic in setting goals for each individual.

Setting up a special clinical service for the pregnant addict

In Leeds, a special service was set up in two specified pre-existing antenatal clinics. This allows all needs to be provided from a single site. The clinic is co-ordinated by a liaison midwife with an obstetrician and an addiction worker in attendance. This ensures access both to the necessary antenatal care and to addiction advice. The service provides a regular clinic available both by appointment and by 'drop in' at the two main hospitals in the city. The non-separation of service provision avoids the potential stigma of a separate clinic and possible loss of confidentiality. The availability of the service is promoted in health centres, hospitals and local relevant organizations.

A close working link has developed between the obstetric and addiction services, with links with the community midwives, primary care doctor, paediatricians, health visitors, child protection nurses, social service departments and general support services such as housing, probation and community care projects. With so many individuals involved, regular monthly meetings are held to exchange information and concerns. Treatment protocols are available for all staff, particularly for those working in shared areas of responsibility with other services.

Regular reviews of the women are important. The Standing Conference on Drug Abuse (SCODA) guidelines are followed. Dates and time intervals for assessments are established at initial presentation and at 32 weeks' gestation, when full assessment should be complete. By that time, a plan should be in place to deal with any outstanding issues and any other professionals, usually social services or the housing authorities who should be involved. This process occurs with the consent of the client unless the baby is thought to be 'at risk', when the authorities need to be involved even without client consent. In cases of significant concern, a full pre-birth assessment may need to be carried out by social services. A post-natal review at three months is also beneficial to assess the progress of the mother and her baby.

Labour and delivery

It is important that the attendant staff have been trained in the care of pregnant drug users and treat them in the same way as other women in labour. On admission, a history of recent drug use (i.e. before admission) is important. Many mothers use heroin prior to hospital admission to help them get through their labour.

There are no specific problems associated with labour or delivery except for maternal analgesia. Methadone should be continued with additional opiate analgesia as required. Since high doses of narcotic may be necessary, epidural analgesia has advantages. Gas and air is also available and may give valuable additional pain relief. At delivery, the baby should not be given naloxone (Narcan) as this would produce a severe withdrawal reaction.

Postnatal care

Post delivery, normal support should be continued and is ideally provided in a transitional care ward. This allows the mother and baby to be together, which is important for bonding and establishment of parenting skills. It is the ideal time for staff both to promote support and assess possible risk. Assessment should be over a minimum of seven days.

The only definite effect of opiate use by the mother is NAS (Hepburn 1993), the incidence and severity of which is partly related to the type and amount of drug used. Poly-drug use can influence this, particularly benzodiazepines and cocaine (Sutton and Hinderliter 1990). The paediatric unit will have been alerted to the potential clinical problems and will hopefully have been involved both in the case discussion and the development of management protocols.

In Leeds, a modified Finnegan scale is used to monitor the baby (Finnegan *et al.* 1975). This is initially carried out four hourly and reduced when appropriate. It is useful for the mother to be involved in these assessments. Many drug-using mothers have strong feelings of guilt, and so it is important to encourage them to feel they are now making a useful contribution. Withdrawal from heroin occurs over one to three days whereas methadone has a longer clearance time and symptoms in the newborn may not occur for up to seven days post-delivery. The classic symptoms are restlessness, jitteriness, failure to feed, tremors, high-pitched cry, arching of the back, yawning, sneezing and sweating. Convulsions can also occur. However, the majority of babies do not have withdrawal problems and can be safely cared for in the transitional care area (Hepburn 1993; Robins and Mills 1993). Of 200 babies born in Glasgow to mothers using illicit drugs or legal methadone, only 7% required treatment for withdrawal, while even fewer required admission to the special care nursery (Hepburn 1993). However, other centres quote incidences of between 10% and 80% of cases depending on the amount of antenatal drug usage and the success of the clinic maintenance programme (Nair et al. 1994; Vanbaar et al. 1994).

Continuing supportive care, including methadone maintenance, may allow the new mother to live a reasonably stable life and to look after her own child. Many studies have demonstrated that infants who remain with their natural parents do better than those who do not (Soepatmi 1994). This requires a continued good working relationship with general practitioners, health visitors, the community paediatricians and the local addiction service. The success of these programmes is varied with more than 50% of those who stop using heroin starting again within six months of delivery. Many of the babies will eventually be in care or cared for by extended family (Fabris et al. 1998).

Breast-feeding

If the mother is stable on methadone, not supplementing and thought to be HIV negative, breast-feeding should be encouraged. The secretion of methadone in the breast milk is variable (Wojnar-Horton et al. 1997) but this could potentially help to reduce withdrawal symptoms. A stable lifestyle helps successful breast-feeding. However, if the mother is still injecting street heroin, is known to be or is at risk of being HIV positive or is using other street drugs such as cocaine, breast-feeding is not advisable.

HIV and other infectious diseases

HIV infection is associated with drug abuse, both because of needle sharing and heterosexual spread from associated prostitution. The danger, particularly in the UK, has been overstated, although, in some areas the incidence of HIV is particularly high. In Edinburgh, out of 290 'at risk' pregnancies, 93 (32%) of the women were HIV positive. However, of these 93 pregnancies, only 8 (8.7%) resulted in an HIV infected child (Ross et al. 1995). Since then, the prevalence of HIV has declined from 0.5% of all pregnancies in 1986 to 0.1% in 1992 and there has been no change since (Goldberg et al. 2000). The risk of vertical transmission has been significantly reduced by the use of anti-viral drugs and obstetric intervention.

Whereas the medical authorities knew most of the HIV positive women in the past, in 1992 only 30% were identified. Therefore, although the number of cases has declined, with most hospitals having only one HIV positive woman a year, the majority of these are now not known to their carers and may be non-users (Johnstone *et al.* 1994; Tappin *et al.* 1995). Since the risk of HIV infection to attendant staff is dependent on the background incidence of HIV in the region and not to specific patient groups, single tier management of all pregnant women is important to reduce the risk of transmission to staff. This also helps to reduce discrimination against substance-misusing women. In the UK, HIV testing is offered to all pregnant women after appropriate counselling. Benefits of testing need to be explained to the mother. Current therapy will not only improve her health but also significantly reduce vertical transmission to the baby.

Hepatitis B and C are also tested for. The most common infection found is hepatitis C. It is generally found in approximately 40–62% of all intravenous drug-abusing women. The evidence to date is that hepatitis C does not adversely affect the pregnancy and the pregnancy does not worsen the viral load or prognosis of the disease. Many women, however, will get a slight rise in levels of ALT post-partum which is not related to viral load (Latt *et al.* 2000). Vertical transmission is around 6% but this can be higher in women with a higher level of HCV–RNA or concurrent HIV infection (Spencer *et al.* 1997). Transmission is also increased in longer labours but breast-feeding does not influence it as HCV–RNA is not detected in breast milk. If babies are found to be HCV positive, they should be followed up for at least a year, as some become negative and others will develop hepatitis. At the time of writing there is no vaccination available.

Less frequently, women are found to be hepatitis B positive. Again, pregnancy does not appear to affect the course of the disease in the mother but vertical transmission without intervention is 80–90%. Of those, more than 85% will become clinical carriers of the virus. Infection in the baby usually occurs at or directly after delivery, so the babies are suitable for post-exposure prophylaxis. In an at-risk baby, it is recommended that it is given HepB immunoglobulin within 12 hours of delivery while concurrently being given the first dose of HepB vaccination. This should be completed with follow-up vaccinations at one month and six months and will provide 90% protection against infection.

Long-term follow-up

Taking a new baby (sometimes still unsettled from withdrawal symptoms) back to possibly difficult family situations is often a time of stress and relapse. Continued support from the addiction and community-based services is required. Long-term follow-up is not encouraging. Many users revert to heroin use and many of their children do not remain in the care of their natural parents. This is partly due to the social environment in which they find themselves and also to the factors that contributed to the initiation of their drug use in the first place.

Long-term outcomes can be assessed by monitoring outcomes of families, the incidence of children being put on the 'at risk' register and the number going into care or being cared for by a member of the extended family. Currently, trying to establish on-going follow-up of these families is difficult due to the chaotic lifestyles, but better links with the community paediatric services are proving helpful in this area.

The future

Substance misuse will be a continuing problem requiring dedicated services (Jones *et al.* 2000). Hopefully better education will improve women's awareness of the risks in pregnancy and encourage early involvement with services. In Leeds, some 1% of the pregnant population is seen in this special service. This is the same percentage as for heroin use in the general population, implying we see the majority of pregnant heroin users. However, the service needs to be further integrated with better long-term follow-up into the community. Dissemination of clear information about drug abuse and pregnancy to staff involved at any level is an important aspect of this work and thought to be helpful in fostering empathy and a non-judgemental attitude.

Because of the complications of the NAS, methadone may not be the best drug for substitution in pregnancy. Studies have shown that buprenorphine may be a better alternative but further investigation is required (Fischer *et al.* 2000). At the time of writing there is a serious lack of data on pregnancy and follow-up. This is a challenge for the future to allow assessment and development of different treatment modalities.

References

Benson, D.S. (2000) Providing health care to human beings trapped in the poverty culture. *Physician Executive,* 26: 28–32.

Boer, K., Smit, B.J., Vanhuis, A.M. & Hogerzeil, H.V. (1994) Substance use in pregnancy – do we care. *Acta Paediatrica Supplement,* 83: 65–71.

Daley, M., Argeriou, M. & McCarty, D. (1998) Substance abuse treatment for pregnant women: a window of opportunity? *Addictive Behaviors,* 23: 239–49.

DePetrillo, P.B. & Rice, J.M. (1995) Methadone dosing and pregnancy: impact on program compliance. *International Journal of the Addictions,* 30: 207–17.

Fabris, C., Prandi, G., Perathoner, C. & Soldi, A. (1998) Neonatal drug addiction. *Panminerva Medica,* 40: 239–43.

Finnegan, L.P., Connaughton, J.F. Jr, Kron, R.E. & Emich, J.P. (1975) Neonatal abstinence syndrome: assessment and management. *Addictive Diseases,* 2: 141–58.

Fischer, G., Johnson, R.E., Eder, H., Jagsch, R., Peternell, A., Weninger, M., Langer, M. & Aschauer, H.N. (2000) Treatment of opioid-dependent pregnant women with buprenorphine. *Addiction,* 95: 239–44.

Fischer, G., Gombas, W., Eder, H., Jagsch, R., Peternell, A., Stuhlinger, G., Pezawas, L., Aschauer, H.N. & Kasper, S.

(1999) Buprenorphine versus methadone maintenance for the treatment of opioid dependence. *Addiction*, 94: 1337–47.

Goldberg, D., Smith, R., MacIntyre, P., Patel, N., Rowarth, M., Allardice, G., Codere, G. & Reid, D. (2000) Prevalence of HIV among pregnant women in Dundee 1988–1997: evidence to gauge the effectiveness of HIV prevention measures. *The Journal of Infection*, 41: 39–44.

Grella, C.E., Joshi, V. & Hser, Y.I. (2000) Program variation in treatment outcomes among women in residential drug treatment. *Evaluation Review,* 24: 364–83.

Hepburn, M. (1998) Drug use in pregnancy: a multidisciplinary responsibility. *Hospital Medicine,* 59: 436.

Hepburn, M. (1993) Drug use in pregnancy. *British Journal of Hospital Medicine,* 49: 51–5.

Jarvis, M.A., Wu-Pong, S., Kniseley, J.S. & Schnoll, S.H. (1999) Alterations in methadone metabolism during late pregnancy. *Journal of Addictive Diseases,* 18: 51–61.

Johnstone, F.D., Brettle, R.P., Burns, S.M., Peutherer, J., Mok, J.Y.Q., Robertson, J.R., Hamilton, B. & Tappin, D.M. (1994) HIV testing and prevalence in pregnancy in Edinburgh. *International Journal of STD & AIDS,* 5: 101–4.

Jones, H.E., Haug, N.A., Stitzer, M.L. & Svikis, D.S. (2000) Improving treatment outcomes for pregnant drug-dependent women using low-magnitude voucher incentives. *Addictive Behaviors*, 25: 263–7.

Kandall, S.R., Gaines, J., Habel, L., Davidson, G. & Jessop, D. (1993) Relationship of maternal substance abuse to subsequent sudden infant death syndrome in offspring. *Journal de Pediatria*, 123: 120–6.

Latt, N.C., Spencer, J.D., Beeby, P.J., McCaughan, G.W., Saunders, J.B., Collins, E., Cossart, Y.E. (2000) Hepatitis C in injecting drug-using women during and after pregnancy. *Journal of Gastroenterology and Hepatology*. 15: 175–81.

Lejeune, C., Ropert, J.C., Montamat, S., Floch-Tudal, C., Mazy, F., Wijkhuisen, N. & Froment, H. (1997) Medical-social outcome of 59 infants born to addicted mothers. *Journal de Gynecologie, Obstetrique et Biologie de la Reproduction*, 26: 395–404.

MacMahon, J.R. (1997) Perinatal substance abuse: the impact of reporting infants to child protective services. *Pediatrics*, 100: E1.

McCarthy, J.E., Siney, C., Shaw, N.J. & Ruben, S.M. (1999) Outcome predictors in pregnant opiate and polydrug users. *European Journal of Pediatrics,* 158: 748–9.

Mello, N.K., Mendelson, J.H., Lukas, S.E., Gastfriend, D.R., Teoh, S.K., Holman, B.L. (1993) Buprenorphine treatment of opiate and cocaine abuse: clinical and preclinical studies. *Harvard Review of Psychiatry,* 1: 168–83.

Nair, P., Rothblum, S. & Hebel, R. (1994) Neonatal outcome in infants with evidence of fetal exposure to opiates, cocaine, and cannabinoids. *Clinical Pediatrics,* 33: 280–5.

Ornoy, A., Michailevskaya, V., Lukashov, I., Bar-Hamburger, R. & Harel, S. (1996) The developmental outcome of children born to heroin-dependent mothers, raised at home or adopted. *Child Abuse and Neglect*, 20: 385–96.

Ottenjann, H. (2000) Drug dependence in pregnancy. Better to substitute than complete withdrawal. *MMW Fortschritte der Medizin,* 142: 16.

Robins, L.N. & Mills, J.L. (1993) Effects of in-utero exposure to street drugs. *American Journal of Public Health,* 83: 1–32.

Ross, A., Raab, G.M., Mok, J., Gilkison, S., Hamilton, B. & Johnstone, F.D. (1995) Maternal HIV-infection, drug-use, and growth of uninfected children in their first 3 years. *Archives of Disease in Childhood*, 73: 490–5.

Schneider, C., Fischer, G., Diamant, K., Hauk, R., Pezawas, L., Lenzinger, E. & Kasper, S. (1996) Pregnancy and drug-abuse. *Wiener Klinische Wochenschrift*, 108: 611–14.

Scholl, T.O., Hediger, M.L. & Belsky, D.H. (1994) Prenatal-care and maternal health during adolescent pregnancy – a review and meta-analysis. *Journal of Adolescent Health,* 15: 444–56.

Siney, C. (1994) Team effort helps pregnant drug users. *MIDIRS Midwifery Digest,* 4: 229–31.

Soepatmi, S. (1994) Developmental outcomes of children of mothers dependent on heroin or heroin/methadone during pregnancy. *Acta Paediatrica Supplement,* 83: 36–9.

Spencer, J.D., Latt, N., Beeby, P.J., Collins, E., Saunders, J.B., McCaughan, G.W. & Cossart, Y.E. (1997) Transmission of hepatitis C virus to infants of human immunodeficiency virus-negative intravenous drug-using mothers: rate of infection and assessment of risk factors for transmission. *Journal of Viral Hepatitis,* 4: 395–409.

Sutton, L.R. & Hinderliter, S.A. (1990) Diazepam abuse in pregnant women on methadone maintenance. Implications for the neonate. *Clinical Pediatrics (Phila),* 29: 108–11.

Tappin, D.M., Johnstone, F.D., Smith, R., Girdwood, R.W.A., Follett, E.A.C. & Davidson, C.F. (1995) Spread of maternal, HIV-infection in Scotland from 1990 to 1992. *Scottish Medical Journal,* 40: 12–14.

Vanbaar, A.L., Soepatmi, S., Gunning, W.B. & Akkerhuis, G.W. (1994) Development after prenatal exposure to cocaine, heroin and methadone. *Acta Paediatrica Supplement*, 83: 40–6.

Wojnar-Horton, R.E., Kristensen, J.H., Yapp, P., Hett, K.F., Dusci, L.J. & Hackett, L.P. (1997) Methadone distribution and excretion into breast milk of clients in a methadone maintenance programme. *British Journal of Clinical Pharmacology,* 44: 543–7.

Wolff, K., Hay, A.W.M., Vail, A., Harrison, K. & Raistrick, D. (1996) Non-prescribed drug-use during methadone treatment by clinic-based and community-based patients. *Addiction,* 91: 1699–1704.

21
Methadone use in young people

Eilish Gilvarry, Jim McCambridge and John Witton

Introduction

This chapter considers the needs of young people involved in illicit opiate use and the role of methadone as one component of a treatment response. These issues are placed in context through examination of data on prevalence and help-seeking among those young people with problems. Arguments for and against the provision of separate services are embraced in the discussion of treatment needs, current policy and practice. In large measure, differing positions in these debates relate to how distinct the needs of young people are, viewed in comparison to the needs of adults, and the implications of these differences for methadone prescribing. The age range encompassed in discussions of the treatment of young people is a source of further complication. For example, the current UK anti-drugs strategy defines young people as those under 25 years old.

Opiate use among young people: from the 1960s to the 1990s

The emergence of mass opiate use since the 1960s has been widely associated with a series of 'epidemics' involving youthful populations. Usually, observations of this type rely heavily on trends in official indicators, including policing and treatment data. Power (1994) describes a stabilization of opiate use in the 1970s following on from dramatic increases in indicator data in the second half of the 1960s. In the years 1980–1985 steeply rising official indicators were accompanied by detailed local studies. From that period, Pearson (1987) and Parker and colleagues (Parker *et al.* 1988) describe a generation of 'new' heroin users. These tended to be young unemployed men in areas of socio-economic deprivation, who often smoked rather than injected heroin. Pearson and Gilman (1994) emphasize local and regional variation in this pattern and Griffiths *et al.* (1994) highlight the significance of the development of heroin smoking. Increases in these official figures slowed down in the latter half of the 1980s.

A later study by Parker *et al.* (1998) reported further 'outbreaks' of heroin use throughout the 1990s in previously unaffected localities and regions.

These involved younger participants from socially disadvantaged back-grounds but included the penetration of heroin use into more affluent communities and those 'from the serious end of recreational drug use'.

Prevalence of opiate use among young people in the general population

It is only since the mid-1990s that nation-wide representative surveys of drug use in the general population have taken place in Britain (Ramsay and Percy 1997). The British Crime Survey has been a biennial survey of victimization that includes a self-reported drug use component among those aged 16 and over. It is the main prevalence instrument with which current prevention policy for England and Wales is evaluated (Ramsey and Spiller 1997; Ramsey et al. 2001). Given the limitations of these data, that which is described below should be interpreted cautiously with an expectation that opiate use preva-lence will tend towards or even exceed the upper estimates given.

Ramsey et al. (2001) reported that, of an estimated 5.8 million young people aged 16–24 in England and Wales, an estimated 46,000 had used heroin in the past year, including an estimated 18,000 who had used heroin in the past month. They further estimated that approximately 1% of all 16–19 year olds had ever used heroin and approximately 2% of all those aged 20–24 had done so. Heroin use within the past year was estimated to be approximately 1% for both 16–19 year olds and 20–24 year olds, with last-month use not registering at this level among young people as a whole. Around 1% of 20–24 year olds had used methadone in their lifetime, and the use of other opiates was relatively rare.

In Britain, heroin use was more common among white ethnic groups than among non-white groups and, in most estimates, more prevalent among men, although the magnitude of the gender difference may be declining over time. Heroin use was also found to be related to socio-economic deprivation via a number of indicators, including neighbourhood housing category, unemployment, household income and poor educational achievement (Ramsey et al. 2001).

In the schools survey of 11–15 year olds, the prevalence counterpart to the British Crime Survey, Goddard and Higgins (2000) found similar levels of life-time opiate use to those found among 16–19 year olds. Among pupils aged 13–15, around 1% reported lifetime opiate use, with 3% of 11 year olds hav-ing ever been offered opiates, rising to 6% by age 15. Regular use of heroin in this age range was found by Balding (1998) to reach 0.2% by age 15.

Evaluation of prevalence data

Existing British population data are limited in many respects. Relatively little is known about the age-related relationships between types of heroin use and other forms of drug use, 'problem behaviours' and other risk factors. Targeted studies of particular groups such as the homeless (Fountain and Howes 2002), and those involved in the criminal justice system (Bennett and Sibbitt 2000), reveal much higher prevalence rates of opiate use than are observed in the general population.

Variations in heroin prevalence rates between geographical areas can be expected in the light of differences in relevant population characteristics and patterns of diffusion of drug use (Parker *et al.* 1988). Where an area is found to have lower prevalence rates than adjoining areas, experience shows this to be a cause for concern as there tends to be a spread from areas of higher prevalence to areas of lower prevalence. The UK government set an ambitious target of a 50% reduction in prevalence of heroin use over ten years (Cabinet Office 1998), but in the first few years of the drugs strategy there is no discernible trend in this direction.

Will new heroin users get any younger?

There is evidence from treatment data that the age of new heroin users has declined over recent years. Comparison with data from help-seekers in the USA suggests that there is potential for further decline. Whilst prevalence rates are broadly comparable for those aged 20 and over, the USA has a two to three times higher rate of lifetime teenage heroin use than is found in the UK (Johnston *et al.* 2000). Lifetime heroin use was reported to have increased consistently since 1991 (0.9% in 1991, 2% in 1998), with the average age of new heroin users reduced from 21.2 years in 1994 to 17.5 years in 1997.

Young people and accidental poisoning

Analysis of deaths from accidental poisoning in the UK from 1985 to 1995 also suggest that opiate use is increasing amongst young people: 436 teenagers aged 15 to 19 years died of an accidental overdose during this period. Twenty-one per cent of these deaths were attributed to accidental poisoning by opiates and related narcotics, making up the largest single category. Whilst the overall death rate attributable to accidental poisoning increased by 8% a year during this period, the death rate from poisoning by opiates and related narcotics increased by 27% per year (Roberts *et al.* 1997).

Young people in treatment

Two UK data sources provide some help in tracking young peoples' treatment-seeking for opiate-related problems over the last decade. The first was the Home Office Addicts Index, established as an attempt to monitor prevalence of drug use and to provide a method for preventing over-prescribing, though its limitations eventually caused its cessation in 1997. Before that date, figures on drug addicts notified showed that in 1988, 214 or 2.8% of the total heroin users reported were 17 years and under. By 1992, the number of 17 year olds and younger had risen to 252, forming the lower 1.5% of the total number of addicts notified for their heroin use (Hansard Society 1994).

The Regional Drug Misuse Databases are the second source of UK data. These databases are used as a treatment-monitoring tool but again their value is compromised by inconsistencies in reporting by the contributing agencies. However, they indicated that 805 people aged 17 and under presented for treatment with a main drug of heroin, methadone or opiates in the six months ending 30 September 2000, with heroin accounting for 97% of the cases. This represents 3.4% of the total presenting for problems related to these drugs and contrasts with a figure of 566 for the six months to 30 September 1996, 3% of the overall group. Ten per cent of this group were under 16 in 1996 but this percentage had risen to 15% by 2000 (Department of Health, personal communication).

There is little published specifically on young heroin users attending treatment facilities. Chien *et al.* (1964), Wiener and Egan (1973) and Noble and Barnes (1971) reported backgrounds of disadvantaged communities, delinquency, frequent and poly-drug use, family dysfunction and greater psychiatric co-morbidity among adolescent heroin users. More recently Crome *et al.* (1998) in the UK reported similar profiles of early initiation, injecting drug use and rapid development of dependence, concurrent poly-drug use and deliberate self-harm. Hopfer *et al.* (2000) in the USA reported on treatment samples of 13–19 year olds, and treatment data for 12 to 17 years are provided by the Treatment Episode Data Set (TEDS). Those using heroin reported earlier age of initiation of any drug use and significantly more diagnoses of poly-drug abuse and dependence when compared with other drug-using youths. The TEDS data showed increases during the 1990s in the absolute number of adolescents in treatment who reported heroin/opiates as a primary or secondary drug. Of adolescents in treatment programmes in the USA, 2.0% had opiate use as a primary or secondary drug problem during 1992–1996 with a rise to 2.6% recorded in 1997. Of those using heroin in the treatment programmes in 1997, almost 80% were white; males constituted 53.4% and almost 60% reported daily use prior to admission. This group reported the highest rate of injecting drug use at 44.6%. Only 8.3% of these youths were treated with methadone.

Service needs

In a number of authoritative policy documents, *'The Substance of Young Needs', Children and Young People: Substance Misuse Services* (Health Advisory Service 1996; 2001), *Young People and Substance Misuse* (Social

Services Inspectorate 1997), *Policy Guidance for Drug Interventions* (Standing Conference on Drug Abuse 1998) as well as the UK Drug Strategy (Cabinet Office 1998), the need for the development of young people's substance-misuse services that are distinct from those designed for adults has been acknowledged. UK government ministers adopted this policy in the *Young People's Substance Misuse Plans* (Drug Prevention Advisory Service 2001), which proposed an integrated approach for the development of substance misuse services within existing children's systems.

Young people's needs are distinct from those of adults, and adults have a responsibility of care. The design and delivery of services need to reflect these intrinsic differences, and work within a developmental model. This demands an understanding of the cognitive, socio-emotional and physical developmental issues in adolescence, issues of motivation, gender and age, academic performance, family involvement, and occasionally multiple needs. Treatments that 'approach young people as "little adults" are bound to fail' (Winters 1999). There is a legislative framework that supports the care and protection of young people and the resolution of multiple problems may be particularly important as lack of such resolution may impede developmental progress and age-appropriate developmental tasks with later effects in adulthood.

A child-centred approach necessitates consideration of parental responsibility, consent to treatment, confidentiality, age of the child and need for protection. Definitions of the age range of youth vary greatly between departments and services with cut-offs described as under 16, 18, 19, 21 and up to 25 years. The UK Drug Strategy refers to young people as those under 25 years of age, with drug prevention and treatment more frequently organized by agencies like the United Kingdom Anti-Drugs Co-ordination Unit (UKADCU) than by children's systems. The term 'child' refers to those individuals under the age of 18 in the UK Children Act (1989) and the United Nations Convention on the Rights of the Child. Generally, those over 18 are considered to be adults, although young people between 16 and 18 years are usually considered competent. Services should operate within the law (in the case of Britain, chiefly the Children Act 1989) and this includes operating within the spirit and intentions of the law. Parental responsibility must be respected and emphasis put on the involvement of the child. The child's view and wishes must be balanced against the age and maturity of the child, the views of the parents and the professionals' assessments of the best interest of the child. The application of adult addiction models of treatment to children and young people should not be considered good practice: for example the attempt to 'empower' premature independence and autonomy from parents, to exclude parents other than in the event of specific child protection matters, is not in the best interest of the child. A young person's drug service containing a 'young person's worker', deployed from adult services, risks the extension of adult models. It undermines co-ordination and consultation with other children's services and may frustrate the appreciation of the ethical and legal framework surrounding children and young people.

Methadone prescribing

The prescription of methadone is a significant treatment requiring a high level of competence from the child to assent to this approach. Services where methadone is prescribed for young people, particularly those under 18, should agree a standard approach to risk assessment, and of working together with other child agencies.

Methadone detoxification and maintenance in adult populations have been extensively studied and reported (Ward et al. 1998) though little systematic data exist in the adolescent population (Gastfriend et al. 1998; Solukhah and Wilens 1998; Weinberg et al. 1998). Adolescent drug programmes do exist (Baer et al. 1998) with outcome measures focusing on domains of functioning such as reduction in drug and alcohol use, crime and school non-attendance (Hser et al. 2001).

One might extrapolate from findings in adults that adolescents may benefit from methadone maintenance for the goals of reduction in crime, reduction in illicit drug use, retention in treatment services and other health benefits. Detoxification, in the few published studies, has resulted in low abstinence rates and poor engagement (Lloyd et al. 1974). Anecdotal evidence suggests that some clinicians consider that adolescents with heroin dependence and other multiple problems might benefit from longer term treatment with methadone alongside ancillary psychological therapies in the way that adults do. In a study of young 'at risk' opiate users, Ward et al. (1996) noted that methadone maintenance reduced the use of illicit drugs and crime as well as conferring positive health benefits. However, the average age of the young person in that study was 25 years.

Anecdotal UK evidence support the finding by Hser that young people in treatment have multiple problems: 58% were involved in the legal system and 63% met diagnostic criteria for a mental disorder (Hser et al. 2001). Further anecdotal evidence suggests that repeated short-term detoxification is not always effective and may reinforce an ethos of failure. Hopfer et al. (2000) comments that the US restrictions on prescribing practices may no longer be sensible as the system necessitates failure with relapse, possibly to injecting practices with the consequent risk of HIV, on at least two occasions.

Ethical and moral dilemmas for methadone maintenance are often voiced, particularly for the younger child or adolescent. Parker et al. (1998) argue that 'the libertarians and critics of methadone will rightly …question whether we wish to submit adolescents… to a chemical cosh, which might in the end act to prolong a dependent drugs career.' He suggests the availability of guidelines and clear advice to avoid entanglement in 'intense debates and disagreements'. One of the key issues in the debate about pharmacotherapy for adolescents is the goal of treatment: is a harm reduction or an abstinence goal to be pursued? The question remains controversial, and highlights the need for further research.

Guidelines

Guidelines on the indications and use of methadone for the adolescent are available in the USA and UK. In the UK, methadone is not licensed for use in children, though a child, for this purpose, is deemed to be aged 12 or under. No specific restrictions are noted for adolescents.

The federal restrictions in the USA on methadone prescribing for adolescents may limit methadone prescriptions, with changes proposed by the Department of Health and Human Services in 1999 (Department of Health and Human Services 1999). The US guidelines refer to treatment standards for both detoxification and maintenance, which encompass areas such as staff credentials, diversion control, patient admission criteria, counselling, initial dose of methadone and 'take home' procedures. They make no comment on any additional expertise or competence required by the prescribing doctor when dealing with adolescents, the ethos of a service for adolescents, the 'mixing' of adolescents and older adults or more distinct therapies for the younger person. These guidelines describe an adult orientated programme with few references to young people. For maintenance treatment for persons under age 18, it is stated that: 'A person under 18 years of age is required to have had two documented attempts at short-term detoxification or drug free treatment to be eligible for maintenance treatment. No person under 18 years of age may be admitted to maintenance treatment unless a parent, legal guardian, or responsible adult designated by the relevant State authority consents in writing to such treatment'.

In the UK, guidelines on clinical management (Department of Health 1999) define young people as those under 18 years old. There is comment on the need to consider the legislative framework for children with all interventions undertaken in accordance with the Children Act 1989 and other appropriate law. Other considerations include comprehensive and developmental approaches to assessment, provision of adolescent services distinct and discrete from adult services, the involvement of families, the adherence to child protection policies and procedures, and the importance of liaison with other child and adolescent services.

Specific guidance is given with regard to the prescribing of controlled drugs, though not necessarily specifying methadone. The recommendations include obtaining explicit consent from someone with parental responsibility for a person under 16. The generalist should only prescribe a controlled drug after assessment and supervision by a specialist; generalists, including child psychiatrists, are warned against prescribing controlled drugs without specific training or formal liaison with an addiction specialist. The guidelines do not recommend maintenance prescriptions and advise protective standards in dispensing and consumption of the controlled drug, though little guidance is given on preferred settings and those process factors such as social and emotional support that should be taken into consideration.

Assessment

The challenges facing services include the need for the assessment to address the legal framework, the role of parents and carers, the role and involvement of schools and other child services and the most appropriate settings for treatment. Treatment-planning decisions should include the competence of the prescriber and the resources available adequately to conduct screening and dose titration.

Guidelines for assessment of the adolescent drug user have been published (Bukstein *et al.* 1997). Necessarily different from that of adults, assessment of children and adolescents should be based on a developmental model with consideration of the developmental age of the child, and his/her ability to understand and consent to the treatment process requiring particular attention. Confidentiality for the young person is important but must be considered alongside parental responsibility, involvement of families and questions of child protection. Involvement of parents coupled with careful risk assessment is advised particularly because of the risk of overdose and premature deaths (Oyefoso *et al.* 1999). With the likelihood of multiple and complex needs, substance-misuse services should be closely linked with all children's systems to ensure an integrated and more comprehensive approach (Health Advisory Service 2001).

Most young people who use drugs will not develop dependence and many may exaggerate their use. Drug testing, usually using urine, helps to confirm use though not dependence. Saliva and hair testing may be helpful. It is important that both parents and child are fully informed of the reasons for these procedures in assessment and continued monitoring.

Including methadone in treatment of young people: is it a good idea?

The evidence in adults increasingly points to the possibility that methadone is successful as a longer-term substitution treatment rather than a shorter-term treatment aimed at abstinence. To the extent that treatment-planning decisions in young people are by definition shorter-term decisions than those taken in the case of adults (shorter history and they will not be young people for ever), decisions regarding methadone treatment will need to be taken with extreme caution. Likely duration of the treatment, though difficult to predict, will be an important consideration. Pharmacotherapy with methadone in young people should be prescribed in conjunction with a comprehensive plan incorporating a variety of individual interventions (education, cognitive-behavioural and other psychotherapies) designed to meet their specific needs (Gilvarry 2000). While this is similar in principle to that of adult services, the nature of treatment is necessarily different, with greater emphasis on family involvement, parental responsibility, school attendance and possible need for protection.

In the UK a variety of settings are used in the community ranging from primary care, adult addiction services and the voluntary sector, with little provision for inpatient methadone detoxification. Most of the prescribing of methadone is either by primary care doctors, specialists in addiction and occasionally child psychiatrists. Settings have developed pragmatically according to perceived local need, availability and willingness of a prescriber. Dose titration occurs in some services, though most review daily with gradual increase of the dose within a few days. Some services have prescribed methadone to a young dependent heroin user who is to be detained in a secure unit or similar situation. Problems can occur in such settings where there is a lack of expertise in identifying withdrawal symptoms and suitable facilities for dispensing and holding a controlled drug on the premises are not available. Alternatives to methadone, such as dihydrocodeine or high dose buprenorphine may be perceived to be safer. Adolescent child psychiatric units and paediatric units (inpatient and day care), though little used for this treatment, may be able to augment their skills with addiction skills and therapies specifically developed for young people (Health Advisory Service 2001) to provide care for this client group.

In summary and in view of the relative lack of evidence and limited experience, the challenges to treating young people with methadone are considerable. These challenges span the domains of ethics, the law and good practice. The particular competencies required of the treatment provider not only include the ability to prescribe methadone safely but the assessment of issues more particular to children, such as consent to treatment, parental responsibility and involvement. While there is minimal research on methadone in young people, nevertheless, a substantial number of doctors are prescribing methadone to people under the age of 18. There is a need for standardization, with prescribing protocols, specified competencies, clarity in the goals of treatment and integral care planning which includes questions of settings for treatment. Comprehensive multi-modal assessment and treatment approaches are required, as prescribing alone without addressing other areas of functioning such as issues of containment and protection, are unlikely to be successful. Of the utmost importance is the area of evaluation and research to inform future good practice.

References

Baer, J.S., MacLean, M.G. & Marlatt, G.A. (1998) Linking aetiology and treatment for adolescent substance abuse: toward a better match. In: Jessor R, ed. *New Perspectives on Adolescent Risk Behaviour.* New York: Cambridge University Press; 182–220.

Balding, J. (1998) *Young People and Illegal Drugs in 1998.* Exeter: Schools Health Education Unit.

Bennett, T. & Sibbitt, R. (2000) *Drug Use among Arrestees.* London: Home Office Research, Development and Statistics Directorate.

Bukstein, O. and the working party on Quality Issues (1997) Practice parameters for the assessment and treatment of children and adolescents with substance use disorders, *Journal of the American Academy of Child and Adolescent Psychiatry*, Supplement 36: 140S–156S.

Cabinet Office (1998) *Tackling Drugs to Build a Better Britain: The Government's 10 Year Strategy for Tackling Drug Misuse.* London: The Stationery Office.

Chien, I., Gerard, D., Lee, R., Rosenfeld, E. & Wilner, D. (1964) *The Road to H: Narcotics, Delinquency and Social Policy.* New York: Basic Books.

Crome, I., Christian, J. & Green, C. (1998) Tip of the iceberg? Profile of adolescent patients prescribed methadone in an innovative community drug service. *Drugs: Education, Prevention and Policy.* 5: 195–7.

Department of Health (1999) *Drug Misuse and Dependence – Guidelines on Clinical Management.* London: The Stationery Office.

Department of Health and Human Services US (1999) *Code of Federal Regulations, Conditions for the Use of Narcotic Drugs: appropriate methods of professional practise for medical treatment of the narcotic addiction of various classes of narcotic addicts under section 4 of the Comprehensive Drug Abuse Prevention and Control Act of 1970.*Title 21, part 291.505. Rockville, MD: United States Department of Health and Human Services.

Drug Prevention Advisory Service (2001) *Young People's Substance Misuse Plans, DAT Guidance.* London: Home Office.

Fountain, J. & Howes, S. (2002) *Home and Dry? Homelessness and Substance Use.* London: Crisis.

Gastfriend, D., Elman, I. & Solhkhah, R. (1998) Pharmacotherapy of substance abuse and dependence. *Psychiatric Clinics of North America: Annals of Drug Therapy,* 5: 211–29.

Gilvarry, E. (2000) Substance abuse in young people. *Journal of Child Psychology and Psychiatry,* 41: 55–80.

Goddard, E. & Higgins, V. (2000) *Drug Use, Smoking and Drinking among Young Teenagers in 1999.* London: The Stationery Office.

Griffiths, P., Gossop, M. & Strang, J. (1994) Chasing the dragon: the development of heroin smoking in the UK , In Strang, J. & Gossop, M (eds) *Heroin Addiction and Drug Policy.* Oxford: Oxford University Press; 121–33

Hansard Society, (1994) *Addicts Index,* (columns 67–70). London: Parliamentary Government 21 June.

Health Advisory Service (2001) *The Substance of Young Needs. Children and Young People: Substance Misuse Services.* London: HMSO.

Health Advisory Service (1996) *The Substance of Young Needs. Children and Young People: Substance Misuse Services.* London: HMSO.

Hopfer, C., Mikulich, S. & Crowley, T. (2000) Heroin use among adolescents in treatment for substance use disorders. *Journal of the American Academy of Child and Adolescent Psychiatry,* 39: 1316–23.

Hser, Y.I., Grella, C., Hubbard, R., Hsieh, S.C., Fletcher, B., Brown, B. & Anglin, D. (2001) An evaluation of drug treatments for adolescents in 4 US cities. *Archives of General Psychiatry,* 58: 689–95.

Johnston, L., O'Malley, P. & Buchman, P. (2000) *Monitoring the Future National Survey Results on Adolescent Drug Use: Overview of Key Findings, 1999.* Rockville, MD: National Institute on Drug Abuse; 56.

Lloyd, R., Katon, R. & DuPont, R. (1974) Evolution of a treatment approach for young heroin addicts: comparison of three treatment modalities. *International Journal of the Addictions* 9: 229–39.

Noble, P. & Barnes, G. (1971) Drug taking in adolescent girls: factors associated with progression to narcotic use. *British Medical Journal,* 2: 620–3.

Oyefeso, A., Ghodse, H., Clancy, C., Corkery, J. & Goldfinch, R. (1999) Drug abuse-related mortality: a study of teenage addicts over a 20 year period. *Social Psychiatry and Psychiatric Epidemiology*, 34: 437–41.

Parker, H., Bury, C. & Egginton, R. (1998) New Heroin Outbreaks amongst Young People in England and Wales; Crime Detection and Prevention Series paper 92. London: Home Office.

Parker, H., Bakx, K. & Newcombe, R. (1988) *Living with Heroin: the Impact of a Drugs 'Epidemic' on an English Community*. Milton Keynes: Open University Press.

Pearson, G. (1987) *The New Heroin Users*. Blackwell: Oxford.

Pearson, G. & Gilman, M. (1994) Local and regional variations in drug misuse: the British heroin epidemic of the 1980s. In: Strang J, Gossop M, eds. *Heroin Addiction and Drug Policy*. Oxford: Oxford University Press; 102–20.

Power, R. (1994) Drug trends since 1968. In: Strang J, Gossop M, eds. *Heroin Addiction and Drug Policy: the British System*. Oxford: Oxford University Press; 29–41.

Ramsay, M. & Percy, A. (1997) A national household survey of drug misuse in Britain: a decade of development. *Addiction*, 92: 931–7.

Ramsay, M. & Spiller, J. (1997) *Drug Misuse Declared in 1996: Latest Results for the British Crime Survey*. London: Home Office Research, Development and Statistics Directorate.

Ramsay, M., Baker, P., Goulden, C., Sharp, C. & Sondhi, A. (2001) *Drug Misuse Declared in 2000: Results from the British Crime Survey*. London: Home Office Research, Development and Statistics Directorate.

Roberts, I., Barker, M. & Leah, L. (1997) Analysis of trends in deaths from accidental drug poisoning in teenagers, 1985–95. *British Medical Journal*, 315: 289.

Social Services Inspectorate (1997) *Young People and Substance Misuse: The Local Authority Response*. London: Department of Health.

Solhkhah, R. & Wilens, T. (1998) Pharmacotherapy of adolescent alcohol and other drug use disorders. *Alcohol Health & Research World*, 22: 123–6.

Standing Conference on Drug Abuse 1998: *Young People and Drugs, Policy Guidance for Drug Interventions*. London: Standing Conference on Drug Abuse.

Ward, J., Mattick, R. & Hall, W. (1998) *Methadone Maintenance Treatment and Other Opioid Replacement Therapies*. Australia: Harwood Academic Publishers.

Ward, J., Van Beek, I., Mattick, R., Hill, P. & Kalder, J. (1996) *A controlled study of methadone maintenance in a primary care setting with young 'at risk' injecting opiate users. NDARC Technical Report No. 41*. Australia: National Drug and Alcohol Research Centre.

Weinberg, N.Z., Rahert, E., Colliver, J.D & Glantz, M. (1998) Adolescent substance abuse: a review of the past 10 years. *Journal of the American Academy of Child and Adolescent Psychiatry*, 37: 252–61.

Wiener, J. & Egan, J. (1973) Heroin addiction in an adolescent population. *Journal of the American Academy of Child and Adolescent Psychiatry*, 12: 48–58.

Winters, K. (1999) Treating adolescents with substance use disorders: an overview of practice issues and treatment outcome. *Substance Abuse*, 20: 203–25.

Section G: Methadone studies

22
Methadone treatment: outcomes and variation in treatment response within NTORS

Duncan Stewart, Michael Gossop and John Marsden

Introduction

The National Treatment Outcome Research Study (NTORS) is a large-scale, multi-site, prospective study of treatment outcome conducted with a cohort of more than 1000 people who entered drug-misuse treatment services in England during 1995. It is the largest prospective study of treatment outcome for drug misusers to be conducted in the UK. The study was commissioned in 1994 by the Task Force to Review Services for Drug Misusers with the specific aim of providing evidence of the effectiveness of existing national drug-misuse treatment services. The design of NTORS is based on a tradition of programme evaluation and longitudinal outcome research developed in the USA, and monitors the progress of clients treated in existing programmes delivering treatment under day-to-day conditions. It is not clear how readily the findings of the US studies can be generalized to the British context. The delivery of methadone treatment in the UK has evolved in a distinctive way and is characterized by decentralized planning and co-ordination and a diverse range of treatment practices. There has also been a relative lack of research addressing the characteristics and outcomes of UK prescribing programmes. However, NTORS has been reporting its findings at a time of heightened awareness from policy planners and service purchasers of the need to accumulate evidence of the impact of methadone treatment in this country.

The 31 methadone programmes in NTORS were selected from both maintenance and reduction treatment modalities. The term 'modality' refers to general defining characteristics and common features, such as the goals of treatment, and the types of treatment services provided. Programmes were classified by programme directors, according to the primary form of treatment delivered. On this basis, 16 programmes were classified as methadone maintenance, and 15 as methadone reduction programmes.

The primary focus of any treatment outcome study is whether an intervention has an observable impact on the psychological, social and behavioural problems of the clients. This question is usually addressed at the cohort level, and studies like NTORS are able to describe such changes in considerable detail. The international literature consistently shows that, on average, methadone treatment is an effective means of reducing levels of substance use and other problem behaviours among drug misusers (Ward et al. 1998). The results for clients treated in the NTORS methadone programmes were also encouraging. However, improvements reported at the cohort level provide only an indication of the overall effectiveness of treatment and are not sensitive to variability between clients in their response to treatment. Not every methadone client is likely to improve. Some clients may show no change in their behaviour after treatment, and others may get worse. Variations in outcome may be explained by a range of factors including pre-existing differences in client characteristics and problems, differences in social and environmental circumstances, and differences in the intensity of treatments received (McLellan et al. 1994). This chapter describes some of the changes in problems and behaviours of clients one year after starting methadone treatment, but also examines variation in outcomes between clients, and over time. Sources of variation in the delivery of methadone treatment are also examined.

Treatment outcomes at one year

At intake to treatment, the NTORS clients reported extensive, chronic and serious problems specifically related to the use of drugs and alcohol (Gossop et al. 1998a). Although the majority of the clients were long-term dependent heroin users, multiple drug use was common. Results from the one-year follow-up showed that clients had markedly reduced their frequency of drug use subsequent to treatment (Gossop et al. 1998b). Regular (weekly or more frequent) use of heroin was nearly halved, from 81% at intake to 49% at one year. Approximately one-third of the clients reported using non-prescribed methadone and non-prescribed benzodiazepines before treatment. Regular use of these drugs was significantly reduced to less than 20% of the sample. A more stringent measure of outcome is abstinence from drugs. At one year, over a quarter of clients were abstinent from heroin. Significant improvements in rates of abstinence were also observed for non-prescribed methadone, non-prescribed benzodiazepines and cocaine.

Although clients were treated primarily for their drug misuse, many also reported problematic drinking patterns prior to starting treatment. Heavy drinking can have serious health consequences for drug misusers, and when alcohol is consumed with illicit drugs there is an increased risk of fatal overdose (Darke and Zador 1996). The outcomes for alcohol consumption among the NTORS methadone clients were disappointing. There were modest reductions in the frequency and quantity of drinking among drinkers at intake, but for the methadone clients as a whole, there was no overall change in levels of alcohol consumption (Gossop et al. 2000a). About a quarter were drinking above the Royal College of Psychiatrists (1986) recommended sensible drinking limits (21 units per week for men and 14 units per week for women) at both intake and one year.

Reduction of substance use (especially illicit opiate use) may be regarded as the primary goal of methadone treatment, but improvements in personal and social functioning are also important elements for the recovery of the client, and have become key concerns from a social and public health perspective. In the UK and many other countries, methadone treatment has played a central role in attempts to reduce the prevalence of risk behaviours associated with the transmission of HIV, and more recently blood-borne hepatitis. It is to be welcomed, therefore, that there were reductions in rates of these behaviours among the NTORS methadone clients. The proportion of clients injecting drugs had significantly reduced from nearly two-thirds at intake to treatment to less than half at one year, thereby reducing the risk of mortality and health problems associated with injecting drugs. Sharing needles and syringes is specifically associated with the spread of infection, and it is widely accepted that eliminating or reducing high-risk drug injecting behaviour is one of the key aims of national treatment services. Rates of sharing for the NTORS methadone clients had fallen from 13% to 5%.

High levels of psychological health problems are common among drug-misusing populations, and as a consequence, a significant proportion of addicts approach treatment services with concurrent substance use and psychiatric disorders, and an elevated risk of suicide. Many of the NTORS methadone clients reported high levels of anxiety and depression at the start of treatment, and a history of contact with psychiatric treatment services. At intake, one-fifth reported having suicidal thoughts (at a moderate or more severe level). One year after starting treatment, there were significant improvements in the overall psychological health of the clients, and the proportion of clients experiencing thoughts of suicide had reduced to 17%. Although this was a statistically significant improvement, levels of suicidal ideation at one year were high enough to remain a cause for concern, especially in terms of the association between suicidal thoughts and drugs overdose (Farrell et al. 1996).

A frequently cited public and policy concern is the strong association between acquisitive crime and the use of drugs such as heroin and cocaine. Many drug misusers commit huge numbers of crimes and a substantial proportion (up to half) of recorded crime is estimated to be drug related. The economic cost to the victims and the criminal justice system of crimes committed by drug misusers are substantial. We estimate that these costs totalled £12 million for the NTORS cohort in the year before starting treatment (Gossop et al. 1998b). The high levels of criminal behaviour reported before treatment had reduced markedly at one year. The proportion of methadone clients committing acquisitive offences had almost halved. In terms of the number of crimes committed, shoplifting and burglary offences were reduced by 70%, robbery by 45%, fraud by 80%. Reductions in acquisitive crime were associated with reductions in frequency of heroin use, particularly among those clients most heavily involved in crime at the start of treatment (Gossop *et al.* 2000b).

Differences in response to treatment

We sought to address the issue of variability in outcome by looking for groups of clients with distinctive treatment response profiles (Gossop *et al.* 2000c). Four groups were identified on the basis of their drug-use outcomes using cluster analysis and are shown in Figure 22.1.

Encouragingly, the majority (59%) of the sample reported substantial reductions in their drug use. Two groups of clients were identified as showing an improved response to treatment. Clients in both groups were frequent users of illicit opiates (heroin and non-prescribed methadone) at intake to treatment, but at follow-up frequency of opiate use had fallen to about one-quarter of intake levels. There were also significant improvements in the frequency of stimulant use, which had reduced to very low levels. The difference between the two improved response groups was related to the use of non-prescribed benzodiazepines. Clients in the first group reported frequent use of benzodiazepines at intake to treatment, and showed a significant reduction in their use at one year. The clients in group 2 were more likely to have confined their pre-treatment drug use to opiates. At follow-up, there

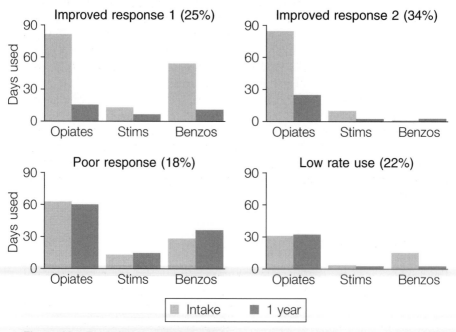

Figure 22.1 Treatment response profiles.

was a statistically significant increase in the frequency of benzodiazepine use, though again this was still at a very low level.

Some clients were characterized by a poor response to treatment. These clients were frequent users of all three types of illicit drugs at intake (though at lower levels than the improved response groups), and showed no overall improvement in their use of any of the target drugs at follow-up. Frequency of benzodiazepine use was significantly higher at follow-up than at intake. In some respects it is encouraging that fewer than one-fifth of the sample achieved such poor outcomes. It is generally accepted that clients need to be retained in treatment long enough for treatment to have an effect and longer terms of methadone treatment have consistently been found to be associated with superior outcomes on a number of measures (Simpson 1997). The outcomes of the poor response group may well reflect the finding that only about a third of these clients remained in their index treatment, compared with over half of clients in the other groups.

A further group of clients were characterized by low frequency drug use at both intake to treatment and at follow-up. For these clients, there were no changes in frequency of opiate or stimulant use, but they did show a significant reduction in their use of benzodiazepines. Compared with the other treatment response groups, these clients were older, and had longer drug-using histories. They also had extensive treatment histories, often involving methadone prescribing. Compared with the other groups, these clients had the highest rates of previous treatment contact. Most reported having been treated for a drug problem in the previous two years, and three-quarters had attended a methadone prescribing service in the three months before the index treatment episode. For this reason, it is possible that their pattern of outcome response had been influenced by the accumulated benefits of prior treatments in addition to the index treatment episode.

The results also show a relationship between changes in drug use and outcomes for other variables. Clients in the two improved response groups showed significant improvements in rates of injecting, physical health, psychological health, and criminal involvement. The poor response groups showed no reductions in these measures. There were significant improvements among clients in the low rate group for physical health, psychological health and crime.

Differences in treatment practices

Relatively little is known about the influence of the structure and operation of treatment programmes on client outcomes. Several research studies in the USA have begun to address this issue. Some of the large-scale treatment outcome studies have described the range of drug treatment services (Ball and Ross 1991; Etheridge et al. 1997; Hubbard et al. 1989). In addition to descriptive analyses, variations in the effectiveness of programmes have been observed, and elements of programme delivery have been linked to improved client outcomes. We have previously reported that clients from some programmes achieved up to three times as great a reduction in heroin use as others (Gossop *et al.* 1998b). Such variation between programmes in client outcomes is obviously of great interest, but it also raises many extremely complex issues, and requires cautious and careful interpretation. Joe *et al.* (1994) found that relapse to opioid use during methadone maintenance treatment was significantly related to programme variables such as methadone dose (higher doses associated with lower relapse rates), urine analysis (increased monitoring related to higher relapse rates), and methadone take-home privileges (more days of take-home related to lower relapse rates). Other studies have shown that variation in client outcomes can in part be attributed to retention in treatment, and the frequency and range of treatment services delivered (Ball and Ross 1991; McLellan *et al.* 1994; Simpson 1997).

The two methadone modalities in NTORS represent fairly broad categories of intervention, within which there is considerable variation in the structure and delivery of treatment between individual programmes (Stewart *et al.* 2000). There were large variations in capacity among the methadone programmes, ranging from 23 to over 800 places. Those with the greatest number of clients were located in large inner city areas. The capacity of some of these services was accounted for by agencies operating shared care arrangements with primary care doctors (GPs). The role of GPs in the treatment of drug misusers is substantial, despite fears concerning the practicality of treating drug misusers in a primary care setting. We have found that clients treated by GPs and specialist clinics made comparable changes in substance use and other problem behaviours (Gossop *et al.* 1999).

The enormous clinical freedom of prescribing practitioners in the UK is reflected in variations in dosages prescribed, frequency of dispensing, the proportion of prescriptions from general practitioners, and the form of methadone prescribed (i.e. liquid, tablets, or ampoules) (Strang and Sheridan 1998). A typical feature of methadone treatment in this country has been the use of prescriptions to be dispensed at a retail pharmacy, to be taken away for consumption. More recently, some clinics have provided methadone treatment in a more structured form, with the consumption of methadone supervised by staff at the clinic. This form of prescribing usually involves daily dispensing in the first instances, but 'take-home' doses can then be prescribed depending on time and progress in treatment. The majority of the NTORS methadone programmes had arrangements for clients to collect their methadone from a retail pharmacy for consumption off the premises. However, at least some of the clients in seven of the maintenance programmes were dispensed methadone on-site under the supervision of staff, though this was much less common in the reduction programmes. Nearly all of the reduction agencies relied on pharmacies to dispense methadone. Daily dispensing was more common in the maintenance programmes, but in both modalities the use of 'take-home' doses of methadone was also reported by the majority of programmes.

There were also considerable differences among the programmes in both modalities in the delivery of counselling and additional treatment services. The frequency of counselling and the range of services provided by methadone programmes have been associated with improved treatment outcomes (McLellan et al. 1994; Ball and Ross 1991), and are thus important elements of the overall treatment package. Weekly individual counselling sessions were reported by a quarter of the maintenance programmes and for a third of the reduction programmes. Only one service from each modality reported weekly group counselling for most or all of their clients. Three-quarters of the maintenance programmes reported treatment services for alcohol and medical problems. The reduction programmes reported the lowest rates of provision of these services (under 50%).

Maintenance of change at two years

Many treatment outcomes studies, including NTORS, have found that changes in drug use and other problem behaviours occur relatively early (i.e. within the first six months) in treatment. For example, in the Treatment Outcomes Prospective Study (TOPS) the lowest levels of heroin use were found at three months in treatment (Hubbard et al. 1989), whilst improvements among the NTORS clients were observed at one month and six months after starting treatment (Gossop et al. 1996; 1997). Also in the UK, a comparison of outcomes of clients randomly allocated to methadone maintenance or methadone reduction treatments found improvements across a range of variables during the first month of treatment (Strang et al. 1997). It is encouraging that changes occur so soon after starting treatment, but this also suggests there may be a limit to the scope of methadone programmes in bringing about further progress over time. A substantial part of methadone treatment, therefore, involves maintaining early treatment gains. Relapses after periods of reduced use or abstinence are a common feature of an addiction career, and drug misusers may well require many years and several treatment interventions to become abstinent. In this regard, it is important to assess the success of treatment interventions in reducing levels of drug misuse and clients' problems over a longer period of time.

Changes among the NTORS methadone clients for a range of outcomes measured over 2 years are shown in Figure 22.2. Following the reduction in the proportion of clients using heroin regularly (weekly or more frequently) at one year, there was a further (statistically significant) improvement at two years. There were also reductions in the use of other drugs, and again these changes were maintained over the two-year period, with no increases in the average frequency of use reported between the two follow-ups (Gossop et al. 2002). Figure 22.2 also shows that after a reduction in regular use of cocaine at one

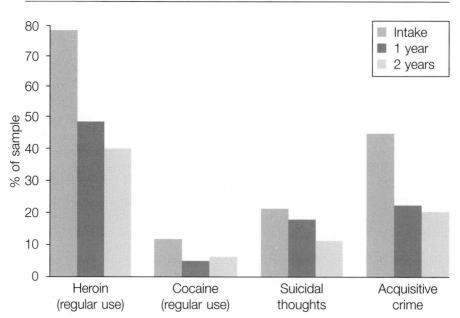

Figure 22.2 Summary of outcomes over two years.

year, regular use remained at half of intake levels at two years. A similar pattern was also observed for other outcomes. The proportion of clients reporting suicidal thoughts (at a moderate or greater level) was significantly reduced at successive follow-up points to about half the level at intake. For acquisitive crime, the large reduction in the proportion of clients committing offences at one year was maintained with a further (non-significant) improvement.

The maintenance of earlier treatment gains is an important and impressive finding, particularly given the severity of the problems with which clients presented to treatment. It is possible that the stability of outcomes over time disguises fluctuations in the progress of individual clients. Good outcomes may be reported by different groups of clients at different follow-up points. For many of the outcome measures, scores at one year and two year follow-ups were significantly correlated (Gossop *et al.* 2002), suggesting that there was some stability in outcome at the individual client level. Interpretation of results for longer-term follow-ups is complicated by the variety of routes through which outcomes are achieved. After two years of the study, many clients had left their original index treatment and had received additional addiction treatment episodes. These included further treatment at methadone programmes, but some clients had been treated at hospital inpatient and residential rehabilitation services. The relationship between multiple treatment episodes and the effectiveness of treatment over time is poorly understood, but it is clear that the outcomes reported here were achieved by fairly intensive use of treatment services.

Implications

The results from NTORS provide useful information about the nature and effectiveness of methadone treatment in the UK. The findings are consistent with those of the large US outcome studies in showing that clients treated in methadone programmes show improvements in their drug use and their psychological and social functioning. Reductions were found in the frequency of use of heroin, benzodiazepines and cocaine. Furthermore, the increases in rates of abstinence for these drugs show that abstinence is a real possibility for clients treated in methadone programmes. In view of the severity of the clients' problems at the start of treatment, it is particularly encouraging that changes were observed across a range of outcome domains, including physical and psychological health, and criminal activity.

The positive message from NTORS is strengthened in two important ways. First, when differences in patterns of treatment response were identified, the majority of clients were classified as showing an improved response to treatment. These clients had the best outcome profile despite starting treatment with some of the highest levels of drug use. Secondly, the improvements reported by the sample were not short-lived. In the US outcome studies, the majority of clients did not revert to levels of drug use reported before treatment (Brown 1998). In NTORS, changes were also largely maintained over a substantial period of time, and for some measures there were further improvements.

Whilst many of the results from outcomes studies tend to emphasize positive changes in behaviour, cases where outcomes are not so good should not be overlooked. Identification of weaknesses in programmes and factors associated with poor performance can be used to improve the delivery of treatment services. Whilst only a minority, some of the NTORS methadone clients did not respond well to treatment, and failed to show improvements on most of the key outcome measures. In addition, the outcomes for alcohol consumption were not satisfactory, and suggest that methadone programmes need to re-evaluate how this important problem is tackled.

References

Ball, J. & Ross, A. (1991) *The Effectiveness of Methadone Maintenance Treatment: Patients, Programmes, Services and Outcomes.* New York: Springer Verlag.

Brown, B.S. (1998) Drug use – chronic and relapsing or a treatable condition. *Substance Use and Misuse* 33: 2515–20.

Darke, S. & Zador, D. (1996) Fatal heroin overdose: a review. *Addiction,* 91: 1765–72.

Etheridge, R.M., Hubbard, R.L., Anderson, J., Craddock, S.G. & Flynn, P.M. (1997) Characteristics of a national sample of drug abuse treatment programmes: implications for health services. *Psychology of Addictive Behaviors*, 11: 244–60.

Farrell, M., Neeleman, J., Griffiths, P. & Strang, J. (1996) Suicide and overdose among opiate addicts. *Addiction,* 91: 321–3.

Gossop, M., Marsden, J., Stewart, D. &

Treacy, S. (2002) Change and stability of change after treatment of drug misuse: two year outcomes from the National Treatment Outcome Research Study (NTORS/UK). *Addictive Behaviors*, 27: 155–66.

Gossop, M., Marsden, J., Stewart, D. & Rolfe, A. (2000a) Patterns of drinking and drinking outcomes among drug misusers: one year follow-up results. *Journal of Substance Abuse Treatment*, 19: 45–50.

Gossop, M., Marsden, J., Stewart, D. & Rolfe, A. (2000b) Reductions in acquisitive crime and drug use after treatment of addiction problems: one year follow-up outcomes. *Drug and Alcohol Dependence,* 58: 165–72.

Gossop, M., Marsden, J., Stewart, D. & Rolfe, A. (2000c) Patterns of improvement after methadone treatment: one year follow-up results from the National Treatment Outcome Research Study (NTORS). *Drug and Alcohol Dependence*, 60: 275–86.

Gossop, M., Marsden, J., Stewart, D., Lehmann, P. & Strang, J. (1999) Treatment outcome among opiate addicts receiving methadone treatment in drug clinics and general practice settings: Results from the National Treatment Outcome Research Study (NTORS). *British Journal of General Practice,* 49: 31–4.

Gossop, M., Marsden, J., Stewart, D., Lehmann, P., Edwards, C., Wilson, A. & Segar, G. (1998a) Substance use, health and social problems of service users at 54 drug treatment agencies: intake data from the National Treatment Outcome Research Study. *British Journal of Psychiatry*, 173: 166–71.

Gossop, M., Marsden, J. & Stewart, D. (1998b) *NTORS at One Year: The National Treatment Outcome Research Study: Changes in Substance Use, Health and Criminal Behaviours at One Year After Intake.* London: Department of Health.

Gossop, M., Marsden, J., Stewart, D., Edwards, C., Lehmann, P., Wilson, A. & Segar, G. (1997) The National Treatment Outcome Research Study in the United Kingdom: Six month follow-up outcomes. *Psychology of Addictive Behaviors,* 11: 324–37.

Gossop, M., Marsden, J., Stewart, D., Edwards, C., Lehmann, P., Wilson, A. & Segar, G. (1996) *NTORS First Bulletin: Summary of the project, the clients, and preliminary findings.* London: Department of Health.

Hubbard, R.L., Marsden, M.E., Rachal, J.V., Harwood, H.J., Cavanaugh, E.R. & Ginzburg, H.M. (1989) *Drug Abuse Treatment: A National Study of Effectiveness.* Chapel Hill: University of North Carolina Press.

Joe, G.W., Simpson, D.D. & Sells, S.B. (1994) Treatment process and relapse to opioid use during methadone maintenance. *American Journal of Drug and Alcohol Abuse*, 20: 173–97.

McLellan T.A., Alterman A.I., Metzger, D.S., Grissom, G.R., Woody, G.E., Luborsky, L. & O'Brien, C.P. (1994) Similarity of predictors across opiate, cocaine, and alcohol treatments: Role of treatment services. *Journal of Consulting and Clinical Psychology*, 62: 141–1158.

Royal College of Psychiatrists (1986) *Alcohol: Our Favourite Drug.* London: Tavistock.

Simpson D.D, (1997) Effectiveness of drug abuse treatment: a review of research from field settings. In: Egertson J, Fox D, Leshner A, eds. *Treating Drug Abusers Effectively.* Oxford: Blackwell.

Stewart, D., Gossop, M., Marsden, J. & Strang, J. (2000) Variation between and within drug treatment modalities: data from the National Treatment Outcome Research Study (UK). *European Addiction Research,* 6: 106–14.

Strang, J., Finch, E., Hankinson, L., Farrell, M., Taylor, C. & Gossop, M. (1997) Methadone treatment for opiate addiction: benefits in the first month. *Addiction Research*, 5: 71–6.

Strang, J. & Sheridan, J. (1998) National and regional methadone prescribing in England and Wales: local analyses of data from the 1995 national survey of community pharmacies. *Journal of Substance Misuse*, 3: 240–6.

Ward, J., Mattick, R. P. & Hall, W. (1998) *Methadone Maintenance Treatment and Other Opioid Replacement Therapies.* Amsterdam: Harwood.

23

Rapid benefit, but what thereafter?
The rush and trickle of benefit from
methadone treatments

Emily Finch

Introduction

It is generally acknowledged that methadone treatment produces improvements in opiate users across many outcome domains. Reductions have been demonstrated in the level of criminal activity (Ball and Ross 1991; Bell *et al.* 1992), injecting risk behaviours (Stark *et al.* 1996; Wells *et al.* 1996) and illicit drug misuse (Ball and Ross 1991; Caplehorn and Bell 1991) with improvements in psychological health (Finch *et al.* 1995). Many reviews have summarized the benefits (Farrell *et al.* 1994; Marsch 1998; Ward *et al.* 1998; Ward *et al.* 1999).

The consensus reached by researchers that methadone treatment is beneficial may, however, hide a complex picture where benefits may be short-lived for some, long-lasting for others and may vary depending on the outcome domain measured. One of the most problematic issues in interpreting research on methadone treatment is to understand what type of treatment is being examined. The philosophy and practice of methadone treatment varies enormously across the world and even within countries such as the USA vast variations are seen (Gossop and Grant 1991; Ball and Ross 1991; see Chapter 1). In much of the USA and in most of Europe, 'standard' methadone treatment is not time limited, but in the UK it is frequently restricted to short-term dose reduction treatments (Farrell *et al.* 2000). This makes time-limited outcome research difficult to interpret.

Most studies of methadone treatment report on benefits at one year and even further on. This is useful in a treatment system where the intervention is expected to last longer than that but less useful in a system where treatment is usually shorter. The interpretation of the findings also depends on whether the sample followed up includes only those who stayed in treatment or also includes those who have left.

This chapter will concentrate on the early improvements seen in individuals in methadone treatment and look at the possible theoretical bases for those changes. It will go on to examine changes across different outcome domains and how these improvements are variable and how understanding them may help clinicians to optimize treatment benefit. In this chapter, early treatment benefits are defined as those within the first six months and longer-term benefits as those seen after one year.

Early changes in methadone treatment

Three theoretical patterns of positive change seen early in clients in methadone treatment

(1) There is an immediate initial improvement which further increases over time, e.g. clients gradually reduced their illicit drug misuse.

(2) There is an initial benefit which is maintained but not improved on, e.g. clients reduce their illicit drug misuse but reach a plateau where no further improvement is seen.

(3) There is initial improvement which gradually falls off as treatment proceeds, e.g. illicit drug misuse initially reduced but gradually returns to pre-treatment levels.

A study of men in a methadone maintenance programme in Philadelphia set out to examine changes that occurred early in methadone treatment (Cacciola *et al.* 1998). A total of 157 subjects were assessed using the Addiction Severity Index (ASI) at treatment entry and two and seven months later (McLellan *et al.* 1992). Regular urine specimens were collected and analysed for illicit drugs. They followed up those who remained in continuous treatment and those who left after the first two months. The subjects were typical of those in other USA methadone programmes with a mean age of 40 years, a mean of 16.4 years of heroin use, 3.6 years of cocaine use and 7.5 years of heavy alcohol use. The results showed that all subjects decreased their illicit drug use from admission to month 2 and admission to month 7 but no reductions in illicit drug use were seen between month 2 and month 7. Severity of problematic alcohol use did not change over the time points. In other problem areas, similar findings were noted with ASI legal composite scores, family/social composite scores and psychiatric composite scores showing improvements between admission and month 2, admission and month 7 but no changes between months 2 and 7. Those who had left treatment had significantly more severe legal and illicit drug problems but those in treatment had more medical problems. Out-of-treatment subjects had spent significantly more time in a restricted environment than in treatment subjects at the seven-month follow-up point. The authors conclude that both for subjects who left treatment and for those who remain in treatment, improvements occur in the initial two months, and then no further improvements or indeed loss of benefit occurs. Thus this study firmly provides evidence for option 2, in which clients in methadone maintenance improve initially but fail to show continuous improvement.

Two studies carried out in the UK have also examined this early benefit from treatment. The National Treatment Outcome Research Study (NTORS) is a prospective longitudinal cohort study of substance misusers in four treatment modalities: inpatient units, residential programmes, outpatient/community-based methadone reduction programmes and outpatient methadone maintenance programmes (Gossop *et al.* 2000; Gossop *et al.* 2002). A total of 1110 clients in treatment agencies across England were included in the original sample. Follow-up interviews were carried out after one month in treatment, after six months in treatment (or two months after leaving treatment) and one year after treatment entry. Subsequently a sub-sample of the cohort has been followed up after two years. The subjects in the study were three-quarters men and had a mean age of 29 years. They were mainly long-term heroin users with an average duration of use of nine years. One in seven reported daily drinking at unsafe levels, 15% had shared syringes and 60% had been involved in criminal activity in the three months prior to treatment.

Unlike many long-term studies, NTORS has published the findings from the early one-month follow-up in the Task Force report to review services for drug misusers (Task Force Report 1996). Those initial improvements are dramatic. Amongst subjects in methadone maintenance, the percentage of subjects using heroin regularly fell from 77% to 44% and in methadone reduction from 90% to 35%. They also report reductions in use of illicit methadone, benzodiazepines, alcohol and crack cocaine. For all those in treatment, the injecting rate fell from 61% prior to admission to 33% following admission with a reduction in sharing from 15% to 5%. Criminal activity also reduced during that first month with the percentage of subjects in methadone maintenance involved in shoplifting reduced from 26% to 19% and in methadone reduction from 36% to 21%.

These initial good outcomes are maintained in the NTORS study with further treatment benefit seen at six-month, one-year and two-year follow-up points (Gossop *et al.* 1997; Gossop *et al.* 2000; Gossop *et al.* 2002). Unfortunately there is no published specific comparison of the changes seen at one month and six months, so the initial pattern of benefit cannot be examined. However, Gossop and colleagues, in a paper specifically addressing stability of changes over time, examined outcome between one- and two-year follow-up points (Gossop *et al.* 2002). They found that, for most outcomes, the benefits seen in the first year are maintained after the second year. This would indicate that initial benefits are maintained and a reduction of benefit is not seen. It is not clear from this analysis however whether the subjects are still in their original treatment episode and whether those interviewed included subjects now out of treatment.

Changes in benefit over time

A separate small study from the same research group has provided further UK data on the benefits seen early on in treatment (Strang *et al.* 1997; Finch 2000). In a randomized clinical trial designed to compare the outcome of subjects in methadone maintenance and methadone reduction treatment, a detailed and frequent follow-up schedule was carried out specifically to examine the early changes seen in treatment (Finch 2000). A total of 119 opiate-dependent subjects were recruited from clients presenting for treatment to a community drug service in South East London. They were randomized to receive either standard methadone reduction treatment delivered by a community drug team or methadone maintenance from a stand-alone daily supervised dispensing programme. They were interviewed at intake, one month, two months, three months, six months and 12 months after entering treatment. Ninety per cent of the subjects were followed up whether they were in or out of treatment. Ninety-three per cent of them were interviewed (both in and out of treatment) after the first month and positive changes were

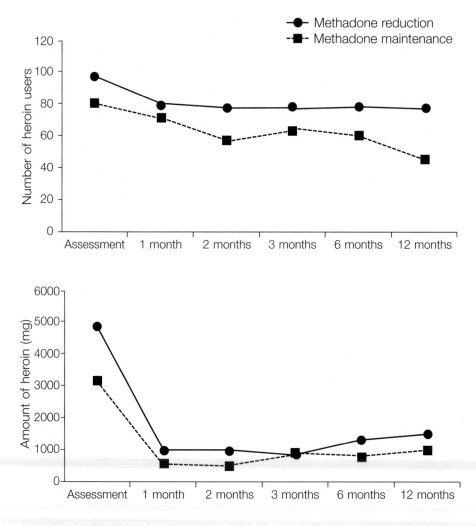

Figure 23.1 Heroin use in methadone treatment: number of heroin users and amounts used.

substantial (Strang *et al.* 1997). They were seen in both groups, whether randomized to methadone maintenance or reduction. Heroin use was reduced from 39.4 g per week at assessment to 7.6 g per week after one month and cocaine use from 10.5 g per week at assessment to 2.6 g per week after one month. Both of these changes were highly significant. The number of injectors fell from 97 to 72 individuals. The mean number of shoplifting incidents per person fell from 13.4 to 1.8. Only the number in employment, which increased from 11 to 19 subjects was not significantly different.

Data collected from this sample have been analysed looking at improvements in key variables at each follow-up point (Finch 2000). Figure 23.1 shows the number of individuals using heroin at each follow-up point and the amount of heroin used by those individuals. There was initially a significant decrease in the numbers using but this was followed by a continued non-significant decrease. When the amount of heroin used was examined at each time point there was a significant reduction initially but this was then followed by a significant increase. This would seem to indicate that the initial reduction in the amount of heroin used was followed by a significant increase. Thus, although in this sample there is an initial highly significant decrease in use after one year, there has been a fall off in benefit, indicating that those who are still using heroin increase the amount they are using and revert back towards pre-treatment levels of use.

Similarly Figure 23.2 shows changes in the amount of crack cocaine use over time. There was an initial highly significant decrease followed by an

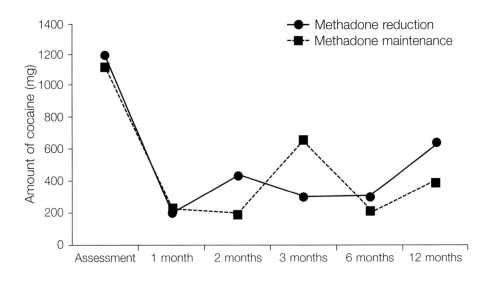

Figure 23.2 Cocaine/crack use.

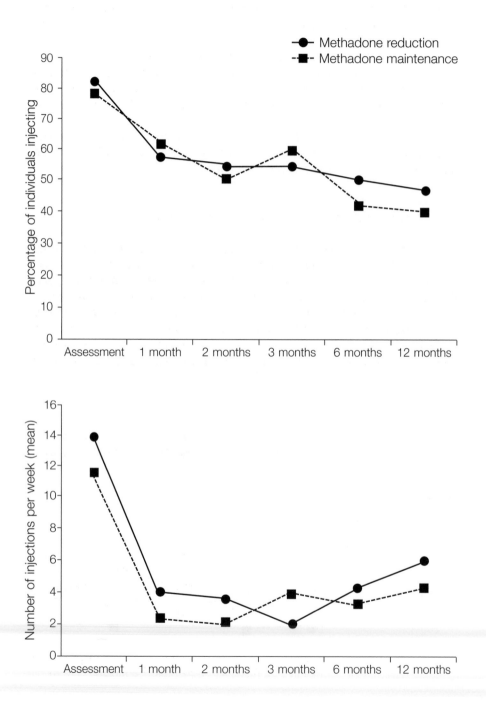

Figure 23.3 Injecting.

increase that is not significant. Thus for cocaine use, although substantial initial benefits in treatment are seen, the changes seen over the subsequent months are no longer significant.

Figure 23.3 shows changes in the numbers of people injecting and in the number of times those who do inject are injecting. The number of people injecting initially reduces substantially and then continues to drop significantly. Thus for injecting, the improvement seems to continue throughout a one-year follow-up period.

Figure 23.4 shows changes in the number of crimes committed at each time-point. For this outcome variable there is a significant initial benefit but this is followed by no further significant benefit.

Why are variations in benefit seen over time?

These results would seem to indicate that some of the improved outcomes seen in methadone treatment might not be maintained over time. The early benefits may be substantial but these benefits are either not maintained and there is a reversion to pre-treatment levels or at best there is no further benefit seen. The explanation for this finding may be a real treatment effect or may be a consequence of the research design. In the above study all individuals were followed up whether they were in or out of treatment. It may be that the reduction in benefit over time is seen because people leave treatment and

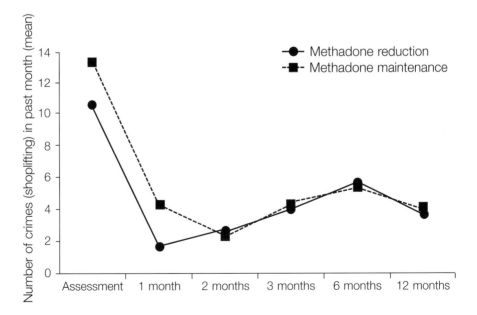

Figure 23.4 Crime.

so these individuals are no longer susceptible to treatment interventions.

Other data on this issue are available from research investigations outside the UK. A study from the USA found that those who had left treatment did use more illicit drugs, injected more frequently and commited more crimes than those who stayed in treatment (Cacciola *et al.* 1998). Therefore these reductions in benefit over time may be a function of the addition of the reduced benefit seen in those who are out of treatment to the improvements seen in those who stay in treatment.

Another explanation may be that treatment philosophies vary between pro-grammes. The above data show aggregated results for two treatment groups, one in methadone maintenance and one in methadone reduction. Although in reality there was little difference in the treatment provided to the two groups, there may nevertheless be treatment differences that result in a larger range of outcome levels especially after a year. This phenomenon of lack of fidelity to detoxification or reduction protocols is also described by Gossop and col-leagues in the treatment agencies participating in NTORS (Gossop *et al.* 2000).

Many longer-term follow-up studies (Simpson 1981) do show improve-ments for subjects who stay in treatment over time. It may be that the full benefits of methadone treatment are only seen after a much longer period of time. This view is supported by evidence from several studies which demon-strate that treatment retention is a crucial element in effective methadone treatment for opiate dependence (Simpson 1990). Thus evidence from short-term follow-up studies is only relevant for individuals who stay in treatment for periods of under one year.

Different outcome variables

Different patterns of outcome are seen for different variables. Figure 23.5 shows changes in the amount of alcohol used in units per week seen at each follow-up point for the sample of 119 individuals described above (Finch 2000).

There is no reduction seen in the amount of alcohol used at any time-point. Other studies have found that there is little reduction in alcohol use in methadone treatment and it may be that alcohol use is particularly resistant to changes in methadone treatment (NTORS one year, Gossop *et al.* 2000). Other variables, for instance employment and housing status may be highly influenced by factors outside the control of the treatment programme and even of the individual client.

Conclusions: implications for clinical management

Many of the benefits of methadone treatment are seen early and most clients can be expected to improve substantially within the first month or two of treatment. However, it is not entirely clear the extent to which these initial

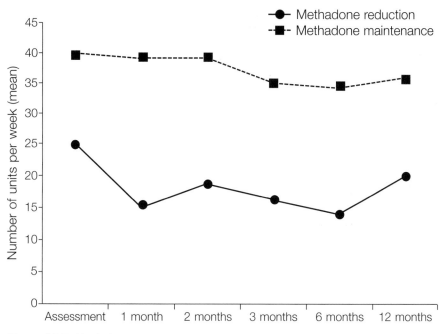

Figure 23.5 Alcohol.

benefits are maintained. For most outcome domains the best that is seen is maintenance of initial improvement and for others the initial benefits may be lost. For the clinician the challenge is to plan treatment interventions which both capitalize on the initial improvements of clients in methadone treatment and maintain those improvements. It is possible that positive initial benefits occur because of the pharmacological effects of methadone itself and that these are relatively easy to achieve. Longer-term benefits may be due to a range of psycho-social benefits which the clinician has a variable ability to influence. These may range from psychotherapy for clients with chronic mood disorders (McLellan et al. 1993) to the provision of adequate housing and employment.

The improvement in some outcome domains is maintained more than in others. Methadone treatment has little effect on alcohol use. Perhaps this is not surprising, as the treatment is not theoretically designed to influence alcohol use. Interventions are needed that specifically address problematic alcohol use in poly-drug users who are receiving methadone treatment. Possible pharmacological approaches could include acamprosate and disulfiram and psychological ones could include specific cognitive behavioural therapy (CBT) interventions or attendance at Alcoholics Anonymous (AA). Similarly specialist CBT interventions may be needed for clients who use cocaine (Carroll *et al.* 1991). Clients who are persistently offending may need programmes directed at offending behaviour in addition to methadone treatment if the reduction in their offending is to be maintained.

There is a substantial degree of heterogeneity in clients attending for methadone treatment. Some may be ready to make changes and maintain those changes but others may not be motivated to do so, resulting in differing expectations. Clinicians need to elicit these differences in clients and be able to react by designing different treatment regimes for the client who is likely to continue to change and the client who will plateau and be unable to improve any more.

Implications for policy

Those who plan and fund methadone treatment need to realize that the benefits may not be easy to achieve and certainly not easy to maintain. Not all clients will improve dramatically and maintain that improvement. Treatment programmes tend to be 'front loaded' in that all the input is to clients at the beginning of a treatment episode and after three months or so clients are expected to need less intense interventions. For instance, keyworker appointments may be less frequent, and dispensing regimes may involve less supervision. Programmes need to address the needs of clients who do not maintain initial improvements both by monitoring potential deterioration and providing continued high intensity input and supervision if it is necessary. Treatment regimes may need to take account of clients with specific needs such as those who abuse alcohol, as conventional methadone treatment may not address all areas of need.

It may also be important to acknowledge that short-term benefits may only be transient and that we cannot expect all clients to maintain dramatic improvements. Failure to acknowledge this may result in problems for both clients and treatment providers with unrealistic expectations of the benefit of treatment which may make them unwilling to continue to make the necessary commitment to treatment.

References

Ball, J.C. & Ross, A. (1991) *The Effectiveness of Methadone Maintenance Treatment: Patients, Programs, Services, and Outcome*. New York: Springer-Verlag.

Bell, J., Hall, W. & Byth, K. (1992) Changes in criminal activity after entering methadone maintenance. *British Journal of Addiction*, 87: 251–8.

Cacciola, J.S., Alterman, A.I., Rutherford, M.J., McKay, J.R. & McLellan, A. (1998) The early course of change in methadone maintenance. *Addiction*, 93: 41–9.

Caplehorn, J.R.M. & Bell, J. (1991) Methadone dosage and retention of patients in maintenance treatment. *The Medical Journal of Australia*, 154: 195–9.

Carroll, K.M., Rounsaville, B.J. & Gawin, F.H. (1991) A comparative trial of psychotherapies for ambulatory cocaine users: relapse prevention and interpersonal psychotherapy. *American Journal of Drug and Alcohol Abuse*, 17: 229–47.

Farrell, M., Howes, S., Verster, A., Davoli, M., Solberg, U., Greenwood, G. & Robertson, K. (2000) *Reviewing Current Practice in Drug-substitution Treatment in the European Union*. European Monitoring Centre for Drugs and Drug Addiction: Insights series 3.

Farrell, M., Ward, J., Des Jarlais, D.C., Gossop, M., Stimson, G.V., Hall, W., Mattick, R. & Strang, J. (1994) Methadone maintenance programmes: review of new data with special reference to impact on HIV transmission. *British Medical Journal*, 309: 997–1001.

Finch, E.J.L. (2000) *A Randomised Clinical Trial of Methadone Maintenance versus Methadone Reduction for Opiate Addiction*. University of London: MD thesis.

Finch, E., Groves, I., Feinman, C. & Farmer, R. (1995) A low threshold methadone stabilisation programme – description and first stage evaluation. *Addiction Research*, 3: 63–71.

Gossop, M., Marsden, J., Stewart, D. & Treacy, S. (2002) Change and stability of change after treatment of drug misusers: 2 year outcomes from the National Treatment Outcome Research Study (UK). *Addictive Behaviors*, 27: 155–66.

Gossop, M. & Grant, M. (1991) A six country survey of the content and structure of heroin treatment programmes using methadone. *British Journal of Addiction*, 86:1151–60.

Gossop, M., Marsden, J., Stewart, D. & Rolfe, A. (2000) Patterns of improvement after methadone treatment: 1 year follow-up results from the National Outcome Research Study (NTORS). *Drug and Alcohol Dependence*, 60: 275–86.

Gossop, M., Marsden, J., Stewart, D., Edwards, C., Lehmann, P., Wilson, A. & Segar, G. (1997) The National Treatment Outcome Research Study: six-month follow-up outcomes. *Psychology of Addictive Behaviors*, 11: 324–37.

Marsch, L.A. (1998) The efficacy of methadone maintenance interventions on reducing illicit opiate use, HIV risk behaviour, and criminality: a meta-analysis. *Addiction*, 93: 515–32.

McLellan, A.T., Arndt, I.O., Metzger, D.S., Woody, G.E. & O'Brien, C.P. (1993) The effects of psychosocial services in substance abuse treatment. *Journal of the American Medical Association*, 269: 1953–9.

McLellan, A.T., Kushner, H., Metzger, D., Peters, R., Smith, I., Grissom, G., Pettinati, H. & Argeriou, M. (1992) The fifth edition of the Addiction Severity Index. *Journal of Substance Abuse Treatment*, 9: 199–213.

Simpson, D.D. (1990) Longitudinal outcome patterns. In: Simpson, DD, Sells SB, eds. *Opioid Addiction and Treatment: A 12 Year Follow-Up*. Florida USA: Robert E. Krieger Publishing.

Simpson, D.D. (1981) Treatment for drug abuse – follow up outcomes and length of time spent. *Archives of General Psychiatry*, 38: 875–80.

Stark, K., Muller, R., Bienzle, U. & Guggenmoos-Holzman, I. (1996) Methadone maintenance treatment and HIV risk taking behaviour among injecting drug users in Berlin. *Journal of Epidemiology and Community Health*, 50: 534–7.

Strang, J., Finch, E., Hankinson, L., Farrell, M., Taylor, C. & Gossop, M. (1997) Methadone treatment for opiate addiction: benefits in the first month. *Addiction Research*, 5: 71–6.

The Task Force to Review Services for Drug Misusers (1996) *Report of an Independent Review of Drug Treatment in England*. London: Department of Health.

Ward, J., Hall, J. & Mattick, R.P. (1999) Role of maintenance treatment in opioid dependence. *Lancet*, 353: 221–6.

Ward, J., Mattick, R.P. & Hall, W. (eds). (1998) *Methadone Maintenance Treatment and Other Opioid Replacement Therapies*. Amsterdam: Harwood Academic.

Wells, E.A., Calsyn, D.A., Clark, L.L., Saxon, A.J. & Jackson, T.R. (1996) Retention in methadone maintenance is associated with reductions in different HIV risk behaviours for women and men. *American Journal of Drug and Alcohol Abuse*, 22: 509–21.

24
Methadone maintenance and reduction treatments: the need for clarity of goals and procedures

Michael Gossop, John Marsden and Duncan Stewart

Programme diversity

Methadone treatments are extremely diverse. All involve the prescription of the same pharmacological agent, methadone hydrochloride. But apart from this common element, they differ in many fundamental respects, and the reasons for this variation are not properly understood. A study of methadone treatment in six countries (Gossop and Grant 1990) found marked variability in the content and structure of programmes. The variation included issues of direct relevance to the nature and probable effectiveness of the interventions. Programmes differed in dose levels, programme entry criteria, time limits for prescribing, frequency of clinic attendance, the manner of dispensing (supervised or unsupervised), and the formulation of the drug used (syrup, tablets or ampoules).

Differences are also found between methadone treatment programmes within countries. In a study of methadone treatment programmes in the UK, Stewart *et al.* (2000) reported differences between 31 methadone programmes. Ball and Ross (1991) found marked differences between methadone maintenance clinics in six US cities. Programmes differed in fundamental ways, including the doses prescribed to patients, provision of counselling services, treatment policies, and not least, in drug use outcomes.

Such marked variation in the provision of methadone treatments is of considerable clinical importance. Ward *et al.* (1998) note that methadone treatments are 'an effective form of treatment for opioid dependence *on average*' (italics in original). It has been suggested that about one in four patients treated in methadone programmes will not respond well to treatment (Gerstein and Harwood 1990). Patient responses may be related to the variation in treatment procedures. An important clinical question, therefore, is how to achieve a more precise differentiation of the ways in which patients respond to the procedures and interventions provided in methadone treatment.

One issue that is of considerable importance to our understanding of methadone treatment programmes concerns the treatment goal itself.

Gossop *et al.* (1989) noted that:

> Insufficient attention has been paid to the manner in which the effective-ness of methadone treatment ... might be maximized .... there remains considerable confusion both about the identification of goals for the treat-ment and management of opioid dependence and also about how such goals are related to treatment methods (pp. 35–6).

Both in the UK and in other countries, there is a tension between the use of methadone as a treatment that is intended to meet a goal of harm reduction, and that in which methadone is used as a device or as an intermediate phase of treatment aimed at abstinence.

The provision of methadone treatments to opiate addicts in the UK has a different history from that in other countries. Methadone treatment became established as an important part of the national response during the early 1970s, but unlike in the USA where methadone treatments were introduced with specific protocols and often with stringent controls, in the UK they have been subject only to the most general controls. As a consequence, the clin-ical delivery of methadone treatment has been extremely variable. Methadone treatments have been provided with wide variation in doses, drug preparations (syrup, tablets and injectable ampoules), treatment dura-tion, and treatment goals. The reasons for this variation have rarely been made explicit, but are sometimes justified in terms of the need to provide an 'individualized' response to meet the needs of each patient.

Methadone reduction and methadone maintenance treatments

Methadone reduction treatment (MRT) has been widely used in the UK for many years. Seivewright (2000) commented that 'it would be impossible to overstate the importance of this form of methadone prescribing in the UK'. Typically, MRT involves prescribing methadone over relatively long periods of time, with the expectation that the dose will gradually be reduced, and that the patient will eventually be withdrawn from the drug and become abstinent from opioids. The move to introduce methadone reduction procedures occurred soon after the establishment of the British clinic system. The pre-scription of opioids was seen as a 'lure' to attract drug misusers into the treatment services so that 'regular contact between the addict and the doctor ... gives the opportunity for a relationship to be built up which may eventually lead to the addict requesting to be taken off the drug' (Connell 1969). Edwards (1969) also noted that clinic attendance was 'not for the continuing handouts of drugs, but for treatment: the patient may not initially be motivated to accept withdrawal but ... motivation will gradually be built [and] dosage gradually reduced'. From the 1970s, clinic policy moved towards 'an attempt to replace indefinite prescribing' and 'a limited stabilization period was followed by reducing prescriptions' (Mitcheson 1994).

During the late1970s and early 1980s, British drug clinics increasingly adopted a form of methadone reduction treatment in which the patient received a relatively short period of dose stabilization at the beginning of treatment. This was to be followed by a series of dose reductions which were often contractually linked to the requirement for the patient to attend the clinic for individual or group counselling sessions targeted at changes in problematic social behaviour, and aimed at abstinence (Strang 1984; Mitcheson 1994). This practice was, however, adopted without formal deliberation (it was never a matter of policy) and without any precise or explicit specification of its procedures.

Methadone reduction should not be seen simply as a detoxification procedure. It is less well-defined, and, in practice, a more complicated procedure. Although not directly comparable, MRT as delivered in the UK, has similarities to certain types of methadone programmes in other countries. A similar procedure has been described in Australia (Capelhorn 1994). It also has some similarities with the gradual methadone detoxification programmes, and with the 90-day, and 180-day detoxification programmes that have been implemented in the USA (Sees *et al.* 2000). The 180-day methadone programmes were made available after Federal Guidelines were revised in 1989 to provide this modality as an 'intermediate' form of treatment between short-term, 21-day detoxification, and long-term maintenance. Despite its widespread implementation, little research evidence is available regarding the delivery and effectiveness of MRT within the UK. There is a lack of information even about the nature and parameters of this form of intervention.

Although forms of methadone reduction treatment are widely used in the UK and in other countries throughout the world, it has been difficult to find any explicit definition. One early attempt to distinguish different forms of methadone treatment differentiated between two forms of MRT, which are described as: short-term detoxification – decreasing doses of methadone over one month or less, and long-term detoxification – decreasing doses over more than one month (Gossop and Grant 1990). These forms of MRT are contrasted with maintenance treatments involving stable doses over various periods of time.

MRT provides a medium-term, abstinence-oriented intervention. In practice, MRT programmes may vary from a few weeks in duration to many months (possibly even years). Reduction schedules may be 'fixed', (i.e. set by the prescribing agency without the patient having any involvement in the duration of the treatment, or the timing or rate of reduction), or they may be 'negotiable', with the patient having some involvement in decisions about the frequency, timing, and amount of dose reductions (Dawe *et al.* 1991). Even where reduction schedules are fixed, alterations may be made to the timing of dose reductions or the duration of the treatment on pragmatic and clinical grounds, because of changed circumstances or crises presented by the patient. Seivewright (2000) has suggested that 'many patients ... wish to gradually reduce' (p. 98), and recent Department of Health Guidelines (1999) note that 'compliance with a drug reduction regimen will only be maintained if patient and doctor both agree that reduction is desirable' (p. 47).

Methadone maintenance treatment (MMT) is such a widely used and well-known treatment that it may seem unnecessary to require definition. However, it is worth explicitly stating that two of its essential features are:

(1) MMT involves the provision of methadone in *stable* doses.
(2) MMT is intended to reduce problematic behaviours associated with illicit drug use (but is not, in itself, an abstinence-oriented treatment and entails continuing use of prescribed methadone).

These features differentiate MMT in important respects from methadone reduction. A basic feature of methadone maintenance is that the drug is prescribed on a stable-dose, non-reducing basis, and following stabilization at a suitable dose level, the patient may be maintained for either a fixed or for an indefinite period.

Owing to the diversity of methadone treatments and their lack of precise definition, the National Treatment Outcome Research Study (NTORS) adopted operational definitions in order to differentiate between patients who received MMT or MRT. These definitions (from Gossop *et al.* 2001) are:

(1) MMT: receiving 70% or more of consecutive methadone prescriptions at the same dose (i.e. dose on occasion $x + 1$ = dose on occasion x).
(2) MRT: receiving 50% or more of consecutive doses of methadone at a reduced dose.

To give a clearer idea of the dose schedules that might be expected for MRT, the Department of Health Guidelines (1999) suggested, as examples, reduction schedules with decrements of 5–10 mg per fortnight. On the basis of the even more conservative reduction rate of 5 mg per fortnight, a patient could be reduced from 60 mg to zero over a period of six months. Similarly, even when allowing for deviations from the ideal reduction curve, a schedule could fail to provide up to 50% of its reductions and still lead to a complete reduction treatment over a 12-month period.

Treatments received and treatment outcomes

In the study of two-year outcomes for the NTORS clients who received treatment in the methadone programmes, we found differences between MMT and MRT both with regard to prescribed methadone doses and treatment retention rates (Gossop *et al.* 2001). The patients in MRT were more likely than the maintenance patients to receive low starting doses (80% received a starting dose of 60 mg or less, and 15% received less than 30 mg). During the course of treatment, the MRT patients were more likely to receive low doses of methadone. Methadone dose has been found to be an important treatment variable, and patients on higher doses tend to achieve better outcomes. In their review, Ward *et al.* (1998) suggested that doses of 60 mg or more were associated with longer stays in treatment and reduced heroin use, and in a randomized, double-blind trial, Strain *et al.* (1999) found that the high-dose methadone group showed greater reductions in illicit opiate use than a low dose group.

In NTORS, patients allocated to MMT were more likely than MRT patients to remain in treatment at six months, at one year, and at two years. To some extent, this is to be expected since some patients receiving reduction treatments might have completed their programmes. However, this is unlikely since there is no evidence of improved outcomes among the MRT patients. Nor is it consistent with the finding that many intended reduction programmes were extended over periods of time well beyond what might be regarded as reasonable. Half of the MRT patients were still in treatment after one year and many had only achieved a slight reduction in dose. Almost a third of them were still in treatment after two years. The finding of lower retention rates among the MRT patients is consistent with the results of the randomized controlled trial conducted by Sees *et al.* (2000), which found that patients receiving 180-day detoxification were less likely to remain in treatment than patients receiving maintenance. For the NTORS maintenance patients (but not for MRT patients), retention in treatment was associated with reductions in illicit heroin use at follow-up.

Treatment retention has been found to be one of the most consistent predictors of favourable treatment outcomes (Simpson *et al.* 1997; McLellan *et al.* 1997). The lower retention rates among the methadone reduction patients in our study may be associated with the lower doses in MRT, or with the dose reductions. They may also be due to the pressure imposed on the patient to accept a reduced dose even when the reducing doses were not subsequently implemented. In practice, the issue of implementing a reducing dose programme can be a frequent (and sometimes acrimonious) topic of discussion within the clinical sessions, with clinic staff pressing for dose reductions and the patient resisting them. This may lead to stressful and difficult sessions for both staff and patients, described in Chapter 4, which may in turn contribute to poor programme implementation and to problems of treatment retention (as well as problems of staff morale). Mitcheson (1994) noted that 'an inordinate and wearisome amount of time was spent in (usually polite) mutual manipulation between staff and patients regarding type of drug and dose'. But whatever the reasons for the higher drop-out rate among the reduction patients, the differences in doses received and in retention rates are important to understanding the outcomes. For the MMT patients, but not for the MRT patients, higher doses and retention in treatment were both associated with favourable heroin use outcomes at two years.

In NTORS, data were first analysed to investigate outcomes for clients classified according to their type of treatment modality. The data were then analysed to investigate outcomes for individual patients classified on an intention-to-treat basis. Both analyses showed significant post-treatment reductions in the use of illicit drugs, psychological and physical health problems, and in acquisitive and drug-selling crime. There were no differences in outcomes for the modality-level comparisons (Gossop et al. 2000), nor for patients assigned to MMT and MRT on an intention-to-treat basis (Gossop et al. 2001).

We were surprised that patients in two such different treatment modalities should, apparently, have achieved such similar outcomes, though others have also found apparently similar outcomes. Strang et al. (1997) compared outcomes of patients randomly allocated to methadone maintenance or methadone reduction treatments. They found no differences between the two methadone conditions, with both treatments showing improvements in a range of substance use and other problem behaviours during the first month of treatment. Studies of shorter-term outpatient reduction programmes have typically found poor outcomes with high drop-out rates, and few patients achieving abstinence (Dawe et al. 1991; Unnithan et al. 1992).

We then explored whether the apparent similarity of outcomes for patients in the maintenance and reduction treatments could be due to the similarities in the treatments received by patients, or to variations in treatment delivery within each modality. We conducted more detailed analyses of the outcomes for the two types of methadone treatment, paying explicit attention to the impact of specific treatment components as delivered to the patient. Ball and Ross (1991) noted that the actual methods and procedures of methadone treatment programmes have seldom been described.

When we investigated the methadone doses actually prescribed to each patient, we found that MRT was frequently not delivered as intended. Whereas the majority (70%) of the patients allocated to maintenance on an intention-to-treat basis received methadone maintenance, only about a third (36%) of the patients allocated to MRT received reduction. Many patients who failed to receive MRT as intended appeared to have received some form of maintenance treatment (Gossop et al. 2001). Examples of different dosing schedules actually provided to patients are shown in Figures 24.1 to 24.6. The dose profiles shown in Figures 24.1 and 24.2 can be regarded as forms of MRT (both in terms of clinical judgement and in terms of their meeting our operational definition), with doses reducing from 70 mg to 15 mg and from 50 mg to 21 mg over a 12-month period. Although some reduction occurs in dose profile 3, (Figure 24.3) this is closer to a form of maintenance, with many stable doses being prescribed over a seven-month period. The dose profiles 4, 5 and 6 (Figures 24.4 to 24.6) are difficult to classify but, despite the clinicians' intentions at the start of treatment, cannot be regarded as reducing schedules.

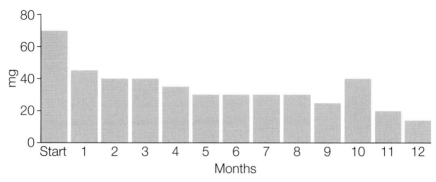

Figure 24.1 Dose profile 1: changing daily dose of methadone over twelve months for patient A.

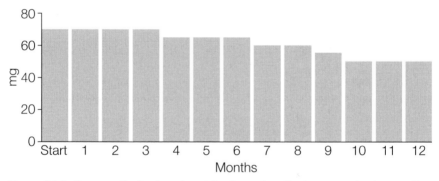

Figure 24.2 Dose profile 2: changing daily dose of methadone over twelve months for patient B.

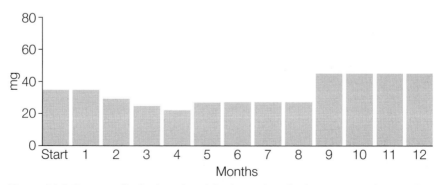

Figure 24.3 Dose profile 3: changing daily dose of methadone over twelve months for patient C.

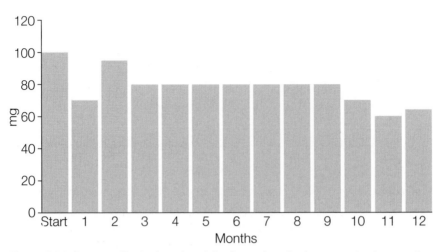

Figure 24.4 Dose profile 4: changing daily dose of methadone over twelve months for patient D.

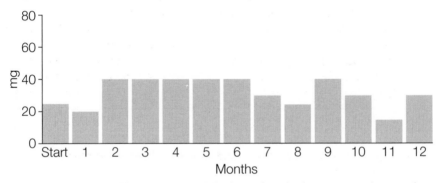

Figure 24.5 Dose profile 5: changing daily dose of methadone over twelve months for patient E.

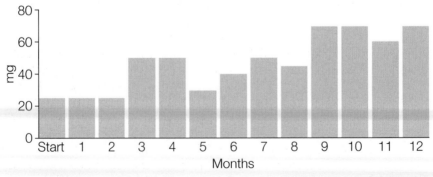

Figure 24.6 Dose profile 6: changing daily dose of methadone over twelve months for patient F.

Implications

The failure of almost two-thirds of the MRT patients to receive reduction treatment as intended raises a number of questions for treatment providers and policy makers. If most of the patients for whom MRT is planned and started subsequently have this treatment changed, the appropriateness of either the initial treatment planning process or the treatment delivery process, or both, are called into question.

Some of the MRT patients may have received other forms of treatment (usually some form of maintenance) because of operational failures to provide treatment as intended or because of changes in treatment goals which led to changes in treatment being deliberately implemented within the clinical service. Alternatively, it is possible that patients were initially admitted onto reduction programmes as an 'entry-level' form of methadone treatment because of the reluctance of staff to put patients directly onto maintenance programmes. This suggestion is consistent with our previous findings that the patients in the methadone reduction modality were, on average, younger, had used heroin for a shorter period, and were less likely to have multiple drug use or alcohol problems (Gossop *et al.* 1998). In some cases, the failure to implement dose reductions probably reflects the fact that some reduction patients resist, or are unable to achieve reductions in their methadone dose, and this leads to the treatment becoming stalled, sometimes permanently. As a result, reduction programmes can 'drift' into something that is very similar to a *de facto* form of maintenance. However, the prescription of a non-reducing dose of methadone when accompanied by disagreements between therapist and patient about the possibilities of reducing the dose level, and without an explicit renegotiation of treatment goals, does not constitute a satisfactory example of a maintenance treatment programme.

The NTORS findings raise other troubling questions about the effectiveness of MRT. Where MRT was delivered as intended, it was associated with poor outcomes. Capelhorn (1994) also found worse outcomes for patients receiving abstinence-oriented rather than indefinite maintenance. For the methadone maintenance patients in NTORS, the primary treatment goal (reductions in illicit heroin use) was associated with higher methadone doses and retention in treatment. The associations between methadone dosage, treatment retention, and treatment outcome are still not fully understood. However, many studies from different treatment settings and in different countries have shown positive associations between higher doses, increased retention and improved outcomes (Ward *et al.* 1998; Strain *et al.* 1999).

For the patients who *received* MRT, the more reducing doses they received, the worse their outcomes. In particular, the more rapidly the methadone was reduced, the worse the heroin use outcomes. This was the only treatment factor which was found to be (negatively) associated with outcome in the MRT group. The finding that the more reducing doses that were given, the worse the outcome, suggests that where MRT patients achieved improved outcomes after treatment, this may have occurred *despite* the specific characteristics of their intended treatment programmes (i.e. reducing doses). The outcomes of the reduction patients may be reflective of some generic treatment effect conferred by receiving a medically prescribed supply of methadone. Alternatively, the outcomes may be reflective of the finding that many of them actually received some form of maintenance.

Despite the apparently quite different aims and procedures of the maintenance and the reduction programmes, comments made to the research team during the inception phase of NTORS suggest that many addiction treatment personnel in the UK do not distinguish between the two types of treatment and believe that the two can, in some way, be alternated and/or provided seamlessly within a single treatment episode. In this respect, the 'crossover' between methadone reduction and methadone maintenance may reflect a conflation of the two treatments, which was deliberately implemented within the programmes. Even in the recent Guidelines the Department of Health (1999) was unable to commit itself on this issue, suggesting that 'withdrawal, detoxification (rapid and gradual) and maintenance, as well as their associated patterns ... overlap' (Department of Health 1999, p. 35) and warned the reader not to expect such clear distinctions in clinical practice.

One differential treatment effect concerned severity of dependence. We found that the more severely opiate-dependent patients achieved better heroin use outcomes when they received MMT, whereas the MRT patients who were more severely dependent on opiates at intake had poorer two-year outcomes. This suggests that where differential allocation of patients to either maintenance or reduction programmes is possible, more severely opiate-dependent patients should be offered methadone maintenance as the outpatient treatment of first choice.

Conclusions

Whereas NTORS reports the impact of methadone treatment programmes in the UK, the results may also have implications for similar treatments provided in other countries. Despite differences in patterns of drug use, in the nature of treatment services, and more generally, in social-environmental conditions, there are remarkable similarities between the NTORS findings and those from the major US treatment outcome studies.

Methadone reduction should be differentiated from, and seen as a different type of treatment to methadone maintenance. In particular, a clearer distinction should be made in clinical practice between the time-limited, abstinence-oriented methadone reduction treatments, and the long-term, stable-dose maintenance treatments that are designed to achieve harm reduction goals.

The different types of methadone treatments not only have different procedures but also, more importantly, have different aims. Some of the uncertainty about appropriate procedures within methadone reduction programmes could be removed if treatment goals were made explicit, and mutual agreement was reached on these between the patient and the clinical staff at the start of treatment. The results from NTORS have particular importance with regard to the findings for methadone reduction treatment about which so little is known. They raise serious questions about the purposes, the delivery, and the effectiveness of methadone reduction treatment, and suggest the need for a critical reappraisal of this widely used form of treatment.

References

Ball, J. & Ross, A. (1991) *The Effectiveness of Methadone Maintenance Treatment.* New York: Springer.

Capelhorn, J.R. (1994) A comparison of abstinence-oriented and indefinite methadone maintenance treatment. *International Journal of the Addictions*, 11: 1361–75.

Connell, P.H. (1969) Drug dependence in Great Britain: a challenge to the practice of medicine. In: Steinberg H, ed. *Scientific Basis of Drug Dependence*. London: Churchill Livingstone.

Dawe, S., Griffiths, P., Gossop, M. & Strang, J. (1991) Should opiate addicts be involved in controlling their own detoxification? A comparison of fixed versus negotiable schedules. *British Journal of Addiction,* 86: 977–82.

Department of Health (1999) *Drug Misuse and Dependence – Guidelines on Clinical Management*. London: The Stationery Office.

Edwards, G. (1969) The British approach to the treatment of heroin addiction. *Lancet,* I: 768–72.

Gerstein, D. & Harwood, H. (1990) *Treating Drug Problems, Volume 1.* Washington DC: National Academy Press.

Gossop, M. & Grant, M. (1990) *The Content and Structure of Methadone Treatment Programmes: A Study in Six Countries.* Geneva: World Health Organization, WHO/PSA.

Gossop, M., Marsden, J., Stewart, D. & Treacy, S. (2001) Outcomes after methadone maintenance and methadone reduction treatments: two-year follow-up results from the National Treatment Outcome Research Study. *Drug and Alcohol Dependence*, 62: 255–64.

Gossop, M., Marsden, J., Stewart, D. & Rolfe, A. (2000) Patterns of improvement after methadone treatment: one year follow-up results from the National Treatment Outcome Research Study (NTORS). *Drug and Alcohol Dependence,* 60: 275–86.

Gossop, M., Marsden, J., Stewart, D., Lehmann, P., Edwards, C., Wilson, A., Segar, G. (1998) Substance use, health and social problems of service users at 54 drug treatment agencies: intake data from the National Treatment Outcome Research Study. *British Journal of Psychiatry*, 173:166–71.

Gossop, M., Grant, M. & Wodak, A. (1989) *The Uses of Methadone in the Treatment and Management of Opioid Dependence*. Geneva: World Health Organization, WHO/MNH/DAT.

McLellan, A.T., Woody, G.E., Metzger, D., McKay, J., Durrell, J., Alterman, A.I. & O'Brien, C.P. (1997) Evaluating the effectiveness of addiction treatments: reasonable expectations, appropriate comparisons. In: Egertson J, Fox D, Leshner A, eds. *Treating Drug Abusers Effectively.* Oxford: Blackwell.

Mitcheson, M. (1994) Drug clinics in the

1970s. In: Strang J, Gossop M, eds. *Heroin Addiction and Drug Policy: The British System.* Oxford: Oxford University Press.

Sees, K., Delucchi, K., Masson, C., Rosen, A., Westly Clark, H., Robillard, H., Banys, P. & Hall, S. (2000) Methadone maintenance versus 180-day psychosocially enriched detoxification for treatment of opioid dependence: a randomized controlled trial. *Journal of the American Medical Association*, 283: 1303–10.

Seivewright, N. (2000) *Community Treatment of Drug Misuse: More than Methadone.* Cambridge: Cambridge University Press.

Simpson, D.D., Joe, G.W. & Brown, B.S. (1997) Treatment retention and follow-up outcomes in the Drug Abuse Treatment Outcome Study (DATOS). *Psychology of Addictive Behaviors*, 11: 294–307.

Stewart, D., Gossop, M., Marsden, J. & Strang, J. (2000) Variation between and within drug treatment modalities: data from the National Treatment Outcome Research Study (UK). *European Addiction Research*, 6: 106–14.

Strain, E.C., Bigelow, G.E., Liebson, I.A. & Stitzer, M.L. (1999) Moderate vs high-dose methadone in the treatment of opioid dependence. *Journal of the American Medical Association,* 281: 1000–5.

Strang, J. (1984) Abstinence or abundance – what goal? *British Medical Journal*, 289: 604.

Strang, J., Finch, E., Hankinson, L., Farrell, M., Taylor, C., & Gossop, M. (1997) Methadone treatment for opiate addiction: benefits in the first month. *Addiction Research*, 5: 71–6.

Unnithan, S., Gossop, M. & Strang, J. (1992) Factors associated with relapse among opiate addicts in an out-patient detoxification programme. *British Journal of Psychiatry*, 309:103–4.

Ward, J., Mattick, R.P. & Hall, W. (eds) (1998) *Methadone Maintenance Treatment and Other Opiate Replacement Therapies*. Amsterdam: Harwood Academic Publishers.

Section H: In conclusion

25
Methadone: achieving the balance

Gillian Tober and John Strang

One of the strengths of health and social policy in the UK addiction field is the centrality of the relative view: there are risks attendant upon any health or social intervention and, in the case of methadone, arguably more than most. The risks attendant upon using heroin for recreation and as a result of dependence form the ultimate benchmark against which to measure the propriety of implementing this difficult treatment, but the contributors to this book have taken us right into the thick of the detail, which reveals a more sophisticated way of assessing the effectiveness of methadone treatment while providing evidence for minimizing the risks inherent in its provision.

It is the diversity of methadone treatment practice in the UK which is perhaps its most distinctive and puzzling feature. This diversity emanates in part from the relative lack of central control on the prescribing and dispensing of methadone, and also in part from the ingenuity, necessity and experience of people working in the field. The goal at the outset was to record that diversity for posterity in a more concrete way; in the event, on collating the material, something more far-reaching has emerged. In assembling the background research which informed the development of practice and then the outcome research which formed the evaluation of practice, the contributing authors have, in fact, produced the evidence upon which to base future practice.

What is the purpose of methadone treatment?

In 1988, the AIDS and Drug Misuse report set out a hierarchy of harm reduction goals starting with the most basic goal of keeping people alive and culminating in the goal of giving up drug use altogether; this hierarchy was subsequently incorporated into the Guidelines for Clinical Management (the 'Orange Guidelines') issued by the Department of Health (Department of Health 1991). For opiate addicts, methadone was well-positioned to make a major contribution towards the achievement of every single one of these goals. With the prescription of methadone, patients have been shown to stop or reduce injecting, to stop or reduce the commission of crimes in order to finance their drug use, to stop or reduce the use of street drugs, to reduce the risk of overdose and to improve social functioning. Thus methadone treatment spans the range of goals from harm reduction to the treatment and reduction of opiate dependence. Huge benefit is to be derived from methadone across the spectrum of treatment goals, and the ways in which such benefit can be maximized have been described in this book. It is as if some flesh has been attached to the bones of the harm reduction hierarchy at the individual level.

Pharmacological, psychological and social attributes

Methadone is a pharmacological agent that, like many drugs both with and without a specific psychoactive effect, also operates at the psychological level as a powerful conditioning agent. Its rapid and predictable psychoactive effects are capable of inducing pleasurable feelings and reducing pain. It therefore creates the expectation of these effects and determines behaviour in the light of their perceived need. The social effects of methadone operate at the level where methadone obviates or reduces the need for heroin and hence potentially reduces the social problems attendant upon heroin use. This affects individuals and their families, and it also contributes to crime prevention and responses to crime at the organizational and economic level. Methadone is a powerful drug, but its strength is expressed not only through pharmacological effects, but also through psychological and social mechanisms.

Opiate use and dependence have long been seen to be the province of both health and criminal justice authorities, but in the latter part of the twentieth century there was a bigger than ever impetus to shift the responsibility for the containment of opiate use into the health arena, resulting in new partnerships and collaborations, with new responses to the growing problem of opiate use by all public services, not just health and criminal justice.

Maximizing the benefits and minimizing the risks

The good of the individual is served in many ways – by reducing the risk of overdose death or damage and the risk of drug-related physical disease and psychiatric disorder, by obviating the need to pursue illicit means of financing drug use, by improving family functioning, by improving the opportunity and capacity for employment and for active involvement in the community in a positive way. The prescribing of methadone, as a substitute for illicit heroin, has been shown to be capable of achieving each of these ends. In general, as a rough rule of thumb, researchers have usually found that the larger the dose of methadone, the greater the likely compliance with methadone treatment, and the greater the compliance with treatment the better the outcome. The risks to the individual are few when the prescription is used in the way it is intended, but there exists an increasing risk of dependence with larger doses and as the prescription continues over time. Methadone treatment might be deemed to have failed, at least in part, where the methadone dose is regularly supplemented or occasionally replaced by heroin, given that the goal of methadone treatment in the first instance will be to substitute for such use. Continued prescription of methadone when the patient carries on 'using on top' incurs its own additional risks, and also exacerbates the problem of increasing dependence.

There is further the matter of the strange paradox that, by removing many of the adverse sequelae of drug use, we might also, possibly, be removing much of the incentive to give up opioid drug use. While harm reduction (with reference to the harms caused by continuing heroin use) may be the ultimate goal for some, it is possible for many to do better than to resign themselves to lifelong use of opioid drugs, even where they do so in a relatively risk-free way. It would almost seem that, with the risk of increasing dependence and reducing the incentive to become opiate free, the effectiveness of treatment in the short term militates against the possibility of short-term treatment. This is a conundrum that remains to be resolved. It is more than just methadone that is required to enhance and maintain a momentum for change towards a drug-free lifestyle, to go beyond the goal of harm minimization.

Individual health gain and the public good

To what extent, in the case of methadone, does individual health gain compromise the public good? Clearly the two cannot be mutually exclusive; to some extent the public good is derived from the greater health gains for individual people, but in the drug misuse arena there may be a tension between the two. The good of the community is served by reducing crime and by reducing or eliminating drug-dealing venues and activities, by reducing the risk of exposure to toxic substances which threaten the lives of people who are unaware of the attendant risks of methadone consumption and by reducing the threat of the spread of infectious disease through the sharing of injecting equipment. Additionally, a community is likely to function better where it contains cohesive families that function well and individuals who are employable and active in the local economy. The provision of methadone as a substitute for heroin is capable of producing all these outcomes at the societal level.

Larger doses of methadone have now been shown repeatedly to be more likely to result in increased attendance for and retention in treatment. The longer the duration of retention in treatment, the greater the opportunity to engage people in psychological and lifestyle changes associated with stable change. Yet larger doses, in addition to being coupled with longer duration, also result in an increased risk of leakage of methadone onto the streets and into the hands of those for whom it was not intended – with the attendant risks of overdose deaths.

We now have convincing evidence that the potential for diversion and the resulting methadone-related mortality can be reduced where distribution and consumption are closely monitored and supervised. In addition, the fact of being able to retain patients in treatment creates the opportunity for the delivery of psycho-social interventions aimed at reducing dependence and working towards drug-free lifestyles over time. In other words, increased risks at the public health level can be reduced by monitoring and controlling the distribution and consumption of methadone, and by providing methadone treatment in conjunction with other interventions. Rather than resigning oneself to some degree of inevitable tension between public and individual health needs, areas of shared objectives have emerged with clear indications of how to achieve health gains at both levels.

Control and regulation: where do we draw the line?

The evidence presented in the foregoing chapters explores the ways which methadone doses and route of administration matter, the method of distribution and dispensing matters, other treatments delivered contemporaneously matter, and the context in which methadone treatment is delivered matters. National policy, based on the evidence of how important it is to get these components of treatment and its delivery right, also matters. In the UK, national policy is implemented as guidelines for good practice in the context of setting outcome targets rather than defining and imposing practice in a legal framework. This results in a degree of scope for flexibility which has afforded the opportunity to try out different methods based upon clinical judgement and subsequently to assemble evidence of good practice and relative outcomes. What emerges is the possibility of improved outcomes given clinical flexibility to address individual needs.

Does the situation in which practice is determined by political consideration and central control, where dedicated methadone specialists working in dedicated methadone programmes with automatic supervised consumption and centrally determined doses, result in better patient outcomes and better public health? If so, on which outcome measures? In such extreme conditions, methadone is treated like a social security pay packet, where amount distributed is determined by a political view of aggregate need; mass distribution is cheaper, can be centrally organized and results in some politically desirable outcomes (notably harm reduction and large numbers attending for treatment). It probably requires far less clinical training, by-passes the need to address local differences and clinical practice variations. This wider availability of lower-impact methadone treatment may be appealing to politicians, perhaps even to the general public, but it will be more questionable and less comfortable to professionals and patients.

The UK guidelines approach with its far fewer legal regulations has undoubtedly resulted in greater flexibility to meet individual needs and to protect the clinical autonomy of the prescribing doctor and her or his freedom to apply clinical judgement. However, from looking at surveys of medical school curricula, it is clear that the average general practitioner, physician and psychiatrist does not have the requisite education and training to practise in this way. Specialist services and training centres go some way to try to address these questions with enhanced shared care arrangements, and there have recently been developments of further specialist training both for the dedicated practitioner and the generalist – but the situation is still unsatisfactory, with the majority of practitioners who find themselves expected to provide methadone treatment feeling inadequately trained, inadequately informed and inadequately supported.

Further problems result from the absence of clearly stated lines of responsibility; in many shared care schemes the boundaries of responsibility between prescribing and non-prescribing staff are laid out in protocols. In law, it is clearly the case that the prescriber is accountable for the safety of the prescription from its delivery to its use; yet the absence of training and current knowledge has resulted in medical practitioners seeking, and sometimes blindly following, advice from sources which may be outside formal shared care arrangements and hold no prescribing authority or pharmacological training. In more extreme situations, prescribing doctors have found themselves subject to pressure, not only from their patients but also from their patients' advocates, to prescribe in doses and regimens that are against their better judgement. A legal framework to the prescribing guidelines would provide a degree of protection against such pressure.

Addiction – a favourite field of practice

In a system which is very tightly regulated, there is little scope for variation in response to individual need but beyond this there is also little scope for the sort of professional job satisfaction that results from the opportunity to use clinical judgement and to carry responsibility for it in practice. In an era when there is growing insistence on the delivery of evidence-based practice and clinical governance measures in place to demonstrate and monitor the way that such practice is delivered, there will still be scope for a degree of clinical judgement within established parameters of good practice. The greater the perceived difficulty of the work, the greater the challenge and the rewards for those considering a career in it.

The message emanating from these chapters is that the constructive use and deployment of controls governing practice, monitored in a framework of clinical governance designed continually to improve that practice combined with creativity and flexibility afforded by the guidelines approach, can result in greater benefit – both for the individual and the public good. In some fields, there is little one can do to effect changes in people's lives or in the life of the community; the field of the treatment of opiate addiction is different. The methadone treatment arena is one in which there is scope for multi-disciplinary practice and diversity of goals, in an environment of continually changing demands resulting both from the changing nature and scope of drug misuse and the changing populations engaged in these activities. Of course, not all heroin users are the same; the population of heroin users is not a homogeneous population, and different perceptions of the existence and nature of problems and of the goals of help-seeking behaviour can result in tension at the coal-face of treatment. Typically the addiction specialist is faced with an array of help-seeking attitudes, ranging from those for whom dependence and problems are beginning to cause unacceptable levels of problems, to those for whom the addiction specialist is probably seen as little more than a source of drug supply. Many conflicts in the clinic room spring from the mismatch between the perceived goal of the practitioner and that of the patient. Those who are 'hit seekers' will, almost by definition, seek to increase the methadone dose in order to go beyond the amelioration of their withdrawal state, will supplement their prescription with other opiates and may well sell their prescription to facilitate the purchase of alternative opiates or other drugs. As such, their 'fit' with the effects of methadone may be very different from the 'fit' of those now mainly seeking 'trough-avoidance' or seeking a 'calm plateau' effect. With this in mind, the preceding chapters have explored the circumstances in which these problems arise and have described the initiatives that have emerged, presented in such a way that they may be adopted in a range of localities as a method and framework for good practice.

The way things are done makes a considerable difference. The foregoing chapters describe a rich range of practice designed to improve treatment outcomes. Careful assessment and dose titration, supervision of consumption including injecting, monitoring use throughout the prescription, providing methadone treatment in different venues, maintaining a therapeutic alliance and providing psycho-social treatments in combination with methadone – all of these will contribute to increasing the benefits that result from our provision of methadone treatment. This should be welcome news for all those who are engaged or interested in the treatment of opiate addiction. There are, however, conclusions that will be less palatable to some, such as the practical implications of policing the distribution and consumption of methadone, using objective means for assessment and monitoring. We have intended to prompt serious review by those providing methadone treatment entirely on the basis of self report, and to prompt critical questioning of automatic acceptance of the client's stated needs as necessarily the best pathway to individual health gain and the greater good of the community. The chapters discussing the practice of prescribing injectable methadone and the difficulty in arriving at a firm conclusion further illustrate the importance of these considerations.

Methadone matters

Methadone matters because, world-wide, more than half a million people take methadone every day, because it has become the most common form of treatment for heroin dependence, because both specialist and non-specialist doctors prescribe it, because it is a treatment actively sought by those caught up in heroin addiction, and also because it is what parents want for their children once they have seen what heroin does to them. But methadone also matters because it is a dangerous drug whose use can result in overdose and death and because continuation of use is likely to result in heightened dependence.

Other drugs, of course, also exist as possible medications for similar pharmacotherapy. These include buprenorphine, and possibly slow-release morphine or codeine (both of which are currently being studied) as well as heroin. But methadone treatment still comprises about 90% of all opiate substitution treatment, and hence it is particularly important to look for ways of increasing the effectiveness of our methadone treatment. Furthermore, the lessons we learn and the improvements we introduce will almost certainly be generalizable and hence transferable in large part to these other drugs. Consequently, we remain convinced of the need for a special focus on methadone treatment.

In spite of increasingly international debate about the proper treatments of drug use and misuse, the systems of controls on such treatment operate quite differently around the world; it is timely to undertake a critical examination of our policies and practices and to search for changes that will result in improved effectiveness of methadone treatment, to the benefit of both the individual and the community. Even when such self-examination has been undertaken and changes are made, important questions will still remain, and we hope that the deliberations in this book will help to frame the necessary scrutiny and re-appraisals which should accompany this treatment.

Reference

Department of Health (1991) *Drug Misuse and Dependence Guidelines on Clinical Management.* London: HMSO.

Index

Sports Personal Injury: Law & Practice

AUSTRALIA
LBC Information Services
Sydney

CANADA AND USA
Carswell
Toronto

NEW ZEALAND
Brooker's
Auckland

SINGAPORE AND MALAYSIA
Sweet & Maxwell Asia
Singapore and Kuala Lumpur